Psychological Staff Support in Healthcare

Every possible effort has been made to ensure that the information contained in this book is accurate at the time of going to press. The publishers and author(s) cannot accept responsibility for any errors and omissions, however caused. No responsibility for loss or damage occasioned to any person acting, or refraining from action, as a result of the material contained in this publication can be accepted by the editor, the publisher or the author.

First published in 2022 by Sequoia Books

Apart from fair dealing for the purposes of research or private study, or criticism or review, as permitted under the Copyright, Designs and Patents act 1988, this publication may only be reproduced, stored or transmitted, in any form or by any means, with the prior permission in writing of the publisher, or in the case of reprographic reproduction in accordance with the terms and licenses issued by the CLA. Enquiries concerning reproduction outside these terms should be sent to the publisher using the details on the website www.sequoia-books.com

©Harriet Conniff

The right of Dr Harriet Conniff to be identified as editor of this work has been asserted in accordance with the Copyright, Designs and Patents act 1988.

ISBN
Print: 9781914110184
EPUB: 9781914110191

A CIP record for this book is available from the British Library

Library of Congress Cataloguing-In-Publication Data
Name: Dr Harriet Conniff
Title: Psychological Staff Support in Healthcare / Dr Harriet Conniff
Description: 1st Edition, Sequoia Books UK 2022
Subjects: R5920 Medicine (general)
Print: 9781914110184
EPUB: 9781914110191

Library of Congress Control Number: 2022914440

Print and Electronic production managed by Deanta Global

Cover designed by Samantha Doe

Psychological Staff Support in Healthcare

Thinking and Practice

Edited by
Dr Harriet Conniff

Consultant Editor
Dr Arabella Kurtz

For Bappy

Contents

An Introduction to Psychological Staff Support   1
Dr Harriet Conniff

Section 1 Thinking   17

1   Making Equality, Diversity, and Inclusion Fundamental to Staff Support Working   19
Dr Raselle Miller

2   Organisational Trauma: An Important Context in Staff Support   47
Dr Karen Treisman

3   Setting up Systems of Staff Support using a Systemic Approach   71
Dr Harriet Conniff and Dr Neil Rees

4   Moral Injury: Why Exploring Novel Terms Makes Space for Talking in Staff Support   96
Dr Esther Murray

5   A Relational Guide to Establish and Maintain a Psychologically Healthier Workplace   107
Dr Adrian Neal and Dr Julie Highfield

6   Reflections on Group Interventions in Staff Health and Wellbeing: The role of psychologists   127
Dr Zoe Berger, Dr Joanna Farrington-Exley, Dr Harriet Conniff, and Dr Sadie Thomas-Unsworth

7   Supporting Staff and Volunteers Delivering Services to People in Crisis   149
Dr Sarah Davidson, Rachel Morley, Paula Aredez Arriazu, and Andrea Wood

8   Research and Evaluation Considerations for Staff Support in Healthcare Settings   166
Dr Matt Hotton, Dr Louise Johnson, and Dr Anika Petrella

CONTENTS

Section 2 Practice — 187

9 Enabling Connection and Compassion through Structured Compassion Practices — 189
Dr Benna Waites, Dr Charlie Jones, Laura Simms, Dr Alister Scott, Andy Bradley, and Dr Rachel Potter

10 Compassion-Focused Staff Support: An Antidote to Empathy Distress — 204
Dr Kate Lucre, Catherine Lacey, and Dr Jon Taylor

11 Using the Professional Tree of Life for Staff Wellbeing and Supervision — 224
Dr Julie Fraser and Dr Liz Matias

12 The Heads and Hearts Model of Reflective Practice — 247
Dr Arabella Kurtz and Dr Joanna Levene

13 Psychological support for healthcare workers in India: Using a reflective lens — 268
Professor Poornima Bhola, Dr Rathna Isaac, and Dr Chetna Duggal

14 Open Dialogue, Dialogical Leadership, and Staff Support — 285
Dr Lisa Monaghan and Cathy Thorley

15 Strategic Working and Supporting Leadership within a Healthcare Context — 301
Dr Julie Highfield and Dr Adrian Neal

16 Brief Interventions with Senior Healthcare Staff during the Pandemic — 317
Dr Penelope Cream and Professor Mike Wang

17 Healthcare Professionals Who Have Experienced Trauma and the Role of EMDR Therapy — 333
Dr Shannon Cullerton and Dr Sherry Rehim

18 Debriefs?: Offering Group Interventions in Response to Difficult Events — 353
Dr Sadie Thomas-Unsworth, Dr Harriet Conniff, Dr Zoe Berger, and Dr Joanna Farrington-Exley

Gathering Our Thoughts — 373
Dr Harriet Conniff

Acknowledgements — 381

Contributor Biographies — 383

An Introduction to Psychological Staff Support

Dr Harriet Conniff

Humans need others to survive. Regardless of one's sex, country or culture of origin, age or economic background, social connection is crucial to human development, health and survival. (Holt-Lunstad et al., 2017, p. 12)

Work can connect us socially, or isolate us, and everything in between. Social isolation is bad for health. It is one more indignity that follows the social gradient – not just more adverse things happening, but fewer potential social supports coming from a variety of sources. (Marmot, 2015, p. 182)

This book is about connection. Connection and good relationships sustain us in our (working) lives and are supportive of wellbeing. Peer support and connection are fundamental to healthcare staff wellbeing and underpin staff support. The ways we connect with healthcare staff in supporting them psychologically are wide ranging and, at times, complex, but, as we shall see, staff support is all about connection. The impact of connection doesn't stop there – there is a symbiotic relationship between staff and patients in their care; caring for our workforce means patients are better cared for.

During the COVID-19 pandemic, we learnt more about the power of connection and coming together. It was also a time when healthcare staff wellbeing was brought to the fore in both the public realm and in psychological working. Prior to this, clinical psychologists and other health professionals commonly provided staff support additional to their clinical roles (particularly those working embedded in medical contexts), but there is little described about the work.

As a consequence of the pandemic, new services and roles were created to lead and develop psychological support for healthcare staff. This has led both to a consolidation of previous work, and creativity and innovation in the field. But who does staff support work? This book brings together contributions from psychologists *and other professionals*, because psychological staff support is not solely the domain of psychologists. In fact, to be effective, the responsibility must be shared by professionals with a wide range of experience in healthcare staff support. Traditionally, for instance, hospital chaplains have carried out a lot of the support for healthcare staff (Stoter, 1997).[1] There are offerings here from those new to the work through the pandemic, those who have been doing it for many years alongside (often squeezed into) their main role and those with designated time to do this work. Throughout, there are examples of psychologists using their unique training and skills to work within staff support at different levels, and instances of collaboration and working alongside other professional groups.

Psychological staff support needs to reside within a tiered system of staff support, of course (Macaulay & Conniff, 2020). This book forefronts the psychological interventions and the role of psychologists within those systems. It showcases psychological staff support work in a broad range of healthcare settings with an emphasis on physical health. It brings together work from psychologists who deliver psychological staff support in different ways such as those embedded in medical specialties, designated staff support psychologists, and those working within Occupational Health. The majority of contributors work in acute physical health settings which present particular challenges to delivery as we shall see. Plus, we will hear from psychologists and other staff wellbeing practitioners who work strategically to design and influence workplace initiatives and think about employee psychological wellbeing.

A variety of psychological models applied to working in staff health and wellbeing are discussed, such as Psychodynamic and Systemic approaches, the Professional Tree of Life, EMDR, and different renderings of compassion practices. Most of the authors do this work in the UK; however, many draw on international theories, practice, and research in this area, so the book will have global relevance.

This book has been loosely divided into two sections. In section 1, 'Thinking', the theoretical and values base for staff support work will be set out. A range of theories and approaches to staff support working is included. The section covers broad principles such as Equality, Diversity, and Inclusion (EDI); being trauma informed; and the importance of relational aspects in order to maintain good staff wellbeing. Organisational level working is captured in a number of chapters

---

[1] Chapter 3 provides an example of this.

and includes setting up of systems of staff support across organisations, service models, and examination of the concepts behind them.

Section 2, 'Practice', sets out the best-established practices and interventions at the individual, team, and organisational level, and descriptions of strategic working such as work with senior leadership. This section charts advances in practice and possible future directions. The chapters in this section broadly move from more 'preventative' aspects of staff support that are offered in an ongoing way, to those held in response to events and trauma. Across the book there will be consideration of the emerging evidence base and the need for evaluation, as well as examination of the contexts and rationale for supporting staff in healthcare. Of course, chapters in the 'Thinking' section discussing theoretical aspects and ideas cannot help but reference practice and vice versa.

Why support healthcare staff?

At a fundamental level, supporting people to do their work makes sense and, as the NHS Constitution for England (Department of Health, 2021) states, 'is the right thing to do'. In a discussion I had with senior leaders about staff wellbeing and whether it was still relevant post pandemic, a nurse leader reflected how we have learnt the importance of personal protective equipment and infection control, and these are not measures we are just going to drop. She went on to say how the pandemic uncovered that many healthcare organisations were not supporting their workforce well and it has taken a pandemic to realise the importance of doing so. She told me that we should "stop calling it wellbeing. It's being – it's normal. It's not an optional extra."

Another significant reason for supporting healthcare staff psychologically is due to the impact of working in healthcare on staff mental health. Healthcare working commonly involves repeated exposure to suffering and pain, death and dying. Sometimes the work has a cumulative negative effect. Although, on the whole, the challenging nature of clinical work does not mean that all healthcare staff are traumatised and need (psychological) staff support. Healthcare staff are motivated to do this kind of work, and often have excellent coping strategies and tolerances to working with high distress. I would argue that the core reasons for the rise in healthcare staff stress and mental health difficulties go beyond the actual clinical work.

The unique pressures of the twenty-first century's healthcare climate have a profound effect on staff. Improvements in medical technology mean that people are not only living longer but those who may have previously died are surviving.

In the main, this should be celebrated; however, in some instances there are difficult questions about quality of life, suffering, and ethical dilemmas which take their toll on all involved. Technology and hospital IT systems can also impact on healthcare staff wellbeing and may not always save time for clinicians (Gawande, 2018). Technological disconnection can occur, affecting the patient relationship and simultaneously healthcare staff who report an 'ache for genuine connection' (Clarke, 2019). Additional challenges that staff report are the role of 'Doctor Google' and the decline of 'experts', with patients and families having more access to information about their health than ever before. Again, the days of the patriarchal 'God-like' doctor whose view cannot be disputed have (thankfully) largely gone with the rise in multidisciplinary team working and involving patients in their own care. But this is a double-edged sword. At the extreme, questioning healthcare opinion to the point of conflict is a modern-day healthcare phenomenon that can impact on staff. Additionally, this century has witnessed increased scrutiny and raised expectations of healthcare providers and their staff by the public and the media which also take its toll on staff wellbeing.

Combined with the pressures above, it is useful to examine the role of power, resources, and systemic issues:

> *Whether health professionals are working in an urban hospital in the United States or a rural health clinic in the mountains of Tajikistan, stress and burnout are ubiquitous ..., even in disparate settings with varying resources, the issues faced by health professionals around the world are similar, including financial stresses, problems with infrastructure, moral stress and compassion fatigue, and difficulties with power and hierarchy among professionals. (Global Forum, 2019, p. 2)*

Pre-pandemic levels of stress and burnout were already high in healthcare staff, having a clear bearing on sickness absence, turnover rates, and staff shortages. Certain groups of staff are likely to be more disproportionately affected by workplace stress than others; systematic inequalities in health outcomes between social and ethnic groups (Marmot, 2015) impact on staff when they are giving care and when they/their family receive care. Institutional and interpersonal racism operate within healthcare organisations too (Olusoga, 2022). A comment by Siddharth Shah, a healthcare leader, is pertinent here: "We are not in a post-racial society, but instead our systems reinforce historical trauma unless we are deliberate about cultivating a more healing and equitable system" (Global Forum, 2019, p. 51).

How might all this play out in supporting staff psychologically and what do we need to consider? We know that healthcare staff who are from ethnic minority/global majority populations are more likely to face discrimination at work, have disciplinaries, and be disproportionately affected by physical and mental health issues. We also know that certain groups of staff in healthcare, such as those on lower incomes, male staff, and ethnically minoritised groups, face barriers in accessing wellbeing and psychological interventions. We must think deeply about how to improve access to staff support services for these groups and how we address issues that healthcare staff experience such as discrimination. We need to consider our role in affecting real change in EDI within staff support so that it is not a tick-box exercise where EDI stands for 'Endless Distraction and Inaction' (Ahsan, 2022). EDI issues are relevant to all staff support working and, as such, many of the chapters consider how we can meaningfully apply them in staff wellbeing. Raselle Miller in chapter 1 'Making Equality, Diversity, and Inclusion Fundamental to Staff Support Working' eloquently draws together some of the central issues when working with healthcare staff, with particular attention to race. She offers useful ways to tackle inequality in staff support working such as how to reflect on our biases and advocate for change, illustrating the work with clear examples from practice.

We know from the psychological safety literature that if employees work in an environment which creates, trust and respects and values staff, this can help improve effectiveness and better team working (Dollard & Bakker, 2010). Compassionate team leadership is necessary for psychological safety (West, 2021, p. 96). It is well established that if we support staff then patient care improves: care becomes more compassionate, fewer mistakes are made, and the overall quality of physical care improves. In other words, there is a direct relationship between staff wellbeing and patient wellbeing.

Lastly, supporting staff in the workplace is important for maintaining our workforce. Increasingly, healthcare organisations are thinking about retention in broad terms, such as bolstering the workforce to retain staff within healthcare broadly, and not just thinking about this within individual organisations. This recognises the fact that people move around more so if healthcare organisations treat staff well when they leave; this may mean that people return and/or recommend the organisation as a good place to work. The pandemic has exacerbated the problem of staff leaving healthcare for good; turnover rates of NHS staff have risen sharply (Collins, 2022) and in America one in five healthcare workers have left their job since the pandemic started (Yong, 2021):

Health-care workers aren't quitting because they can't handle their jobs. They're quitting because they can't handle being unable to do their jobs. Even before COVID-19, many of them struggled to bridge the gap between the noble ideals of their profession and the realities of its business. (Yong, 2021)

This highlights resource and systemic issues, as well as the reality of modern healthcare being all about big business – a far cry from the motivations and training of most clinical healthcare staff, psychologists included. Other than looking after the healthcare workforce being the right thing to do, if we follow in the business vein, surely supporting staff to work well saves money in days lost through sickness absence, recruitment, and the organisation also benefits from the positive impact of maintaining patient activity. Consequently, it is crucial that we evaluate what we do, making sure it fits with the aims of individuals, teams, and organisations. Chapter 8, 'Research and Evaluation Considerations for Staff Support in Healthcare Settings', by Matt Hotton, Louise Johnson, and Anika Petrella, explores ways to do just this. There is some emerging qualitative evidence from the pandemic suggesting the importance of having psychological staff support within stepped models of psychological care (Daniels et al., 2021). However, there is still little research on whether the work is effective generally, for instance, can it usefully impact on workplace metrics like staff turnover and sickness rates? This chapter looks at ways we might remedy this by appraising the effectiveness of our practice, whether it be by seeing if we can make a difference to symptom outcomes for individuals or improve team morale and team working, and thereby ultimately impact positively on patient care.

The changing profile of staff support

We have all started marking time with the words 'before the pandemic'. In the realm of staff support there is a striking difference between the profile of professionals working in staff health and wellbeing before and after the pandemic. Before the pandemic, people were interested, sure. Some organisations had already placed staff wellbeing more centrally to their work than others, and in some hospitals, there were dedicated staff psychologists or those with allocated time to do this work. However, this was not commonplace and certainly many psychologists and other professionals struggled to find the time (and managerial and system backup) to do this work. Time and again I have heard that supporting staff is not direct clinical care and not income generating, so a luxury use of precious psychology time. In my experience, leaders and the system not valuing staff support can in itself become a stressor by denying that staff are experiencing stress or mental health decline.

Yet at the same time, discussions about staff wellbeing and the 'human factors' associated with healthcare have become more commonplace. We have also seen a rise in 'author clinicians' writing books on their experience of working in healthcare which inevitably touch on the impact on their own wellbeing (Clarke, 2017; Marsh, 2014) and on being on the receiving end of care (Gawande, 2014; Kalanithi, 2016). In talking with the fantastic chapter authors who have given their time to write here, I kept hearing that this is a book that is long overdue. There is a wealth of literature in Organisational Development (OD) and organisational psychology related to teams and organisations. But what of staff support working involving psychologists (and other wellbeing practitioners) who work clinically in healthcare?

Since the turn of the century there have been many articles researching the wellbeing of healthcare staff in acute physical health contexts looking at burnout, PTSD, coping, and resiliency (for intensive care settings in the UK, see various articles by Gillian Colville and Julie Highfield). Such findings tend to point to the importance of having time for staff to connect in huddles or use supervision/reflective practice although there are few publications that explore the effectiveness of this, one example is D'Urso et al. (2019). Specific interventions in healthcare have been outlined, such as Wallbank's (2016) model of restorative supervision and in the UK, some have written about working in organisations and healthcare broadly (Obholzer & Roberts, 1996; Campbell, 2000; Wren, 2016). Lately (no doubt spurred on by the pandemic's pressing need) we have seen several books on healthcare staff wellbeing, including nurturing maternity staff (Smith, 2021); looking at healthcare staff mental health (Murray & Brown, 2021); wellbeing and spirituality of health and social care professionals (Aris et al., 2021); trauma-informed organisations (Treisman, 2021); and reflective practice in healthcare (Kurtz, 2020).

So, it seems true that prior to the pandemic there was not much published about staff support in (acute) physical healthcare settings despite the work having gone on for years. Why is this? We have touched upon how general staff wellbeing has been largely undervalued due to the priority of clinical (seeing patients) activity and focus on (direct) income generating work. This means that in some areas psychologists are simply not allowed to do this work. Sadly, this not only demonstrates that staff support is not highly regarded in some health organisations but also reflects a short-term view of workplace wellbeing. This lack of value and short-sightedness can mean that even if there are staff support measures in place, staff are not released to attend or there are not sufficient structures backed up by senior leadership and resources to scaffold the work.

Staff support not being valued or prioritised can also be linked to stigma in help-giving professions; clinical staff may feel the need to act with bravado, may have concerns about career progression or having their fitness to practise questioned if they admit they need help (Mildenhall, 2021, p. 55). Staff may be influenced by narratives such as how can heroes ask for help or heroes don't need to ask for support:

> *Traditionally, doctors [read any healthcare staff] have been resistant to the idea that they might benefit from or need support. 'Not being able to cope' was seen as a sign of weakness; asking for help was 'giving in'. There had been a misguided notion that, because they are trained and qualified to look after others, they should not need to be looked after, mentally and emotionally, themselves.* (Morrison, 2021, p. 96)

Sometimes staff and organisations do not see the work as serious; in one place I worked staff support was referred to as 'fluffy'. Some talk about generational differences and sometimes this is described in polarised negative terms with staff support seen as something needed more by the younger, touchy feely, or 'snowflake' generation. Conversely, the older 'battleaxe' generations' approach to workplace and organisational stress as something they went through so junior colleagues must also endure them.

However, with the pandemic we have seen a shift in this, with those individual staff and areas who previously may not have considered staff support seeking it out for themselves and staff in their teams. To borrow the words of Cream and Wang (chapter 16), we have seen 'COVID-19 as proxy' which as everyone was affected helped reduce stigma about help-seeking – the COVID-19 context gave permission to seek help. Has staff wellbeing truly become more commonplace though? The pandemic has highlighted its need but will the attention and support for it wane? It will be interesting to see what remains in place in organisations currently 'well resourced' for psychological staff support as we move further away from the peaks of the pandemic.

Further reasons for the changing profile of staff wellbeing include the (fair) concerns about the impact of any staff interventions. There can be fears around creating 'bitching or moaning arenas' and/or uncovering problems or even causing trouble. Such concerns do need to be considered and signify the importance of working systemically and setting up the work well. Some types of staff support work, for example, debriefs, have had a narrative about them causing harm which, even though this has now been found to be misguided, has meant that psychologists offering support and healthcare staff seeking it have understandably kept away from them. Chapter 18, by Sadie Thomas-Unsworth, Zoe Berger, Joanna Farrington-Exley, and myself, is about offering debriefs/group interventions in response to difficult events (such as crash calls and patient deaths). We explore the history of and evidence for psychological debriefs and present a model to deliver these in a psychologically safer way.

One of the main reasons for there being little published about psychological staff support is that many psychologists are doing this work but barely have the time to do so, let alone write about it. This book aims to redress this balance: to chronicle and celebrate the excellent thinking and practice that is out there already and to spur practitioners on to develop this field.

What is staff support? Working definitions and terms

As an emerging speciality, defining what staff support and wellbeing is, and importantly what it is not, is tricky. Staff support has many dimensions; it is important that we don't just focus on the psychological but consider practical and spiritual elements too. All the chapters here have slightly different takes on staff support work. When I try and explain psychological staff support, I often come back to the refrain 'staff support is not therapy'. This could be misunderstood to mean that it is not skilled. Let us explore why it is not traditional therapy. The loose premise of staff support is that staff have been affected by their work or that their ability to work has been affected by something. In practice this is not an easy distinction to make, as the work may involve supporting individuals and teams related to a distressing incident on the ward, but it may also be that something outside work is combining with workplace stress to have an impact. This was certainly the case in the pandemic where healthcare staff were affected both at work and at home.

The focus of the work is broader than individual, and team concerns though. It is necessarily strategic and operates at an organisational level, and therefore cannot ignore systemic and workplace issues that cause stress and mental health problems for staff. Consequently, it is critical to consider language used to describe our interventions and how some terms can become 'dirty words'. Resilience is a case in point; I would say it is essential to reflect on the ethics of delivering 'resilience training' to individuals when there are systemic issues such as resource or staff shortage at the root of staff stress. Instead, we need to think about how we support our organisations and practices to be more resilient and provide decent working conditions to better serve their patients and staff.

Associated with this, staff I have spoken with have also started to react badly to 'kindness' initiatives telling me they need more than platitudes and feel patronised when told to feel kind: "I don't feel kind when I am stressed and overworked" one staff member told me and "being told to be kind, in these instances, just has the opposite effect". In the UK, the NHS has Civility and Respect Programmes with initiatives to put kindness into action via kinder leadership to develop kinder cultures. These are all noble aims but how they are put into practice may place the onus on individuals (leaders, team members) to be civil and kind whereas often little is said about examples of 'unkindness' and 'incivility' at a societal and/or organisational level such as chronic underfunding and poorly resourced systems. Michael West (2021) clarifies that the term compassionate leadership does not only relate to individuals but is applicable to institutions or political leaders. How much organisations value compassion, he argues, will influence the 'value fit' between staff: "The stronger the alignment of individual and organisational values, the higher the levels of staff members' commitment, engagement and satisfaction" (West, 2021, p. 63). Several chapters reflect on how language is used in staff wellbeing. In chapter 4, 'Moral Injury: Why Exploring Novel Terms Makes Space for Talking in Staff Support', Esther Murray considers the vocabulary of the staff support arena and whether we construct certain labels to enable emotional talking in healthcare settings where traditionally staff are supposed to be 'strong' and care for others.

Furthermore, staff support is different to therapy because it involves a collegiate relationship[2] rather than a client/patient therapist relationship. In some instances, we may support staff at the same time as working together with patients and families. So, we may experience similar stresses from our shared workplace. This throws to light questions and dilemmas around the boundaries of confidentiality and how we protect this. Linked to this, not only are we part of the same organisation as the staff we see, we also may operate in that system in different ways beyond working directly with staff and consider issues at an organisational level. Karen Treisman writes (chapter 2) about organisational trauma related to staff wellbeing and integrates narrative, compassion practices, and ideas from community psychology. The chapter condenses her book on trauma-informed organisations which suggests that organisations can be like living organisms and display trauma behaviour within their systems, processes,

---

[2] This is mainly the case for those of us doing the work from within the same organisation, but we may still have a near collegiate relationship as healthcare professionals regardless of our place of work.

and behaviours. Her chapter illustrates what patients and staff may experience when a system or organisation is traumatised, and thankfully offers some brilliant ways to counteract this and help organisations to become more trauma informed.

Clearly thinking systemically and relationally is vital. Adrian Neal and Julie Highfield (chapter 5) encourage us to reflect on our work at different levels (individual, team, and organisational) and propose a relational guide to aid us to do so. Particularly useful aspects of their guide are contemplations on the tension of delivering compassionate care alongside self-compassion as well as applications of the concept of intelligent kindness on ourselves in supporting others.

Lastly, we might say staff support is not therapy because it is often short term and does not involve many sessions – it could involve just a one-off meeting.[3] Does this mean it is akin to 'downgraded therapy' which is a term applied to therapies with fewer sessions and online automated therapy? I would argue not as it requires a different skill set where the work is informed by psychological models and interventions and is carried out at multiple levels. If it is not therapy, does this mean that anyone can do it? Well yes and no – it depends on what training people have and what they are setting out to do. Ideally any staff wellbeing support will exist within a tiered framework with trained mental health practitioners who can be in a position to support and consult with others.[4]

Subsequently, the work requires a wide range of skills that are psychologically informed such as rapid and complex assessment skills and triaging, sign posting, coaching, group facilitation, psychological first aid, connecting people to their own effective wellbeing strategies, psychoeducation, and risk management. This involves distilling an extensive psychological evidence base from areas as wide ranging as stress and anxiety management; sleep hygiene; and individual, group, and organisational trauma; as well as getting up to speed on workplace policies such as those within occupational health and human resources.

---

[3] I recognise that an important exception to this claim is Solution-Focused therapy which can be short term and may involve just one session. This is why I think it fits so well with staff support work.
[4] An example in the UK is supporting restorative supervision carried out by Professional Midwifery and Nursing Advocates.

Approaches to staff support

Traditional therapeutic models and practice have been adapted with new applications emerging relevant to staff support. Some are described in this book including chapter 10 by Kate Lucre, Catherine Lacey, and Jon Taylor which runs through the theory and neurobiological basis for compassion and considers the debate around vicarious distress before presenting a model of Compassion-Focused Staff Support. In chapter 11, Julie Fraser and Liz Matias write about the Professional Tree of Life applied to working with healthcare staff, which has been adapted from Tree of Life and Narrative practice. Their chapter describes how staff can use this approach to work on their own and their team's wellbeing (the forest). Additionally, they argue that this work can nurture understanding in teams and mark the diversity of staff's backgrounds and experiences. Chapter 17 by Shannon Cullerton and Sherry Rehim discusses how working in healthcare can be potentially triggering for people with previous trauma history from outside work and/or from past work experiences. They go on to outline how they have used EMDR with staff working in acute physical health settings to good effect. As we have seen already, there are many different types of staff support which operate at different levels. Let us look more closely at what we mean by group/team staff support and support at the organisational level.

Group and team level

As most healthcare staff work in teams of some description, and as we have established that social connection and peer support are important factors (alongside decent working conditions) in staff wellbeing, it will come as no surprise that we have lots of chapters describing work at a group and/or team level. Some I have introduced already and others I will detail here. Before I do so it is useful to reflect on this quote from Neal and Highfield (chapter 15):

> *Within the workplace, groups of people who cooperate are often called 'teams' (e.g., on a shift or within the same department or sharing a physical space). Especially in healthcare they may not meet the specific criteria needed to be a 'true team'. True teams rely on their ability to sustain relationships and cooperation to achieve their shared aims and objectives.*

Chapter 6 by Zoe Berger, Joanna Farrington-Exley, Sadie Thomas-Unsworth, and myself centres around types of interventions that can be offered to teams and groups (and leadership) beyond those in response to adverse events. It reflects on the role of psychologists in providing staff wellbeing input to 'teams' and how they may do so in direct and indirect ways. It considers whether psychologists are always best placed to offer these interventions and the importance of careful commissioning of the work. In chapter 9, Benna Waites, Charlie Jones, Laura Simms, Alister Scott, Rachel Potter, and Andy Bradley demonstrate the power of connection to positively support staff through structured compassion practices which maximise peer support even in a one-off meeting. This chapter describes cross-professional collaboration between psychology, nursing, and colleagues in OD in the development of different kinds of spaces for staff groups drawing on compassion principles, including taking care giving care rounds, compassion circles, and care spaces.

Elsewhere group interventions can be ongoing such as those charted in the two chapters concentrating on reflective practice. The first, 'The Heads and Hearts Model of Reflective Practice' (chapter 12) by Arabella Kurtz and Joanna Levene, builds on the model outlined in Arabella's book (Kurtz, 2021) with particular adaptations for shorter-term reflective interventions. This model draws on a range of influences including psychoanalytic concepts of emotional containment and the social defence system, as well as research on effective supervision and psychological safety within the supervisory relationship, to produce a model that is both clear and adjustable to different contexts. The chapter discusses dilemmas such as group membership, attendance, and organisational support for reflective practice groups. The second chapter championing reflective practice, chapter 13, is written by three esteemed psychologists, Poornima Bhola, Rathna Isaac, and Chetna Duggal, and discusses creative ways to use a reflective practice lens in planning and delivering support when resources are scarce and thinly spread. It presents a range of reflective practice innovations taking place in India with healthcare workers, including programmes in general hospital settings and in rural communities, independent practitioner initiatives, and those related to pandemic/disaster work. This chapter ties nicely with chapter 7, 'Supporting Staff and Volunteers Delivering Services to People in Crisis', by Sarah Davidson, Rachel Morley, Paula Aredez Arriazu, and Andrea Wood which depicts work by the psychosocial and mental health team of the British Red Cross. Their extensive experience shines through as they describe the importance of cultural humility, especially when working for a humanitarian organisation in order to provide culturally appropriate interventions with diverse staff groups. They present the CALMER model as a key structure to their work and outline some of the ways they support staff and volunteers such as reflective practice, their peer supporter programme, and workshops.

Strategic and organisational working

Having said all of this, the nature of staff support means that a lot of the work does not actually relate to a set group intervention or individual staff support, and as mentioned previously, this makes it hard to describe in a concise way. What we do may take up a lot of time, but we may not have something tangible (a consultation or debrief) to show for it as it is about building relationships and strategic working. So if, like me, you sometimes feel the work is a bit slippery and vague, turn to Julie Highfield and Adrian Neal (chapter 15), 'Strategic Working and Supporting Leadership within a Healthcare Context'. This chapter beautifully outlines the various roles psychologists can have working in staff wellbeing in different ways across an organisation. Highfield and Neal introduce the concept of influence as a practitioner psychologist, comparing and contrasting formalised roles of staff wellbeing and authorised influence versus other more traditional roles for psychologists and informal influence. This leads us to contemplate how our work is commissioned and what permissions we have to do the work. Furthermore how wellbeing generally is positioned?

Thinking about positioning and commissioning of the work is central to setting up the work which Neil Rees and I consider in our chapter 'Setting up Systems of Staff Support Using a Systemic Approach' (chapter 3). We chart how we applied systemic principles in building a comprehensive system to support the healthcare workforce in our organisation and argue that collaboration and developing relationships with key players is paramount. Another chapter that centres on relational aspects in approaching the work is chapter 14 where Lisa Monaghan and Cathy Thorley describe their innovative application of the Open Dialogue approach to staff support interventions. Here they build the case for using Open Dialogue because of its positive impact on staff wellbeing – whether that is indirectly through working with clients or directly supporting staff in supervision-type sessions.

While I was keen for this book not to focus solely on the pandemic, we cannot ignore the lasting and wide-ranging influence of COVID-19 on healthcare staff. It continues to affect our energy levels and psychological wellbeing, as we continue to ride waves of infections while trying to balance the continuing ongoing demands of regular clinical care. Some chapters document the possibilities opened up by the pandemic and excellent staff support initiatives formed as a result. Penelope Cream and Mike Wang outline the Association of Clinical Psychology's (ACP-UK) response in chapter 16: 'Brief Interventions with Senior Healthcare Staff during the Pandemic'. They give us a fascinating account of setting up this work at national level and reflect on how we generalise the learning from this into ongoing psychological staff support working, including addressing the needs of psychologists doing staff support work. This is an essential and often neglected component of the work.

I have been fortunate in the editing role to connect meaningfully with chapter authors and contributors, some of whom I have never met in person. I have learned a great deal from the content of these chapters and been hugely impressed by the authors who wrote them. I hope the same will be true for you.

References and further reading

Ahsan, S. (2022). 'EDI' endless distraction and inaction. *The Psychologist*, April 2022, 35, 23–26.

Aris, S., Garraway, H., & Gilbert, H. (2021). *Mental health, spirituality and wellbeing*. Hove: Pavilion.

Campbell, D. (2000). *The socially constructed organization*. London: Karnac Books. (The systemic thinking and practice series – work with organizations).

Clarke, R. (2017). *Your life in my hands: A Junior Doctor's story*. London: Metro Books.

Clarke, R. (2019). Medicine for the soul – Thoughts from dotMD conference 2019. *BMJ blog*. https://blogs.bmj.com/bmj/2019/09/19/rachel-clarke-medicine-for-the-soul-thoughts-from-dotmd-conference-2019/ (Accessed 18/10/2021).

Collins, A. (2022). More than 7k resignations every month as NHS staff seek better work-life balance. HSJ. https://www.hsj.co.uk/workforce/more-than-7k-resignations-every-month-as-nhs-staff-seek-better-work-life-balance/7032351.article (Accessed 31/3/2022).

Department of Health. (2021). The NHS constitution for England. https://www.gov.uk/government/publications/the-nhs-constitution-for-england (Accessed 22/4/2022).

Dollard, M., & Bakker, A. B. (2010). Psychosocial safety climate as a precursor to conducive work environments, psychological health problems, and employee engagement. *Journal of Occupational & Organizational Psychology*, 83, 579–599.

D'Urso, A., O'Curry, S., Mitchell, L., et al. (2019). Staff matter too: Pilot staff support intervention to reduce stress and burn-out on a neonatal intensive care unit. *Archives of Disease in Child Fetal Neonatal Edition*, May; 104.

Gawande, A. (2014). *Being mortal: Medicine and what matters in the end*. London: Profile Books.

Gawande, A. (2018). Why doctors hate their computers. *The New Yorker*, November 12th Issue.

Global Forum. (2019). 1.5-day workshop for global healthcare leaders called 'a systems-approach to alleviating work-induced stress and improving health, well-being, and resilience of health professionals within and beyond education'.

Kalanithi, P. (2016). *When breath becomes air*. London: Bodley Head.

Kurtz, A. (2020). *How to run reflective practice groups: A guide for healthcare professionals*. London: Routledge.

Macaulay, C., & Conniff, H. (2020). Developing a programme of staff support in a children's hospital. *Archives of Disease in Childhood British Medical Journal*, June, 106(6), 523–524.

Marmot, M. (2015). *The health gap: The challenge of an unequal world*. London: Bloomsbury.

Marsh, H. (2014). *Do no harm: Stories of life, death and brain surgery*. London: Weidenfeld & Nicolson.

Mildenhall, J. (2021). Paramedics lived experiences of post incident traumatic distress and psychosocial support. In: Murray, E. & Brown, J. (Eds.), *The mental health and wellbeing of healthcare practitioners: Research and practice*, 54–72. London: Wiley Blackwell.

Murray, E., & Brown, J. (2021). *The mental health and wellbeing of healthcare practitioners: Research and practice*. London: Wiley Blackwell.

Morrison, L. (2021). *The wellbeing toolkit for doctors*. London: Watkins.

Obholzer, A., & Roberts, V. Z. (1996). *The unconscious at work: Individual and organizational stress in the human services*. London: Routledge.

Olusoga, D. (2022). Much as we love the NHS we can no longer ignore the ethnic inequalities that beset it. *The Observer*, 47 (Accessed 20/02/2022).

Smith, J. (2021). *Nurturing maternity staff: How to tackle trauma, stress and burnout to create a positive working culture in the NHS*. London: Pinter & Martin.

Stoter, D. J. (1997). *Staff support in healthcare*. London: Blackwell.

Tavistock & Portman. (2019). Workplace stress and the supportive organisation: A framework for improvement through reflection curiosity and change. Health Education England Commissioned service from the Tavistock & Portman NHS Foundation Trust's National Workforce Skills Development Unit.

Wallbank, S. (2016). *The restorative resilience model of supervision: A reader exploring resilience to workplace stress in health and social care professionals*. Hove: Pavilion.

West, M. A. (2021). *Compassionate leadership: Sustaining wisdom, humanity and presence in health and social care*. Swirling Leaf Press.

Wren, B. (2016). *True tales of organisational life*. London: Karnac.

Yong, E. (2021). Why health-care workers are quitting in droves. *The Atlantic* (Accessed 16/11/2021).

Section 1
Thinking

1 Making Equality, Diversity, and Inclusion Fundamental to Staff Support Working

Dr Raselle Miller

'Were you asked to write a chapter to make an "ethnic-diversity" quota?' asked a colleague, when they learnt I was contributing to a book.

At the time of writing this chapter, I do not know the identity characteristics of other authors and yet I find myself wondering if any of them have been asked a similar question, or if their expertise is assumed and unquestioned. As a Black female psychologist, am I seen as being in the 'valued expert' in-group or the 'ethnic-diversity quota' out-group? In these seconds, I am reminded of why this particular chapter needs to be written.

Language disclaimer

Language powerfully shapes the sense we make of experiences and sets parameters that guide our understanding of what is, or is not, possible. For a long time, I felt uncomfortable with the language used in discussions around equality, diversity, and inclusion (EDI). In my ongoing attempts to name and explain the dynamics of inequality, oppression, and marginalisation, like others, I have been guilty of using limited terms that maintain the very status quo that should rightly be dismantled. In my search for a greater understanding, I was relieved to come across others grappling with this dilemma, such as Dr Muna Abdi (2021) who is also on a quest for alternatives to words such as 'ethnic minorities', 'privilege', and 'allyship'. I do not use the word 'minority' in recognition of multiple experiences people come with and acknowledge that people are 'marginalised' due to social mechanisms of power and structural dominance.

In this chapter, the language I use represents language that has evolved with my learning and feels to me in the context of this moment, closer to comfortable. I note that language is not fixed, and as the perceptions of the world change, our language, including my own, will change too. As such, there may come a time when the words used here may no longer fit with the new sense we have made of the world. I remain eager and ready to learn.

In this chapter I present some ideas and an example to support the reader in thinking about EDI in staff support working. The people, settings, or scenarios described are an amalgamation of experiences I, and others, have witnessed or experienced since joining the healthcare profession in 2009. All identifiable details have been changed to maintain confidentiality.

Introduction and key points

We do not live in an equal world. Social inequalities are all around us. News stories, conversations, and perhaps our own experiences remind us of differences in income and poverty levels, health access and outcomes, educational and employment opportunities. These differences are further influenced by cultural or social group status such as gender, age, sexual identity, sexual orientation, having a disability, or being from a particular racial or ethnic group – to name just a handful.

Chronic exposure to inequalities such as socio-economic disadvantage, stigma, marginalisation, and discrimination can be directly linked to differences in physical health, psychological and emotional wellbeing, and even life expectancy (Anderson, 2013; Assari and Moghani Lankarani, 2018; Brondolo et al., 2009; Fujishiro, 2009; Thornicroft et al., 2016). The COVID-19 pandemic emphasised rising health inequalities for marginalised and under-represented communities (Marmot et al., 2020). Those identifying as being from Black and Asian ethnic communities, people living with disabilities and long-term health conditions, and people migrating to the United Kingdom (UK) and the United States (US) have all faced mounting hardship and barriers to good health. The global Black Lives Matter movement (BLM) further heightened public consciousness of race inequality and the impact of race-based trauma in people's day-to-day lives, although the content was not new to many experiencing such distress.

Despite evidence revealing direct links between our social experience and physical and emotional health, we continually fail to give social experience the weight it deserves (Taylor, 2020). We spend a significant amount of our adult lives as 'staff', working in organisations and services. These organisations are embedded in society and are influenced by the tides of the times (Kinouani, 2021). Understanding these influences and the context in which they are being experienced are key to thinking about how we support people in the workplace.

Within health settings across the UK, Europe, and the US, research demonstrates that a workforce that feels valued, included, and motivated supports the delivery of high-quality patient care and increases both patient safety and patient-reported satisfaction (Aiken et al., 2012). Supporting and valuing staff – not only for *what* they do, but for how they *feel* while doing it – is the right thing to do.

Despite decades of surveys, rhetoric, reports, and policy change, health providers such as the National Health Service (NHS) continue to perform poorly across many measures of staff health and wellbeing, and EDI outcomes (Royal College of Physicians, 2015). EDI can sit on a spectrum from non-existent to an overused common phrase or process constant use of the term that does nothing more than virtual signal. In some cases, it is a tick-box exercise rather than actioning a set of words that represent everything a meaningful society should have as its foundation. EDI should be as fundamental as breathing is to living. In the workplace, we must be prepared to make real changes to challenge our own private thoughts, attitudes, and beliefs about individuals we work with who may be of different ethnicities to our own. We must support everyone's right to be treated with respect. Everyone deserves to have access to fair and equal opportunities so they can flourish and succeed in an environment that uniquely enables them to do so. Organisations must recognise that 'diverse' identities all belong and must create an environment where 'diverse' thought and experience is celebrated, and each person's contribution is seen and valued.

Staff support for the workforce can be defined by the health and wellbeing ethos of an organisation. Much of the focus of staff support initiatives in recent years has been on the organisational cost of impaired wellbeing, such as absenteeism and staff retention rates, rather than the experience of individuals (Litchfield, 2021). 'Wellbeing' is in danger of becoming a buzzword linked to processes and procedures. For me, wellbeing is about the safety that comes with feeling included and with having a purposeful life (Nikolova and Graham, 2020). Safety encompasses the physical (environment and body), psychological/emotional, spiritual, social, and financial. Within the workplace, this might be asking how a colleague is and genuinely meaning it; seeing people for who they are and what they need and sharing experiences.

There are many forms of oppression and inequality faced by marginalised groups. Examples include racism, sexism, and ableism, all of which involve a form of power and control, and result in people being separated into hierarchical groups (David and Derthick, 2017; Hwang, 2021). Some examples include superior/inferior, dominant/dominated. Also see Iris Young's (2009) 'Five Faces of Oppression' for further reading beyond the -isms. This chapter will use race and cultural inequality as its main example.

In all Western nations where data is collected, Black people and those from marginalised ethnic groups continue to experience hostile workplaces (Kinouani, 2021). This is the case when they are in the minority or have a sense of being the 'out-group'. Numerous research studies in the UK and US demonstrate that people from ethnically marginalised groups are significantly less likely to be offered wellbeing or emotional support when reporting distress, and face increased barriers when trying to access support from numerous organisations, including those in the health sector (Bignall et al., 2020), educational institutions (Haque and Elliot, 2017), and the police (Smith Lee and Robinson, 2019). Individuals are often called upon to improve their physical and psychological resilience, rather than recognise the challenges are due to deep-rooted structural organisational processes (Litchfield, 2021).

When behaviours, structures, and systems that maintain inequality and oppression are unchallenged, they become the norm. If we are going to truly support employees, we must address racial inequalities for staff, and for the patients and families they support. We must have open and honest conversations with ourselves and others about the impact of inequality, discrimination, and racism, and work together to create change. From small steps to big efforts, every single person's contribution will count towards reducing inequalities and support a culture where wellbeing matters for all.

A focus on ethnically marginalised groups is rarely given and is thus the focus of this chapter. Defensive manoeuvres and distractions often deflect to other intersecting areas of oppression that frequently centres 'Whiteness' (Ahsan, 2022). Race is often seen as an insignificant topic within organisations (Kandola, 2020). It is time that the experience of those racially marginalised is allowed a platform to be understood. This chapter aims to provoke thinking and conversations around racial inequality, and to serve as a springboard for supporting individual distress and organisational change. I hope it will support readers to consider the varying needs of staff within their own practice areas, from a corridor conversation to the design and implementation of new approaches within their organisations that can move us towards true equality, fairness, and inclusivity.

The meaning of EDI

Nowadays it is hard to find a workplace or institution that does not have some form of an EDI statement, policy, or working group. At the time of writing (February

2022), for example, all 227 NHS Trusts in the UK (NHS, 2021) give some reference to 'equality … treating people fairly …' and/or 'with respect'. But what does this actually mean? The broadness of the term has allowed room for confusion. If we are suggesting that EDI is all fundamental to staff support working, it feels important to start by defining what we mean by the terms that are so often used in this triple tandem.

Equality is a person's right to equal opportunity and treatment, and not to be discriminated against because of their identified characteristics. In the UK, the Equality Act 2010 (Figure 1.1; *UK Government, 2022*) highlights the unlawful ways to treat someone and legally protects people from discrimination in the workplace and wider society.

Equality cannot be achieved without considering equity. Equity means recognising that people do not start from the same place, and sometimes adjustments for imbalances are needed to ensure genuine access to opportunity (to learn more, see the Equality and Human Rights Commission, EHRC, 2022).

To be diverse is to be different or varied. **Diversity** is taking account of the differences or variety within people or groups, to explore these differences and to place a positive value on those differences.

Inclusion is to feel respectfully included, to have a sense of belonging and to be embraced as part of something.

These words are not static. They depend on people, reflection, challenge, and change. In the workplace, diversity is what makes people unique, while inclusion refers to the social norms and behaviours that support people in feeling welcome, valued, and essential to the success of the organisation.

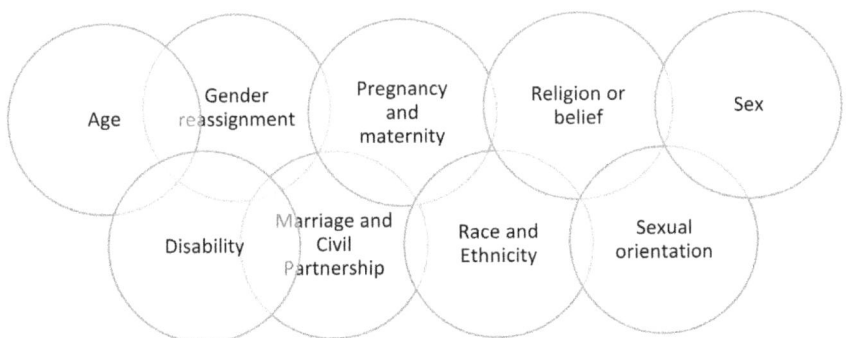

FIGURE 1.1: Protected characteristics under the UK Equality Act (2010).

Organisations may have commissioned an EDI team or individual who is allocated the mammoth task of somehow transforming inequality within an institution. However, this does not guarantee an institution is willing to be transformed (Ahsan, 2022). It is not the task of one named person to do the work of a whole institution. We are all stakeholders in the move towards a diverse and inclusive workplace. The risks to individual wellbeing and quality of experience are too high for it to be otherwise. As such, everyone has a responsibility to contribute. This may be through participation, leadership, and/or solidarity. These positions may create different emotional 'burdens' and therefore require different acknowledgements and support.

Data

When we think of staff support, data is not the first thing that comes to mind. Furthermore, there are a number of challenges when collecting data – for example, survey fatigue, a lack of contextual understanding, reluctance to offer time when there is doubt about the possibility of meaningful change, and the fear of repercussions if answers are honest. However, equality data collection can be a powerful tool by proving discrimination and exclusion that would otherwise be invisible in general anonymous surveys (European Network Against Racism, ENAR, 2018; 2022). If data collection is carried out in an environment where people feel safe, it can allow an individual to share their experiences and help to evaluate and improve legislation, policies, and practice. Since 2015 in the UK, NHS and independent healthcare providers are required to demonstrate how they are addressing race equality issues through the Workforce Race Equality Standard (WRES) (NHS England, 2021). Data from 2020 to 2021 show that 63% of healthcare staff within England reported experiencing discrimination at work based on their ethnicity/race, significantly higher than any other protected characteristic (see Figure 1.2).

Ethnically marginalised staff also consistently report lower levels of equality of opportunity in the workplace than their White counterparts (Equality and Human Rights Commission, EHRC, 2022).

The ENAR has highlighted that the UK is the only country (previously in the EU) that routinely collects equality data on race and ethnicity. There is no **European-wide data available** to indicate how many persons experience unequal treatment because of their racial or ethnic origin (ENAR, 2022).

A report from the EHRC stated that more than 50% of organisations face barriers when collecting equality data. Thirty-two per cent of those surveyed

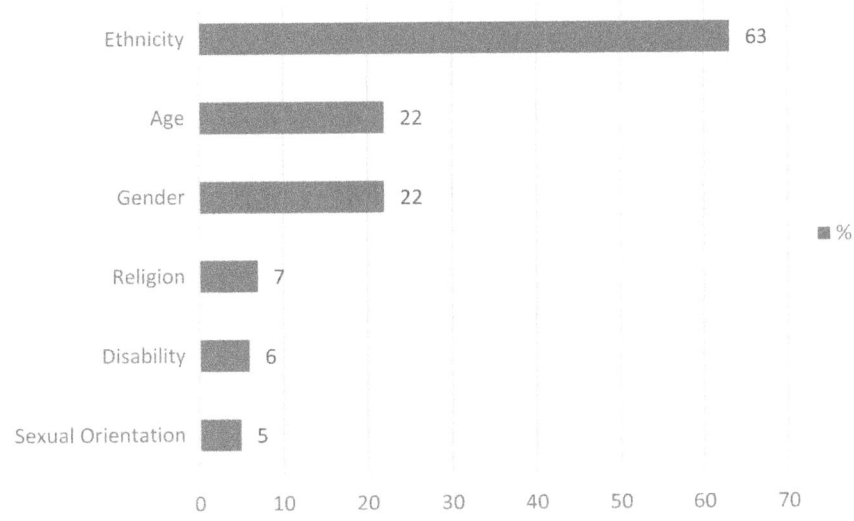

FIGURE 1.2: Reported discrimination by healthcare staff in the NHS (2020–2021).

reported concern about questions being too intrusive or believed employees would not want to share (Adams et al., 2018). These concerns and assumptions could be argued to be a form of discrimination themselves. By not recording data, either in the form of surveys or lived experiences, these organisations are making it difficult to recognise problems that will impact critical areas such as recruitment, job progression, and employee experience. This in turn puts marginalised groups at even more of a disadvantage. Without data-based insights, organisations cannot meaningfully tackle the underlying causes of inequality.

> *In collecting data, do you understand and agree with what you are asking? Secondly, can you explain these reasons to others with conviction? If you can't – can you adapt or change the data measure? Consider the needs of those being asked – what do you need to do to make people feel safe or brave enough to honestly share their lived experiences?*

The multi-dimensions of racism

Racism is manifested in many forms and can be understood using a multi-dimensional model as shown in Figure 1.3, and with a staff support example later in this chapter. Racism is a form of oppression and can be characterised as both a

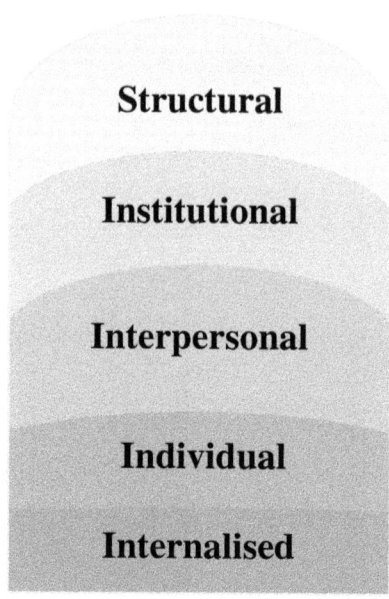

FIGURE 1.3: The multi-dimensions of racism.

process and an outcome (Griffith et al., 2007). Please see Shelly Harrell's (2000) paper – which is still strikingly relevant after 22 years – to better understand how the constructs of race and racism can be defined, as well as the detailed descriptions of racism-related stress.

- **Structural racism:** the overarching system of racial bias across institutions and society, and over time. *For example, a Black staff member is placed on a formal disciplinary notice for lateness for while a White staff member is not. The Black staff member is sometimes late due to the disproportionate number of identity and belongings checks by security staff on entering the building.*
- **Institutional racism:** the policies and practices at an organisational or sector level that perpetuate oppression and result in inequitable outcomes. *For example during interview shortlisting, a potential candidate is disqualified because the manager does not recognise the country or name of the institution where they trained.*
- **Interpersonal racism**: where individual views are brought into the public realm, occurring between individuals, both within and across difference. *For example, a White staff member favours a shift partnership with someone*

of the same race or ethnicity, voicing their unhappiness when partnered with someone different. In my case, the belief of one person that I could have only been asked to write a chapter because I am Black and can meet a quota, not because of my knowledge or the respect I have from the editors.

- **Individual racism:** the beliefs, attitudes, and actions of individuals that support or perpetuate racism in conscious ways and equally damaging, unconscious ways. This is what people typically think of when they think of racism. Examples include overt social avoidance or exclusion, discrimination, stigmatisation, harassment or threat (Brondolo et al., 2009). It can also take less perceptible forms, such as 'micro-aggressions' – the subtle attitudes and beliefs against people due to their colour/look/race (Sue et al., 2007). *For example, telling a joke in the staff room that is based on racial categorisation and telling someone not to be so sensitive if they try to voice offence.*
- **Internalised racism:** acceptance by members of the stigmatised racial group of negative messages and stereotypes, leading to the doubt and devaluation of their own abilities and the intrinsic worth of people of their own race (Jones, 2000; Pyke, 2010). *For example, a person attempting to change the characteristics that they believe makes them racially distinct. Not associating with colleagues of a similar race or ethnicity.*

Countless empirical studies document the association of racism with the experience of physical stress and/or emotional distress. Global research demonstrates everything from disproportionately high levels of common colds, diabetes, and blood pressure issues to lifetime cardiovascular disease (Brondolo et al., 2009; Anderson, 2013). People who identified as being from a racially marginalised group were disproportionately affected by COVID-19. For example, in England, they were far more likely to die: approximately 62%–75% of healthcare staff who died up from COVID-19-related causes were from racially marginalised communities (*statistic reflects data up to April 2020*) (see Phiri et al., 2013).

Studies also show that incidents of racism are linked to higher levels of stress, depression, anxiety, and trauma (Brondolo et al., 2009). There is also a strong body of evidence emphasising the neurological and cognitive impact of racism, inequality, and oppression. One such example is a longitudinal study of women in the US which revealed that experiences of racism are linked with decreased memory and cognition later in life (Coogan et al., 2020).

There can be numerous benefits in organisations recognising these implications. However, there are also some risks. One is in a form of 'diagnostic overshadowing'. For example, a needle phobia can just be a needle phobia and not the unconscious fear of medical experimentation stemming from ancestors who were enslaved in eighteenth-century Caribbean colonies. It is important to recognise not all individuals experience their cultural or racial marginalisation as disadvantage (Anderson, 2013). While everyone has a culture and has been subjected to socially constructed racial categorisation, no one person's experience is representative or generalisable to others. Each individual's embodiment of their culture will be different. While the evidence of such human distress is overwhelming, we must be careful not to limit narratives around race and ethnicity exclusively through a lens of disadvantage and deficit. This overlooks the richness and variety in experience of joy, ability, achievement, and strength held by individuals and within racially marginalised groups. Tadmor, Galinsky, and Maddux (2012), for example, show that bicultural individuals and those who have lived in a country with a different cultural context have significant increases in problem-solving creativity, perhaps as a result of added experience reconciling their different cultural identities and social norms.

The role of intersectionality

It is widely accepted that the opportunities any individual is offered in life are greatly impacted by their race, gender, sexual orientation, and disability status, along with many other aspects of their identity. These elements in turn can be consistently associated with varying determinants of health inequalities, wellbeing, and access to services (Marmot, 2005, 2020).

Within research, practice, and the development of policy, there has been a tendency to recognise each element in isolation and respond to them as separate entities, rather than as one piece of a puzzle (Muirhead et al., 2020). Crenshaw (1989) recognised the need to name the interrelationship among them and coined the term 'intersectionality' to describe how aspects of a person's social and political identities combine to create different experience and life chances. Some elements of identity are associated with privilege and hierarchy dominance, while others are disadvantageous. Intersectionality opposes systems that treat each oppressive factor in isolation (Crenshaw, 1989). There may be simultaneous interactions, but these are not synonymous. For example, economic oppression is not synonymous with racial oppression. Take the example of a staff member who describes herself as a doctor, of Ghanaian heritage, a female, mother of two, and a homeowner. This person may experience heterosexual, educational, and socio-economic privilege, while also simultaneously enduring the oppression associated with membership of marginalised gender and marginalised racial groups. The ways in which a person can identify can be vast, with people claiming distinct and overlapping identities at different times (Goclowska and Crisp, 2014). So how does this relate to staff support? When people identify as being from multiple oppressed or marginalised groups, there can be a cumulative negative impact on wellbeing. For example, studies in Black-American and Black-Caribbean populations show the dual stigma of homophobia and racism is predictive of higher instances of depression and suicidal ideation (Couzens et al., 2017).

> *"As a Black, Muslim man, I am more than twice as likely to experience discrimination at work from a colleague as white staff, and more than twice as likely to experience discrimination as staff of no religion. I'm 27% less likely than White staff to become a 'very senior manager' – you think work is a nice place for me to be?"*

In supporting staff, take a moment to reflect on your own experience. When working with staff, *are there particular identities you notice or find yourself prioritising over others? Notice these and reflect on what has come up, and why.*

An **identities chart or map** can be a helpful way of supporting an individual to connect to words they use to describe themselves – sibling, runner, holder of faith, survivor, poet, father, or nurse – as well as noticing the labels that the community or society may give them.

Burnham's social graces mnemonic (2012) may also be a supportive reflexive tool to help identify the visible and invisible aspects of identity that may impact our lives.

Staff support example

Ayọ̀bámi walks past a staff support information stall in a work corridor and stops for a moment as she is early for her shift. She[1] doesn't enquire about

---

[1] These are the staff member's chosen pronouns.

wellbeing support or therapy. She asks if there is somewhere she can learn about training and work progression opportunities outside of her appraisals with her manager.

> *What are your initial thoughts or assumptions about what is happening for Ayọ̀bámi? In hearing her name, pronouns, and request? What is Ayọ̀bámi asking for and how might you go about helping her?*

Ayọ̀bámi

I have worked in healthcare for eight years. I love my work but some colleagues who started after me, some that I trained, are progressing faster than me. They are invited to attend meetings, are given time to shadow or go to training days, but I am not given these opportunities. When I speak with my managers, and let them know I too want to progress, I am told it is not the right time due to budget or staffing shortages. I wait patiently for my turn hoping they see I can be different and am ready, trying not to push – I don't want to be seen as demanding or aggressive – but then see someone else has again gone ahead of me. It's as if they are in the right place at the right time to be seen by our managers. I wonder what I am doing wrong. My husband jokes that they talk when they get their sandwiches. I usually heat my food in the staff kitchen. I keep thinking of ways to fit in that could help. I remember a time when a colleague told me my hair was 'too big' for work, so I take time now to straighten it and tie in a similar way to my White colleagues for workdays. I feel ashamed that I am still in this junior role, and not earning more money for my family here and back home. I feel down a lot of the time, and tired of working so hard to prove myself when no one seems to notice how much harder I am working than others. My family tells me to keep going in. I don't feel valued here but feel stuck. Maybe I am not good enough. What if I can't get a different job? Maybe if I know what training or support to ask for, they will see I am serious?

Read more about her experience below.

> *What do you feel in reading this passage? How quickly did you come to the conclusion that race and difference play a role in her experience? Did you want there to be other reasons first? Did you question her job capability? Is there a déjà vu sense in your reading? Why might Ayọ̀bámi not ask for support, only information?*

Let's try to break down some common feelings here around this experience. (Note: These may differ depending on a person's racial and ethnic characteristics and lived experiences of racism.)

I will start with a reader's possible reactions. Firstly, 'I've heard something similar to this before' feeling. Kinouani (2021) reminds us that experiences of racism at work usually revolve around a similar script, and therefore evoke that déjà vu sense of past events and historical configurations related to what she terms 'micro-colonialism' (p. 117). For example, the frequent daily intrusions, breaches of physical or psychological boundaries, and invasions of privacy and personal space (e.g. feeling she is treated differently than her peers, comments on her hair) experienced by Black people. It can be this familiar feeling that stops us from connecting with our emotions and recognising the negative impact it can have for that individual and ourselves.

> *Did you identify with some of the struggles Ayọ̀bámi described but not connect with its significance?*

Let's look at some further common emotional reactions. Perhaps you felt some sadness, surprise, anger, or guilt. DiAngelo (2011, 2018) describes how people racialised as White can have a low ability to tolerate racial stress and develop strategies to protect their 'racial comfort' when hearing experiences like Ayọ̀bámi's. Where race-based discrimination is even subtly alluded to, people (particularly those racialised as White) may deny the prevalence of racism and look to find another reason, segueing perhaps into discussions about capability, educational status, gender, or class (Brown, 2019). This internalises the problem as that individual's particular experience rather than a structural or systemic societal issue that requires action. Alternatively, or maybe in addition, they might experience such emotive reactions – sadness, guilt, shock, shame, and so on – that they inadvertently silence the person who is sharing their experience. DiAngelo (2011) terms some of these reactions as examples of 'White fragility' (see DiAngelo's work to learn more).

> *Are there times when you can recall White fragility being centred in your work or workplace?*

People from ethnically marginalised groups may notice a familiar narrative and feel anger, loss, burnout/tiredness, or shame. People from ethnically marginalised groups are more likely to be in low paid, insecure jobs and are more likely to face discrimination and formal disciplinary processes. In addition, there is the misconception that they themselves are meant to manage such inequality. Next, let's consider what might be going on for Ayọ̀bámi.

Ayọ̀bámi is confused by her experience. She asks for information, not help or emotional support for experiences of racism, discrimination, and exclusion. There may be a number of reasons why she asks for support in this way. Her approach may relate to a previous experience of 'helping services'. We know people from ethnically marginalised groups are significantly less likely to be offered wellbeing, emotional support, or talking therapies when reporting distress (Memon et al., 2016). This could be a result of biased assumptions about therapies not being for certain cultural groups, and that certain groups are 'not psychologically minded' or are 'hard to reach'. A dominant narrative within supportive work is 'how capable someone is to engage in the work', rather than thinking about what a therapist or service is doing to be open and increase the chances of people feeling able to engage. People also report feeling misunderstood in supportive or therapeutic work. Culturally different verbal and non-verbal communication styles, and the misinterpretation of a person's intent by therapists, such as descriptions of physically embodied experiences, expressive gesturing, or lack of eye contact, can create misunderstandings and a low therapeutic rapport. Another reason is the erasure of important aspects of someone's identities, including their religious or spiritual beliefs, as they are believed to be incongruent with psychological interventions or talking therapy. This is often based on a therapist's interpretation of a model or reliance on more manualised forms of therapy. It may also be a protective strategy driven by a fear of damaging the therapeutic relationship. For example, it is better not to ask than get it wrong. As a result, people from ethnically or racially marginalised groups can feel that talking spaces and therapy are not for them.

Ayọbámi may have asked for support in this way because she wants to avoid triggering negative stereotypes about people of her heritage and/or the impact of intergenerational racism and employer bias. Ayọbámi may be reacting to her perceived value, related to stereotyping and internalised racism. Multi-dimensions of this include the belief or acceptance in a biased representation of history, internalising negative stereotypes about Black people (such as the negative myth of the 'angry Black woman' [Ashley, 2014]), and 'code-switching' – altering characteristics or appearance, conscious or unconscious, to fit a Eurocentric/Westernised aesthetic (Cokley, 2002; Parmer et al., 2004). 'Code-switching' can be a means of professional and/or personal survival but can lead to low esteem, anxiety, emotional exhaustion, and overall, a lowered sense of wellbeing.

Intergenerational trauma can be seen in the protective messaging Black families share with their children: to succeed despite racially based inequality and discrimination, they must 'work twice as hard … be twice as good … twice as smart'. Ayọbámi may have been subjected to contextual narratives from the family or community that suggest her personal struggles are not to be shared in public, and that she must be strong, resilient, and 'get on with it'. In the workplace, research from the US demonstrates that employer bias interferes with perceptions in job performance (Cavounidis and Lang, 2015). They show that Black employees are likely to receive more scrutiny (e.g. direct observations) from their managers than their White colleagues, meaning that small errors are more likely to be noticed. As a result, Black colleagues are more likely to be referred to performance review, disciplinary, or termination of employment for such errors. Therefore, to keep a job, Black employees must reach a higher bar. Is Ayọbámi trying not to show errors for fear of scrutiny? Is she worried that she will be penalised rather than supported? If you do not identify with others around, you are less likely to think that people will step in and have your back (Taylor, 2020).

Finally, Ayọbámi could be fatigued from having to navigate the emotional turmoil and energy required to fight daily inequality. She may want to protectively deny that racism and discrimination is a cause of this differential treatment as a form of respite. Many struggle emotionally with profound levels of awareness of structural racism and its implications for racially marginalised communities and find themselves worn out (Blaisdell, 2016). Chen and Gorski

(2015) use the term 'activist burnout' to describe when stress levels, emotional and physical health become so affected that an individual's abilities to remain effective and engaged in their activism are compromised.

Currently in the UK and US, many organisations are attempting to train their employees to recognise bias and are actively trying to attract people from racially marginalised groups into senior positions. However, ascending to an executive position does not end a person's struggles with racism, and sometimes increases those challenges (Thomas-Breitfeld and Kunreuther, 2022). Thomas-Breitfeld and Kunreuther's (2022) extensive research on non-profit executives in the US further highlights the burdens placed on 'leaders of colour' who follow a person racialised as White. With these positions often comes the powerful but silently enforced expectation of the person to 'dress in Whiteness'. This means being silent when subjected to micro-aggressions or racism, thus allowing the dominant group – White people – to remain comfortable (Kinouani, 2021). It may also mean the person is tasked with speaking up about inequality and actioning change – and is held responsible for failure when such changes are not seen.

So what next for Ayọ̀bámi? I will go on to share some of the possible options of support for people similar to Ayọ̀bámi, from individual support and sensitive group spaces. I will also share possible indirect systems level support and the power in influencing wider EDI practice. But I first ask how we can actively support EDI work.

How can we support EDI of ethnically and racially marginalised groups?

Self-care and setting boundaries

As a facilitator of staff support, there are times when we collaboratively share ideas and other times when we need to take our own advice. Setting your boundaries is one such time. Acknowledging and honouring that there must be time for rest is key to maintaining your own physical and emotional health.

If you are a person from a racially marginalised group, you may feel that you must have an opinion, that you must be able to respond to requests to share and educate and that you must continually be responsible for 'doing' in order for there be change. This is not the case. Drawing on Chris Iron's self-compassion work, how can you 'warm-up' your mind and body ready to have conversations that might feel threatening and trigger you? (Or to say 'no' that day?!) What helps you to 'warm-down' after those conversations? How can you be open and accepting of the support, care, and compassion – from yourself and others – that you need to do this work? Rest, recharge, connect, and celebrate yourself, as well as helping others to do the same.

Being a wider 'ally' is part of the support

Privilege based on racial grouping can be the difference between being able to choose whether you engage with race or not (Brown, 2019). When supporting or supervising others, it is crucial to address your own racial self-awareness by engaging in reflection on your personal experience as a racial being (Pieterse, 2018).

"The privilege of pondering the ramifications of race and racism, when it's convenient, is vastly different from the experience of walking around in the shoes of someone who can't, for a second, forget about their skin colour when it becomes inconvenient" (Sliwa, 2017:1 cited in Lloyd and Polland, 2019).

Many times have I heard phrases along the lines of: 'that training/work doesn't apply to me – my partner is from X', 'I am not racist because I lived in …', 'I have mixed race children so …' More recently it has been 'how can you think about racism when there is a war in …?' In the words of Angela Davis: "In a racist society, it is not enough to be non-racist, we must be anti-racist." It is not COVID-19 or racism, war or racism, disability or racism. It is always *and*.

Brown (2019) writes that failing to name race as a source of anxiety or conflict leaves the person alone in carrying what should be a shared commitment and silences their thinking about unjust realities.

While you may be in a formal supporting role, you are also a stakeholder in a fair and equal society. If you recognise yourself as someone who holds a form of ethnic or racial privilege, being an active accomplice to change means amplifying the voices of marginalised people, not using your position to speak for them. Following are some suggestions for indirectly supporting individuals through learning and being an active accomplice to change.

Get to know the issues

Like learning anything new, start by reading, listening, and educating yourself about the complexities of the issues you will be confronting. A search engine is a great resource for any question you might have (and you don't have to worry about how offensive it might sound). If you do have an opportunity to speak to colleagues about their experiences as part of your learning journey, listen and be compassionate about the challenges they face. If you are asking them to support your education, remember you are not entitled to their stories, time, and energy. Let them know they can decline.

Use your therapeutic relationship skills

Remind yourself of what creates a supportive and respectful relationship. An awareness of your own culture and biases (we all have both), letting go of any assumptions, being curious, and open to learning about the person and their experience (including allowing them to teach you) are key to building trust (Ade-Serrano et al., 2017).

Take considered risks

Be aware of the language you use. If you are unsure how to pronounce a name, having a go shows trying. You can also ask what someone would like to be called. Ask how someone identifies – whether this is their nationality, ethnicity, race, or language. Perhaps you can share your identity too. This sends a clear message that you haven't made an assumption and it creates the opportunity for someone to open up if they wish to.

Notice your interpretations or assumptions around the intent of a person's behaviour or communication style – for example, eye contact or use of gestures. Take a risk by being curious about how you are understanding or being understood by a person, or within a group.

Make your commitment visible to (the right) people

If you have learnt something, don't feel the need to prove what you know to your friends and colleagues from marginalised ethnic groups (this then becomes performative virtue signalling, not solidarity). Instead, send the information, book, podcast, article, and event details to someone who has a smaller knowledge base than yourself. Your new knowledge will speak for itself to those who are already committed to change.

The value of an individual space

Ayọ̀bámi's experience aims to highlight the complexities that come with each staff support request, and the potential value in offering someone a space to further explore what they feel they require. While some people may require signposting, others may value a different experience of support, particularly those who are influenced by feelings of fear, mistrust, or shame alongside their distress. One-to-one support can also be valuable for people who may not feel safe enough to voice issues in a team or group meeting, even with supportive peers.

Giving choice is a helpful place to start. Do not assume someone wants support, or that they can only be supported by someone who is from the same ethnic group or community as them. Some people may not want to talk about race-related trauma and distress. Let them know you are open and able to make space for talking about racism and inequality, discrimination if they want to.

> *How might you invite people to share marginalised aspects of their cultural and racial identities?*

> *"I was a bit taken aback when he shared that systemic racism may have a role to play in my experience and that he hoped this could become a safe space to discuss. I didn't even know talking about that would be on the table in a wellbeing meeting. The relief I felt in this person not being colour-blind was phenomenal."*

There are an array of client/practitioner dyads at play in any support space. Acknowledging power within the dynamics of the relationship and co-creating permission to speak about those dynamics can build trust and rapport.

When we belong in our environment

Taylor's (2020) writings on race and wellbeing in organisations highlight the unique influence of our working environment on health and wellbeing. He outlines the evidence showing that interactions, however brief, can reinforce our sense of belonging and feeling of connection to others. He demonstrates that identifying with those we interact with is a significant factor in enhancing self-esteem, wellbeing, and sense of control (e.g. Greenaway et al., 2015; Jetten et al., 2015). Furthermore, receiving support from others with whom you identify can counter the effects of stress within the workplace. Identification with a positive group supports strength, purpose, and motivation, even in demanding times.

When putting this into practice, naturally one of the quickest ways to identify with people is to look for visible and surface-level characteristics that rely on personal judgement – for example, a person's age, gender, or race. However, there is also value in shared beliefs.

The value of group spaces

Supportive group spaces such as reflective practice groups, Balint Groups, Compassion Circles (see chapter 9 for more on these), and organisation-wide Schwartz Rounds can be helpful in supporting people to feel connected in a shared experience, as well as having the potential to improve self-awareness and increase knowledge through learning about others' experiences. Reflections about inequality, discrimination and/or marginalisation may come up in general supportive spaces, such as a ward-based reflective practice group. Other group spaces may include the topics as an embedded discussion point, where wellbeing is considered through a lens of solidarity and active anti-racism. There may also be requests for groups to be created, named and protected, and facilitated. Here are some examples:

Group one: A reflective learning space

There is something powerful in not being alone in learning and the recognition of feelings. Setting up a regular reflective and educational space for people who want to act in solidarity with racism/EDI can be a useful place for people to come together to learn.

Group two: Creating an action-based anti-oppression group

Key to any group is its inclusive membership. Being part of a shared collective voice can be valuable for individual wellbeing as well as holding the organisation accountable to making change.

Group three: 'Safe' spaces for ethnically marginalised groups

To heal from and terminate the cycles of racial trauma, people require safe spaces to voice their stories and express their outrage (Mangum, 2010). As the human mind is storied, therapeutic storytelling with validating listeners can be a helpful way of coping with the psychological impact of racism (White and Epston, 1990).

Afiya Mbilishaka (2018) writes about the mismatch that can occur in Westernised forms of healing, for example meeting with a stranger in an unfamiliar or sterile space for 50 minutes a week, compared with a community-based space with collective healing at its heart. She notes that health professionals have been slow to match therapeutic techniques with community-based social movements such as BLM. Healing and storytelling are central tenets of BLM. Social media and shared physical spaces have offered space for Black people to tell their emotional stories about racism and to organise empowering collective grassroots resistance (Mbilishaka, 2018). Having a positive racial identity within a group can be a significant protective factor against the negative mental health effects of racism-related stress (Neblett and Carter, 2012).

The Association of Black Psychologists and the Community Healing Network jointly developed a facilitated group space they call Emotional Emancipation Circles. These aim to be safe cultural spaces for people of Black ancestry to come together to share their stories, including historical trauma and counteractive stories of joy, and to critically reflect on their experiences within the community.

In a London NHS Trust, I developed the 'hear me meeting' – a monthly drop-in reflective group for all staff who identify as being from a racially marginalised group. It is not driven by action or agenda, but is an inclusive space encouraging expression, celebrating culture, and allowing people to be seen and heard by others who have similar experiences, regardless of their job role. The group aims to combat the feelings of exclusion, difference, and loneliness in the workplace. It also breaks down some of the hierarchy that can be present in health settings.

Group narrative therapy approaches such as the 'Tree of Life' (Ncube-Mlilo, 2006) (see chapter 11), 'narratives in a suitcase' (Ncube-Mlilo, 2013), as well as narrative and cognitive analytic therapy style 'multi-local life story mapping' (Selasi, 2014; Potter, 2020) can be helpful ways to support a person or people in telling neglected stories from their point of view.

There is also value in creative therapies such as art drawing with socially marginalised groups. A creative therapy can be an indirect, but deeply communicative, symbolic vehicle with which to express pain and struggle (Huss and Cwikel, 2008). Some London-based city farms are opening their spaces to 'eco-therapy groups for people of colour'. They describe these as nurturing spaces to explore woundings and find healing around experiences of racism and belonging through a deepening relationship with the natural world.

Influencing the system

As psychologists and leaders, we are trained to assess, formulate, and share understandings. Use your psychological skills and language tools to look critically in team meetings and organisation-led training sessions to highlight where there is a lack of commitment to EDI, or where there are gaps in understanding (your own or others). Request avenues for racial dialogue.

In the UK, racial diversity in key positions within organisations remains low. Senior teams are not representative of the communities they serve and the staff they lead. If people from ethnically marginalised backgrounds get to these most senior levels, they may need to contend with being the only one in a space – an experience that can be more distressing and more dynamically complex than experiences of overt discrimination or racism (Kinouani, 2021).

People from ethnically marginalised groups are over-represented in the NHS workforce. However, there are notable differences in their types of employment, pay and banding, as well as representation within senior positions within their organisations. In the UK, the March 2020 WRES data showed only 13 of the 227 NHS Trusts could report that up to 25% of their senior board contained people from Black, Asian, or other ethnic groups. Ninety-three of the 227 trusts reported more than 91% of its board identified as White. Thirty-three of 227 trusts reported 100% White identifying boards. Taylor (2020) writes: "If we do not feel an affinity with the people we work with, we do not benefit from their presence."

How do people feel safe, know they belong, or know their perspectives relating to diversity and inclusion are being considered and addressed if there is no diversity of opinion, experience, or background in the boardroom?

Support the system in its responsibility to be racially responsive and culturally sensitive.

Key practice points

In order to be truly inclusive of the diverse needs of the staff you are supporting, you should promote holistic wellbeing. This includes physical (environment and body), psychological/emotional, spiritual, social, and financial wellbeing.

There is a renewed rhetoric around cultural competence and an increased commitment to work effectively and inclusively around issues of diversity. However, many people continue to find conversations around diversity and difference challenging, particularly in public forums, training environments, and in supervision (e.g. Ellis and Cooper, 2013). Regardless of our own racial and ethnic background, it can be helpful for everyone to consider what support and resources we might need to increase our sense of safety, and our ability to offer quality support to others.

Questions for yourself when approaching EDI in staff support

- When you approach any staff support task – individual, team, or department consultation – are you actively considering the constructions of power, hierarchy, and inequality dynamics that could be at play?
- Data, data, data. What formal equality data, both qualitative and quantitative, are you actively collecting and why?
- For each request, ask yourself whether you are genuinely going to be the most helpful person to support this task in this moment. Reflect on your reasons. Do you notice yourself closely identifying with the stories shared? Are you fearful of difference or do you recognise your potential to unintentionally cause harm? Are you able to notice any personal barriers to exploring marginalised identities? Theoretical models such as the Coordinated Management of Meaning (Pearce and Cronen, 1980) can support reflexivity around one's position and communication.
- Supervision and reflective spaces: are you using your own clinical supervision or management meetings to reflect on, or consider, EDI? If you feel unable to discuss difference and diversity, why is that? What might you need to feel safe to reflect on these issues? What space are you holding for people you are supervising to consider EDI?
- What training modules or sessions are being offered from the organisation that will enhance your understanding? For example, conscious and unconscious bias, cultural humility, allyship, and anti-racism. Are you making time to engage with these?
- Team meetings: notice who is in the room. Have a variety of voices been heard and valued? Who might be trying to speak but cannot do so because they are in the minority? Whose safety and comfort might be taking priority over everyone's ideas being heard?
- Action-based learning – can you join your organisation's EDI action or working group, or can you become an advocate or representative on matters of EDI? Can you request mentoring from a colleague, or staff member, to support your learning?

Internal organisational and external resources

- Support a staff member to learn about the resources within the organisation. For example, is there a support network, a 'speak-up' team, a wellbeing team, or reflective practice and peer support group spaces that they can use? Spaces for informal conversations and shared rests enable connection and time to recharge.
- Acknowledge that support can come in different forms. For many people, religious or spiritual faith is deeply important. Support people who would like to bring these views into the workplace. Connect with any spiritual care team or chaplaincy support that exists. There may be people who are willing to share the importance of faith, or you could find external organisations that you could signpost to.
- Staff networks can also be instrumental in promoting inclusion and belonging through a connecting collective voice. Share information and encourage staff members to join staff networks (e.g. Ethnicity Network, Woman's Equality Network, LGBTQ Staff Network) that provide individual empowerment, group peer support, solidarity, and signposting.
- Help staff to know their rights and access further information and legal advocacy via professional bodies, such as the Health and Care Professions Council, the Nursing and Midwifery Council, or from a trade union.
- Recognise that some people may not feel safe or may not trust internal resources. Support them in finding similar offers externally. Consider the financial implications if funding is required.
- Acknowledge the value of a person's social community and what support they may also be able to access there. For example, community centres; spiritual, religious, and faith organisation; and natural storytelling spaces that bring people comfort in challenging times.

Conclusion

This chapter has considered the importance of EDI and active anti-racism when supporting staff at different levels, from individual working to organisational practices. I hope that readers will have these priorities at the foundations of their daily and professional lives. US poet and civil rights activist Maya Angelou said: "I did then what I knew how to do. Now that I know better, I do better."

References

Abdi, M. (2021) Language is important: Why we are moving away from the terms 'allyship' and 'privilege' in our work. https://ma-consultancy.co.uk/blog/language-is-important-why-we-will-no-longer-use-allyship-and-privilege-in-our-work. Date accessed: 3.1.2022.

Adams, L., Luanaigh, A. N., Thomson, D. and Rossite, H. (2018) *Measuring and reporting on disability and ethnicity pay gaps*. Manchester: Equality and Human Rights Commission.

Ade-Serrano, Y., Nkansa-Dwamena, O. and McIntosh, M. (2016) *Race, culture and diversity: A collection of articles*. Leicester: BPS Division of Counselling Psychology.

Ahsan, S. (2022) 'EDI': Endless distraction and inaction. *The Psychologist*, 35, 22–27.

Aiken, L. H., Sermeus, W., Van den Heede, K., Sloane, D. M., Busse, R., McKee, M., et al. (2012) Patient safety, satisfaction, and quality of hospital care: Cross sectional surveys of nurses and patients in 12 countries in Europe and the United States. *British Medical Journal*, 344, e1717.

Anderson, F. K. (2013) Diagnosing discrimination: Stress from perceived racism and the mental and physical health effects. *Sociological Inquiry*, 83(1), 55–81.

Ashley, W. (2014) The angry Black woman: The impact of pejorative stereotypes on psychotherapy with Black women. *Social Work in Public Health*, 29(1), 27–34.

Assari, S. and Moghani Lankarani, M. (2018) Workplace racial composition explains high perceived discrimination of high socioeconomic status African American men. *Brain Sciences*, 8(8), 139.

Bignall, T., Jeraj, S., Helsby, E. and Butt, J. (2020) *Racial disparities in mental health: Literature and evidence review*. London: Race Equality Foundation.

Blaisdell, B. (2016) Schools as racial spaces: Understanding and resisting structural racism. *International Journal of Qualitative Studies in Education*, 29(2), 248–272.

Brondolo, E., Gallo, L. C. and Myers, H. F. (2009) Race, racism and health: Disparities, mechanisms, and interventions. *Journal of Behavioural Medicine*, 32, 1.

Brown, H. (2019) Owning privilege and acknowledging racism. In Lloyd, J. and Polland, P. (Eds.), *Cognitive analytic therapy and the politics of mental health*, 210–221. Oxon: Routledge.

Burnham, J. (2012) Developments in social GRRRAAACCEEESSS: Visible – invisible and voiced – unvoiced. In Krause, I.-B. (Ed.), *Culture and reflexivity in systemic psychotherapy: Mutual perspectives*, 139–160). London: Karnac.

Cavounidis, C. and Lang, K. (2015) Discrimination and worker evaluation. National Bureau of Economic Research, October 2015, Working paper 21612.

Chen, C. and Gorski, P. (2015) Burnout in social justice and human rights activists: Symptoms, causes, and implications. *Journal of Human Rights Practice*, 7(3), 366–390.

Cokley, K. O. (2002) Testing cross's revised racial identity model: An examination of the relationship between racial identity and internalized racialism. *Journal of Counseling Psychology*, 49(4), 476–483.

Coogan, P., Schon, K., Li, S., Cozier, Y., Bethea, T. and Rosenberg, L. (2020) Experiences of racism and subjective cognitive function in African American women. *Alzheimer's & Dementia: Diagnosis, Assessment and Disease*, 12(1), e12067.

Couzens, J., Mahoney, B. and Wilkinson, D. (2017) "It's just more acceptable to be white or mixed race and gay than Black and gay": The perceptions and experiences of homophobia in St. Lucia. *Frontiers in Psychology*, 8(947), 1–16.

Crenshaw, K. (1989) Demarginalizing the intersection of race and sex: A Black feminist critique of antidiscrimination doctrine, feminist theory and antiracist politics. *University of Chicago Legal Forum*, 1(8), 139–167.

David, E. J. R. and Derthick, A. O. (2017) *The psychology of oppression*. New York: Springer.

DiAngelo, R. (2011) White fragility. *The International Journal of Critical Pedagogy*, 3(3), 54–70.

DiAngelo, R. (2018) *White fragility: Why it's so hard for White people to talk about racism*. Boston: Beacon Press.

Ellis, E. and Cooper, N. (2013) Silenced: The Black student experience. *Therapy Today*, 24(10). https://www.bacp.co.uk/bacp-journals/therapy-today/2013/december-2013/the-black-student-experience/. Date accessed: 3.1.2022.

European Network Against Racism (ENAR). (2022a) Combating inequality and discrimination in employment: Data collection as a necessary step to plan action. UK Government. Equality Act, 2010. https://www.legislation.gov.uk/ukpga/2010/15/section/4; https://www.gov.uk/guidance/equality-act-2010-guidance

European Network Against Racism. (2022b) Equality data collection: Facts and Principles. https://www.enar-eu.org/Equality-data-collection-151.

Equality and Human Rights Commission (EHRC). (2022) https://www.equalityhumanrights.com/en.

Fujishiro, K. (2009) 'Is perceived racial privilege associated with health? Findings from the behavioural risk factor surveillance system'. *Social Science and Medicine*, 68, 840–844.

Greenaway, K. H., Cruwys, T., Haslam, S. and Jetten, J. (2016) Social identities promote well-being because they satisfy global psychological needs. *European Journal of Social Psychology*, 46(3), 294–307.

Griffith, D. M., Childs, E. L., Eng, E. and Jeffries, V. (2007) Racism in organizations: The case of a county public health department. *Journal of Community Psychology*, 35(3), 287–302.

Goclowska, M. A. and Crisp, R. J. (2014) How dual-identity processes foster creativity. *Review of General Psychology*, 18(3), 216–237.

Haque, Z. and Elliot, S. (2017) *Visible and invisible barriers: The impact of racism on BME teachers*. The Runnymede Trust. London: Communications Department of the National Union of Teachers.

Harrell, S. P. (2000) A multidimensional conceptualization of racism-related stress: Implications for the well-being of people of color. *American Journal of Orthopsychiatry*, 70, 42–57.

Huss, E. and Cwikel, J. (2008) Embodied drawings as expressions of distress among impoverished single Bedouin mothers. *Archives of Women's Mental Health*, 11, 137–147.

Hwang, W.-C. (2021) Demystifying and addressing internalized racism and oppression among Asian Americans. *American Psychological Association*, 76(4), 596–610.

Jetten, J., Branscombe, N., Haslam, S. A., Haslam, C., Cruyws, T., Jones, J. M., Cui, L., Dingle, G., Liu, J., Murphy, S., Thai, A., Walter, Z. and Zhang, A. (2015) Having a lot of a good thing: Multiple important group memberships as a source of self-esteem. *PLoS ONE*, 10(5), 1–29.

Jones, C. P. (2000) Levels of racism: A theoretical framework and a gardener's tale. *American Journal of Public Health*, 90(8), 1212–1215.

Kandola, B. (2020) *Free to soar: Race and wellbeing in organisations*. Oxford: Pearn Kandola.

Kinouani, G. (2021) *Living while Black: The essential guide to overcoming racial trauma*. London: Ebury Publishing, Penguin Random House.

Litchfield, P. (2021) *Wellbeing guardians: Guidance for introducing the role in healthcare*. Organisations. Publication approval reference: B0189. London: NHS England and NHS Improvement.

Mangum, A. M. (2010) Race self-complexity and emotion: "How does it make you feel" to be Black in American society and culture? (Unpublished doctoral dissertation). Howard University, Washington, DC. Cited in Mbilishaka, A. (2018) Black lives (and stories) matter:

Race narrative therapy in Black hair care spaces. *Community Psychology in Global Perspective CPGP*, 4(2), 22–33.

Marmot, M. (2005) Social determinants of health inequalities. *Lancet*, 365(9464), 1099–1104.

Marmot, M., Allen, J., Goldblatt, P., Herd, E. and Morrison, J. (2020) *Build back fairer: The COVID-19 marmot review. The pandemic, socioeconomic and health inequalities in England.* London: Institute of Health Equity.

Mbilishaka, A. (2018) Black lives (and stories) matter: Race narrative therapy in Black hair care spaces. *Community Psychology in Global Perspective CPGP*, 4(2), 22–33.

Memon, A., Taylor, K., Mohebati, L. M., et al. (2016) Perceived barriers to accessing mental health services among Black and minority ethnic (BME) communities: A qualitative study in Southeast England. *BMJ Open*, Vol 6, Issue 11, e012337.

Muirhead, V. E., Milner, A., Freeman, R. Doughty, J. and Macdonalds, M. E. (2020) What is intersectionality and why is it important in oral health research? *Community Dentistry and Oral Epidemiology*, 48, 464–470.

National Health Service, (NHS). (2021) https://www.nhs.uk/servicedirectories/pages/nhstrustlisting.aspx. Date accessed: 7.9.2021.

Ncube-Mlilo, N. (2006) The tree of life project: Using narrative ideas in work with vulnerable children in Southern Africa. *International Journal of Narrative Therapy and Community Work*, 1, 3–16.

Ncube-Mlilo, N. (2013) Narratives in the suitcase. Video Presentation. Retrieved from https://dulwichcentre.com.au/narratives-in-the-suitcase-by-ncazelo-ncube-mlilo/.

Neblett, E. W. and Carter, S. E. (2012) The protective role of racial identity and Afrocentric worldview in the association between racial discrimination and blood pressure. *Psychosomatic Medicine*, 74(5), 509–516.

Nikolova, M. and Graham, C. (2020) The economics of happiness. Global labour organization GLO, GLO discussion paper series 640.

NHS England. (2021) Wellbeing guardians guidance for introducing the role in healthcare organisations. NHS England and NHS Improvement, Publication approval reference: B0189.

Parmer, T. A., Arnold, N., Natt, H. R. and Janson, L. (2004) Physical attractiveness as a process of internalized oppression and multigenerational transmission in African American families. *The Family Journal: Counselling and Therapy for Couples and Families*, 12, 230–242.

Pearce, W. B. and Cronen, V. E. (1980) *Communication, action and meaning: The creation of social realities.* New York: Praeger.

Phiri, P., Delanerolle, G., Al-Sudani, A. and Rathod, S. (2021) COVID-19 and Black, Asian, and minority ethnic communities: A complex relationship without just cause. *JMIR Public Health Surveill*, 7(2), e22581.

Pieterse, A. L. (2018) Attending to racial trauma in clinical supervision: Enhancing client and supervisee outcomes. *The Clinical Supervisor*, 37(1), 204–220.

Potter, S. (2020) *Therapy with a map: A cognitive analytic approach to helping relationships.* London: Luminate.

Pyke, K. (2010) What is internalized racial oppression and why don't we study it? Acknowledging racism's hidden injuries. *Sociological Perspectives*, 53(4), 551–572.

Royal College of Physicians. (2015) Work and wellbeing in the NHS: Why staff health matters to patient care. https://www.rcplondon.ac.uk/file/2025/download.

Selasi, T. (2014) Don't ask where I'm from, ask where I'm a local. October 2014. TED Global. https://www.ted.com/talks/taiye_selasi_don_t_ask_where_i_m_from_ask_where_i_m_a_local. Date accessed: 07/09/2021.

Sliwa, M. (2017) Understanding the relationship between poverty and White privilege. https://goodmenproject.com/featured-content/understanding-relationship-poverty-White-privilege-wcz/. Also cited in Lloyd, J. and Polland, P. (Eds.). (2019) *Cognitive analytic therapy and the politics of mental health*. Oxon: Routledge.

Smith Lee, J. R. and Robinson, M. A. (2019) "That's my number one fear in life. It's the police": Examining young Black men's exposures to trauma and loss resulting from police violence and police killings. *Journal of Black Psychology*, 45(3), 143–184.

Sue, D. W., Capodilupo, C. M., Torino, G. C., Bucceri, J. M. Holder, A. M. B., Nadal, K. L. and Esquilin, M. (2007) Racial microaggressions in everyday life: Implications for clinical practice. *American Psychologist*, 62(4), 271–286.

Tadmor, C. T., Galinsky, A. D. and Maddux, W. W. (2012) Getting the most out of living abroad: Biculturalism and integrative complexity as key drivers of creative and professional success. *Journal of Personality and Social Psychology*, 103(3), 520–542.

Taylor, J. (2000) Why our social environment matters: Out need for connection and belonging. In Kandola, B. (Ed.), *Free to soar: Race and wellbeing in organisations*. Oxford: Pearn Kandola.

Thomas-Breitfeld, S. and Kunreuther, F. (2022) *Trading glass ceilings for glass cliffs: A race to lead report on non-profit executives of colour*. New York: Building Movement Project.

Thornicroft, G., Mehta, N., Clement, S., Evans-Lacko, S., Doherty, M., Rose, D., Koschorke, M., Shidhaye, R., O'Reilly, C., and Henderson, C. (2016) Evidence for effective interventions to reduce mental-health-related stigma and discrimination. *The Lancet*, 387, 1123–1132.

White, M. and Epston, D. (1990) *Narrative means to therapeutic ends*. New York: W. W. Norton.

WRES NHS England. (2021) https://www.england.nhs.uk/about/equality/equality-hub/equality-standard/. Date accessed: 3.9.2021.

Young, I. M. (2009) Five faces of oppression. In Henderson, G. L. and Waterstone, M. (Eds.), *Geographic thought: A praxis perspective*, 55–71). New York: Routledge.

> # 2 Organisational Trauma
An Important Context in Staff Support[1]

Dr Karen Treisman

Organisational trauma is an area beneath the trauma umbrella that is often not named, acknowledged, or discussed. A central part of becoming more adversity, culturally, and trauma informed, infused, and responsive at an organisational level, is around understanding and reflecting on organisational trauma, and on how an organisation itself can become traumatised, trauma inducing, dysregulated, and trauma soaked. This includes how an organisation and system can add trauma and stress to the people who use the service. But also, how trauma and loss can impact the people working within the organisation, for instance through organisational adverse experiences, secondary trauma, vicarious trauma, compassionate fatigue, burnout, and work-related stress/strain.

Moreover, understanding system, secondary, community, and organisational trauma and dynamics is often not prioritised in people's training and in professional development training. The focus tends to be on other people's trauma, rather than one's own, and the impact on an individual level, rather than from an organisational or community lens. An organisation cannot meaningfully become more trauma, adversity, and culturally informed, infused, and responsive without shining a spotlight on organisational trauma, organisational processes and dynamics, and the organisation-in-mind.

Some key concepts related to organisational trauma will be briefly presented in this chapter, such as thinking about an organisation as alive with signs, signals, and symptoms of trauma. This will include insight into organisational

---

[1] This is a chapter adapted from Treisman, K. (2021). *A Treasure Box for Creating Trauma Informed organizations: A Ready-to-Use Resource for Trauma, Adversity, and Culturally Informed, Infused, and Responsive Systems*. London: Jessica Kingsley Publishers.

memory and amnesia, and mirroring and parallel processes. There will be an introduction to secondary and vicarious trauma within organisations, as well as re-traumatising and trauma-inducing practices and processes, alongside organisational adverse experiences. This chapter is central to implementing adversity, culturally and trauma-informed, infused, and responsive practice. However, this is part of a larger puzzle. To learn about the other pieces, see my complete work on trauma-informed organisations (Treisman, 2021).

An organisation, like a person, is alive with thoughts, feelings, values, and much more

Organisations can be emotional and relational places. They are made up of people, who come from their own families and a variety of systems, including other organisational families (e.g. other jobs, workplace, and educational climates). Systems and organisations, just like people, are not machines or blank slates. Instead, it can be helpful to see organisations as being alive and having a collective brain (Bloom, 2010). Like people, organisations develop, grow, change, and adapt. Organisations, systems, and individuals are bidirectional which means they are dynamic, and interact, influence, shape, and flow with, to, through, and in between each other. Like a person, an organisation:

- Has a personality, a culture, and different aspects of identity.
- Has protective factors, strengths, and resources.
- Has values, attitudes, beliefs, expectations, and assumptions.
- Has a range of feelings. An organisation, or a team within an organisation, can feel anxious, vulnerable, happy, sad, stressed, confused, stuck, attacked, conflicted, angry, helpless, hopeless, and so on.
- Has a memory, has travelled a journey, and a history of experiences.
- Can be unhealthy or have a compromised immune system.
- Can experience and be impacted by stress, trauma, distress, dysregulation, and dissociation.
- Can have signals and signs when they are distressed, struggling, or dysregulated.
- Might have had to operate in survival mode, and, so, develop ways and responses to cope, protect itself, and navigate through these experiences.

> - *What parallels and comparisons can you see between people and organisations?*
> - *If you were going to describe the feeling of your organisation or describe its personality using three words what would you say? How does the organisation/ services leave people feeling? If the building could talk, what would it say?*
> - *Take a moment, what would this mean and feel like if you responded and formulated about the organisation like a person? What if you thought about the organisation as the 'client'? (This is where therapeutic skills can be so useful to apply at an organisational level).*

If an organisation can operate in survival mode and be impacted by trauma, like a person, it can also become consumed, flooded, and overwhelmed by the trauma, adversity, and stress. The organisation itself, or a team within it, can become trauma organised and trauma soaked. It can be dominated by survival needs. Dr Sandy Bloom, a trailblazer and leader in this field, defines what being trauma organised is: "When an individual, family, organisation, system, or culture becomes fundamentally and unconsciously organized around the impact of chronic and toxic stress, even when this undermines its adaptive ability" (Bloom, 2010, p. 29).

Trauma, loss, dissociation, dysregulation, and toxic stress can spread like a wildfire throughout an organisation. It can interrupt the organisation's flow, and the ripple effects can be felt through multiple layers. If it isn't attended to, like a fire, it can continue to spread and intensify. The word trauma itself comes from the Greek word 'traumata', which means to pierce. This feels apt when thinking of trauma and organisations as trauma can wound, pierce, be soaked in, and permeate through individual, family, organisational, and societal layers. Erik de Soir (2012) talks about how the organisation's protective emotional membrane can be pierced by trauma. Trauma can also be absorbed; and at the same time, it can seep, leak, and spill out. Shohet and Shohet (2019) describe how without reflection, processing, and so forth, it is like swallowing food, which is not ingested properly and may have to be vomited out later.

Although these concepts can be applied to any organisation, they are even more important to consider when the main work of an organisation is around trauma, distress, and stress, for example social services, prisons, residential care, services for those in emotional distress, and acute physical healthcare settings.

What we might see when an organisation is in a place of trauma, stress, dissociation, and dysregulation

Often when faced with painful feelings, anxieties, uncertainty, threat, danger, dysregulation, and so forth, organisations, like people, try to find ways to guard, shield, protect, and defend against these. When in survival mode or in toxic stress, organisations often respond, cope, and function through fight, flight, freeze, feign, and flop responses. They often cope and respond by going into either rigidity or chaos or oscillating between the two.

Importantly, these anxieties and survival responses often flow and travel. They can get passed down the system, from leadership. If they are not acknowledged, named, and processed, the pain, hurt, trauma, dissociation, and stress can be pushed deeper into the fabric of the organisation.

- *Stop for a moment and think about the common presentations, and signals of trauma and toxic stress at an individual level* (e.g. a child who has experienced domestic violence). This might include hypervigilance, dissociation, dysregulation, changes in eating and sleeping patterns, and avoidance.
- *Now consider how many of these can also show themselves at an organisational level – in individuals, teams, in the wider organisational culture, and/or between different organisations?* There are many similarities, overlaps, and mirroring processes between individuals and organisations.

Here are some ways that the people within organisations, or the organisational culture/team as a whole, can react to pain and anxieties:

- Be reactive and/or crisis driven. Including being in quick-fix mode, and/or doing and acting without thinking. Reacting instead of reflecting. Being in survival mode where it can be harder to think and reflect, and use more abstract cognitive and executive functions, such as attention, concentration, problem-solving. Bloom (2010) refers to this as organisational learning disabilities. It can be harder to make simple decisions when feeling full up and overwhelmed. People can have their 'minds full' rather than being 'mindful'.
- Fight/attack/defend. People can respond in more 'bullying, authoritarian, and/or aggressive' ways. People, teams, or organisations can go into 'attack', 'defend', or 'fight' modes. In shark-infested waters,

people learn to act like sharks themselves, following the notion that it is better to attack rather than be attacked, to be feared rather than fearful, to be powerful instead of powerless.
- Hyper-aroused, on edge, hyper-alert, and hyper-vigilant. This can show itself as major reactive responses to something 'minor' like when the milk runs out in the kitchen. It can manifest as: people feeling criticised and attacked so responding as such; increased conflict and people feeling spoken about and unsafe to be themselves. We might also see much more limbic, emotionally driven responses, or the opposite as an attempt to avoid emotions. This might include people or the organisation feeling attacked, under siege, or persecuted.
- Avoidance, withdrawal, numbing, retreating, detaching, or dissociating. For example, an organisation may become detached from its mission and its purpose or an organisation or person may become detached from feeling, thinking, and reflecting. This might present as someone burying their head in the sand and not talking about the important stuff like power, racism, trauma, and political and financial drivers. It can also include people or teams checking out, withdrawing emotionally or physically, with people actually leaving, or people just keeping their heads down.
- Too busy to think or feel, for example, where thinking and feeling is timetabled out or where people are super busy like moving darts. This might include when organisations don't stop, like overwhelming changes in a short space of time. This has implications for attendance at staff support interventions.
- Physically and emotionally unwell. We can see people, teams, and the organisation become unwell physically with more sickness and a compromised immune system, as well as increased levels of stress, emotional dysregulation, and distress. This can include impacted sleep, eating, and alcohol consumption.
- Confused, lost, alone, and disoriented. This might include the team or organisation feeling like it has a fragile sense of identity (e.g. who are we, why are we here, what are we doing, where are we headed?), and not feeling grounded or anchored to a purpose or their mission.
- Rigid and inflexible (including striving for perfectionism). This can include very black and white thinking with little room for curiosity and being open to other possibilities. This can mean ideas and beliefs can be clung to and new ideas are discounted, disbelieved, or attacked. This rigidity stems from trying to search for stability and certainty but can

show itself as a lack of humility and reflection. This includes responses such as 'we have done trauma', 'we know this all', 'we are trauma informed'. This extends to holding on to processes or ideas even when feedback and new evidence suggests otherwise, for example, concepts around the links between emotional wellbeing and adversity, oppression and social exclusion.

This is by no means an exhaustive or prescriptive list, and the examples given of course vary depending on the context (for more examples, see Treisman, 2021).

> - *As you were reading which ones resonated? What reflections did you have?*
> - *What else would you add, or have you observed/felt/learned about?*
> - *How does your team or organisation show its survival and coping responses? What does this look like? Can you think of examples of these responses?*

Here are some individual examples of survival and coping responses to traumatic workplaces:

> *Talia was allocated a new case and upon reading graphic details of neglect said, "It's not that bad, I've seen much worse." Her threshold has become too high and for a range of reasons, including protective dissociation and feeling uncared for herself, she has become desensitised, disconnected, and hardened to the work. This could have a range of concerning effects on the work she may do with the family.*
>
> *David had become so emotionally full and consumed by work that he defended against these feelings by making fun of the people he worked with, distancing himself emotionally from them, and widening the 'Them and Us' gap.*
>
> *One social worker felt so overwhelmed by the hostility a birth mother displayed towards her, and by the pain that the child was facing, that she responded to these feelings by emotionally withdrawing and disconnecting from the mother. This crushed her ability to empathise with the mother's trauma throughout her life and of having her child removed, and to see the hurt and scared person behind the 'anger'. Instead, at times she dehumanised the mother, positioning her in polarised, negative terms.*

These consequences and survival responses are naturally more likely to have ripple effects on things such as staff wellness, commitment, morale, spirit, energy, productivity, turnover, and retention as well as on the decisions made, on the feelings shared, on the culture felt, and on the 'outcomes' achieved.[2]

Organisational memory and amnesia

Developing the concept that organisations are alive, like people, organisations also have their own influencing events/people, journey, embedded stories, roots, and history. Organisations can have their own historical trauma, their own ghosts (Fraiberg, 1975), haunters, scars, wounds, and shadows of the past as well as having their own angels (Lieberman et al., 2005), guiders, lighthouses, inspirers, and protectors. We need to find a way to honour, reflect, and understand this history, as this not only supports us to understand the cultural and wider context of the organisation, but also allows us to learn from the past, inform the future, and honour the distance already travelled. This is especially important where there is a lot of staff turnover, because this crucial tacit knowledge can be easily lost.

Lack of learning and reflecting from the past can feed into what many people refer to as 'organisational amnesia'. In this case, we can see history repeating itself, and the same difficulties returning in a cyclical nature. An example being in serious case reviews where the same recommendations appear again and again, yet they are not acted on. Organisations can re-enact the past and get stuck in a loop.

Organisational amnesia can lead organisations to forget why they are there in the first place; their mission and vision become blurred and diluted. Just like a traumatised person, an organisation can feel fragmented, uprooted, and have a fragile sense of identity. This resonates with many of the organisations I support, for example a head teacher in a place of distress told me, "I came into this to make a difference, I loved kids, I wanted to inspire, I wanted to create a place where my teachers could do that too; but somehow we have lost our way, we are in a sea of firefighting, and paperwork, and the love and vision seems to have dissipated, or is hanging on by a thin thread."

Organisational memory and history will inevitably shape and guide people and the culture, both positively, negatively, and all of the shades in between. The weight of these is likely to be more impactful if these are not addressed, acknowledged,

---

[2] For more information and insights around the impact of traumatised organisations, please see work by Dr Sandra Bloom, Philippe Bailleur, Vega Zagier Roberts, and Anton Obholzer.

and processed. For example, when an organisation experiences something traumatic like a child death, funding cuts, and a shame-based leader, the experience is felt, but things are left unarticulated and unspoken. This mirrors what happens in trauma; trauma is often silenced, unspoken, invalidated, ignored, and avoided. Then it can seep and leak out in other ways: in someone feeling strong feelings but not knowing why, or becoming dysregulated, or learning to minimise or shutdown their own feelings. Or knowing something has happened because they sense and feel it, but haven't had it confirmed or processed, so their imagination can go wild and they may catastrophise or internalise it. Organisations are similar: these memories and influencing factors, often unsaid, or avoided, can be consciously and unconsciously present and imprinted into the fabric of the organisation; their ripples felt bubbling under the surface. This fragmented and unresolved memory and experience can come out in other ways.

We can think about amnesia in wider society: what things come and go, are forgotten or pushed underground, for example, HIV, coronavirus, incest, famous people who have abused, child abuse, abuse among the disabled, famines, and war. Dr Judith Herman (1992), a leader in the trauma field, shared, "the knowledge of horrible events periodically intrudes into public awareness but is rarely retained for long. Denial, repression, and dissociation operate on a social as well as an individual level. The study of psychological trauma has an 'underground' history. Like traumatized people, we have been cut-off from the knowledge of our past. Like traumatized people, we need to understand the past in order to reclaim the present and the future. Therefore, an understanding of psychological trauma begins with rediscovering history" (p. 2).

Mirroring and parallel processes

Due to its piercing nature, trauma can be passed from an individual, to a family, to an organisation, to a society, in multiple directions. This means that we can sometimes see parallel, echoing, and mirroring processes occur between the work itself, families, and the organisation. Britton (1994, pp. 79–80) uses a theatre metaphor to reflect this, "The cast changes, but the plot remains the same" and this is especially true when teams mirror the groups with whom they work.

Additionally, we all come from a primary group, our family. Sometimes our family dynamics and roles can be (usually unintentionally) re-enacted, mirrored, and echoed at work. These processes are crucial to understand, as they can reinforce family trauma and stress. For example, within social services, a traumatised system supporting a traumatised family further compounds the trauma – it creates a triple deprivation (Emanuel, 2002). This can be trauma inducing and re-traumatising which is the opposite of what healing and reparative systems should be doing. Some examples of mirroring and parallel processes, as well as some survival responses follow:

- Mission mirroring is where an organisation can replicate the difficulties which they are trying to change or solve. For instance, an organisation designed to advocate for social injustice and unfairness, instead somehow mirrors the very thing they were designed to oppose, resulting in high levels of injustice and boundary violations which leave employees feeling treated in an unfair and unjust way.
- When a team feels on edge and scared due to fear-based leadership, this anxiety and fear can pass onto clients. The team, as a defence to the anxiety, might respond in lots of ways, such as becoming more fearful, less containing and more dysregulated, or more 'controlling or authoritarian' towards families.
- We can see 'victim, persecutor, rescuer, and bystander' roles played out throughout the system. If the service positions themselves as the rescuer, then families are often in the position of 'victim'. If families, such as in social services, are positioned as the 'persecutor', the person supporting, or the organisation might take the position of 'victim'. This can be even more powerful if it is re-creating other dynamics which people have felt in other times and in their own relational experiences.
- Additionally, feelings, themes, experiences, and processes can ripple or permeate through multiple layers of a system; neglect can get neglected, or dissociation can make people/systems dissociate. For example, Niamh presented with symptoms of depression, her child with low mood, their social worker as hopeless and depleted, and the overarching organisation as deflated, with a collective sense of helplessness and stuckness.

> - *Take some time to think about what mirroring or parallel processes you might have seen, felt, and/or experienced?*
> - *Why do you think it is important to consider, name, and reflect on these? What might be the hazards of not considering them, on you, the team, and on the work?*

Mirroring family dynamics and role positioning

Additional to being 'live' systems, organisations and team dynamics can be likened to a family group. Like families, there are unique systems and coalitions within them, and we all can take and be positioned within different roles. For example, effective leadership is crucial for effective teamwork, which parallels the pivotal role parenting plays within a family.

Similarly, when a valued manager leaves a team, this can trigger feelings of abandonment and loss within its members, even more so if a team member themselves has a history of abandonment. Building on this, leaders, like parents, are commonly polarised, for example they can be seen as all-knowing or impotent, idealised, or denigrated. Furthermore, these roles can get entangled; a leader might be looked to by an employee to meet a need which was not met in their life, or to re-enact a relationship they previously had with someone in authority, like a parent, for example, feeling not good enough. Or colleagues, managers, and their employees can re-enact rivalrous sibling relationships.

Because of the powerful and permeating nature of stress and trauma within health and social care, and the personal nature the work often involves, this mirroring and positioning can be profound.

> This exercise can be triggering and powerful. So as with all the exercises in this chapter, please think about your safety first.
>
> *What was your experience and role within your primary group (family of origin)? How and why did/do you play these roles? How has this impacted your role in teams and groups in the past and currently? Have these roles changed over time?*
> *What roles do you currently hold within your team?* (e.g. mediator, nurturer, and peace maker)
> *What other roles within your team do you align with or find trickier? Do certain team members represent roles in other areas of your life and relational experiences?*

Re-traumatising, trauma-inducing, and triggering experiences within the system

A central tenet of adversity, trauma, and culturally informed, infused, and responsive systems is that we acknowledge that the environments and systems we operate in, including the system itself, can be (often unintentionally) re-traumatising, trauma inducing, re-triggering, dysregulating, and re-activating. They can mirror, parallel, be reminiscent, and/or reinforce experiences of trauma, and the related feelings and associations to the trauma/s. If we are committing to working in a trauma-informed way, we need to find ways to actively reduce these, and work towards increasing feelings of safety and trust, and being trauma reducing instead of trauma inducing. This again is a key part about moving from knowing (i.e. having the information) to actually doing and being – actively responding to the information and doing things differently (table 2.1).

- *What else might you add to this list?*
- *Which resonate with you, or jar with you?*
- *Take one and think about how it might be or feel from a trauma lens? What could be done to increase people's feelings of safety and decrease their feelings of danger or threat?*

Following are some real-world examples of practices within services which could be re-traumatising, triggering, and trauma inducing (names and any identifiable information has been changed). For additional examples, please see Treisman (2021).

These are not intended to blame or shame services, we all have done things that we would do differently with the information we now have, and we all are on a learning journey. These examples are intended to make people stop and think and become more aware of system trauma, and the harm caused by the system (mostly unintentionally). As you are reading, think about power, privilege, fear, safety, trust, the multi-sensory experience, communication, injustice, oppression, humility, relationships, collaboration, and much more.

- A hospital ward placed Laura, a woman who had just delivered a stillborn baby, on a busy ward of women and their new, healthy babies.
- Lola was in treatment for a diagnosis of anorexia. She found eating very triggering and difficult. She was never asked about her trauma history while on the eating disorder unit. Turns out that every time she ate, she was catapulted down a time hole to a memory of being forced to give a relative oral sex.

TABLE 2.1: Examples of re-traumatising, trauma-inducing, and triggering experiences within the system.

1. Being treated, reduced, and/or feeling like a number, statistic, label, or behaviour. This includes not seeing the person within the context of their experiences. As well as when people are reduced to a behaviour or the worst thing that has happened to them. Not seeing the person behind the behaviour and behaviour as communication, with ways of responding as creative coping and survival skills.

    This includes diagnosis overshadowing, where people just see the diagnosis, and explain everything by connecting it to the diagnosis.

2. Being in a depriving, bare, or stark environment which can be reminiscent of past experiences of neglect, relational poverty, and deprivation.

3. Being in a relationship where expressions of distress or dysregulation are seen as 'dangerous', 'naughty', 'intolerable', 'manipulative', 'attention-seeking', and so on. So, people do not feel safe to show or express their emotions or contained when expressing them. This can mirror previous experiences where emotions have been ignored, denied, invalidated, minimised, misinterpreted, or silenced.

4. Feeling blamed, shamed, punished, or humiliated which may be apparent in responses to professionals who ask for help or make a mistake or in the blaming and shaming responses towards a person who has self-harmed, or around 'victim blaming' following a crime.

    This can also include people feeling their dignity and integrity has been violated, which can mirror the dignity and integrity violation which often takes place when there is a trauma. For example, privacy not respected, trauma-inducing assessments and examinations.

5. The lack of choice, voice, collaboration, and agency and within this, feeling done to/silenced/ignored/minimised. This can mirror the powerlessness and misuse of power within trauma and includes where they are clear othering, splitting, divides, and Them and Us processes.

6. A hostile and trauma-inducing environment and atmosphere (including a lack of feeling human, not maintained and not warm).

7. Constant retelling of one's story or graphic details when not necessary or the opposite – a lack of confidentiality and details of someone's information being overshared.

8. Institutional racism, exclusion, stigma, social injustice, and inequalities and this includes micro-aggressions and inaccessible services.

9. Services not taking into account people's intersection of identities and multiplicity of narratives – for staff and people using the services. This also includes power, privilege, and accessibility.

10. The lack of supervision or reflective spaces. This also includes the lack of meaningful high-quality debriefing spaces.

(These are by no means exhaustive and of course there are multiple interplaying factors involved. These include practices that impact on staff wellbeing).

- In Rwanda, Imaculee was raped several times by men who identified themselves as being Hutu. While in a UK psychiatric hospital, the interpreter hired was a man who identified himself as Hutu. Upon seeing him, she, understandably, became very distressed and went down a time hole to the time she was raped. The ward said she was 'overreacting and being dramatic'. The staff had unintentionally assumed that an interpreter from Rwanda would be sufficient and had not considered her trauma experiences and wider contextual factors. Moreover, she was pathologised as an individual, without the possible impact of historical, cultural, and racial trauma being explored. This compounded Imaculee's reported experience of discrimination and feeling misunderstood within systems.
- Billie, who was sexually abused as a child, was admitted to a psychiatric hospital and placed on one-to-one observations. She was re-triggered by being constantly watched and feeling invaded by male staff. They walked into her room without knocking and peered through the glass window on her door.
- Each time Tom (a man with learning disabilities) showed his distress, he was told to 'settle down' and 'calm down'. When he tried to communicate what had happened to him, the response was that he didn't have the capacity to understand what abuse was and that he had gotten confused. He described often feeling people spoke to him like he was stupid or spoke about him rather than to him.

- *How do you feel physically, emotionally, and from a sensory level when reading these?*
- *How are these from a power, privilege, fear, safety, trust, the multi-sensory experience, communication, injustice, oppression, humility, relationships, collaboration, and much more lens?*
- *How can you apply the feelings and themes to other contexts and areas?*
- *What can be done in your own practice, team, and in the wider organisation to become more aware of these, including our own blind spots, and to reduce and try to avoid them?*

Organisational adverse experiences, organisational trauma and stressors, and work-related stress and strain

Staff may also have experienced trauma, toxic stress, and adversity from the work itself or from the work context/climate/culture. Remen (1994) writes: "The expectation that we can be immersed in suffering and loss daily and not be touched by it is as unrealistic as expecting to be able to walk through water and expecting not to get wet."

In addition to the nature of the work, there can be an array of other organisational aspects which can create stress, strain, and trauma. Particularly if these are ongoing, and if people have a steady diet of fear and stress at work, these can have a cumulative chipping away effect. These are also more likely to be felt if the organisation is in a place of stress, fragility, dysregulation, and trauma; and conversely, more likely to be buffered should there be more protective factors in place. Examples of organisational adverse experiences and organisational stressors follow (for more, see Treisman, 2021):

- Staff, particularly those working with people in distress, often have to cope with a high level of unpredictability, ambiguity, and uncertainty within the work – both on a daily basis and longer term. This might be uncertainty as to what will happen each day or what they will be faced with, legal changes, system changes, and working in emotionally charged contexts.
- People often have to manage the high pressures and a high sense of responsibility, including where there are complex decisions to be made with a human cost. This can be even more stressful if there are not sufficient or available services around to signpost to; and/or if these are available, if people don't feel ready or able to access these services.
- Staff may have to make decisions which conflict with their own values, gut instinct, and wishes; and therefore, may be in a double bind. For example, not having enough staff or resources to give proper care in physical health settings, especially during the pandemic. Or having to deliver therapy in six sessions, even though one's training and gut says this should be longer.
- Bullying, conflict, sexism, racism, (other forms of discrimination) and harassment in the workplace, between colleagues, and in the wider organisation. Including indirect or direct abuse, assault, or aggression.

- Criticism, blame, and negative discourses from external agencies, the media, the public, and so on. Including allegations, threats, serious complaints, or being sued.
- Trauma-inducing supervision, team meetings, and emails.
- Tricky IT systems.
- Physical environment. For example, unsafe, oppressive, triggering environments and/or a physical move to a different building.
- Feeling done to, ignored, minimised, and/or silenced. Including poor or ineffective communication.
- A lack or blurred vision, mission, meaning, or purpose, including not having something to anchor on to.
- Unrealistic deadlines and timelines.

> *This is not an exhaustive or prescriptive list.*
>
> - *What else would you add?*
> - *Which of these resonate with you?*
> - *Which of these jar with you?*

Wellbeing leads to well doing: The importance and centrality of safety and trust

Having explored some of the key themes around traumatised and trauma-soaked organisations, and additional traumas and stressors which can occur during the work, we will now discuss the potential impact this can have on staff wellbeing and the work itself, including secondary trauma. We know that when an individual is feeling unwell, it is harder to be their optimal self, and that is the same for an organisation. When organisations are unwell and traumatised, they are not going to be able to deliver the high-quality care people need and deserve. If we want to deliver and improve relationships, high-quality care, effectiveness, productivity, and decision-making, as well as finding ways to decrease staff turnover, dissatisfaction, sickness, and so forth, we need to invest in staff wellbeing and wellness.[3]

For people to do their job to the best of their ability, employees need to be treated in a way that supports and models staff wellbeing. People are better able

---

[3] Please see my 2021 book *Trauma-informed organizations* for more on staff wellness, supervision, reflective practice, and the physical environment.

to think, be reflective, play, innovate, explore, and be healthier when they feel safer, and are not dysregulated, and/or operating out of a place of fear, toxic stress, and trauma. It is about reflecting instead of reacting, and about being in our thinking brains instead of our survival brains.

As shared earlier, a loss of sense of safety may result in a range of different responses from anxiety and dysregulation through to someone/the organisation becoming more authoritarian and directive (Harris and Fallot, 2001). In therapy, trust, safety, and stabilisation are paramount and foundational, and this is the same in organisations. People need to be and feel safe emotionally, physically, relationally, morally, and so forth. We know that the more regulated, organised, and grounded children are, the more able they will be, to be able to learn, be creative, explore, and engage. The more regulated, contained, and grounded staff feel, the more able they will be to think, reflect, be creative, innovate, explore, and so on. How can staff model the model or be the co-regulators if they are not having this modelled?

- *How well can you perform, think, and flourish under unsafe, unsupportive, or unthinking situations?*
- *In what environments do we best thrive, develop, think, create, and grow?*
- *What do we internalize, absorb, breathe in, and feel each day in our work environments? ('Positive', 'negative', and all the shades in between).*

Secondary trauma, vicarious trauma, compassion fatigue, and burnout

Care and support for all staff is crucial. Even more so as we know there is a common prevalence and occurrence of trauma and adversity in our communities and societies, which means that many staff themselves may have experienced trauma and adversity in their own childhoods and lives. From the literature (Thomas, 2016; Dykes, 2011; Bride, 2007) we know that this can be higher for those who choose to go into the helping/caring professions. The previously mentioned complexities, pressures, organisational stressors, and the nature of the work itself often mean that professionals working within these contexts are more likely to experience secondary trauma (Perez et al., 2010; Kadambi et al., 2004; Stamm, 1999), work strain/stress, vicarious trauma (McCann and Pearlman, 1990), compassion fatigue (Figley, 1995), and burnout. Here are some additional factors to consider:

- Professionals who go into the caring professionals are more likely to have a rescue valency (e.g. want to help, want to be liked, want to rescue others, and want to care and look after people) which can be tricky to manage when this is challenged. This can create lots of conflicting situations, such as going into the work with the hope of wanting to support and keep families together, and then being responsible for removing a child; or working with someone for a year to improve their adherence to medication to treat a long-term health condition and they suddenly stop taking it and have to be admitted to hospital. This can also extend to having to function in limbo or uncertainty, and make very complex and multilayered judgements and decisions, such as the many shades involved in whether parenting is 'good enough', or if a child is 'safe'.
- Working with complex trauma inevitably evokes powerful feelings and often triggers professionals' own hotspots and vulnerabilities. Therefore, the worker's own unresolved losses and traumas such as abandonment, injustice, and helplessness may resurface.
- Professionals are often the containers for difficult feelings, and in order to be effective, they need to connect with the person, perspective-take, and empathise. However, connecting in this way can open one up to facing parts of human nature and society which are painful and difficult, and understandably avoided.
- Often professionals working in health and social care have heavy, complex, and trauma-dominated 'caseloads', which means having daily trauma exposure with little recovery time or respite. These experiences get stacked up and are exacerbated further if cases feel in crisis or stuck.
- Organisations are increasingly driven by performance indicators, financial implications, and paperwork/policies; this can neglect accounting for and acknowledgement of the complex nature of the work and lose sight of the 'patient/client', the underlying motivation for being in the caring profession, and the human costs. Working in a system where a practitioner does not feel valued or appreciated, and where the overarching vision or purpose of work becomes diluted, makes them more vulnerable to consequences such as compassion fatigue or secondary trauma. These conflicts are compounded by wider systemic issues such as public opinion, the media (naming, shaming, and blaming), and changing political agendas.

In essence, secondary trauma, vicarious trauma, compassion fatigue, and burnout can lead to higher levels of staff dissatisfaction, turnover, sickness, and levels of stress (Bride et al., 2007; Sprang et al., 2011). Moreover, the presence of secondary trauma, vicarious trauma, compassion fatigue, and burnout can permeate into various areas of the professional's spiritual, physical, emotional, and cognitive life, and impact on their ability to do their job to the best of their ability.

A growing body of literature describes how stress impacts on one's judgement, and the ability to effectively perform tasks (Baginsky, 2013), difficulties with thinking and reflecting, and difficulties with decision-making. The effects of secondary trauma, vicarious trauma, burnout, and compassion fatigue are far reaching but may include a loss of interest, weakened empathy, agitation, feeling cynical, emotionally depleted, exhausted, anxiety, low mood, withdrawal, anger, avoidance, hypervigilance, mistrust, frustration, hopelessness, and detachment. These responses can also show themselves in different ways, ranging from crushed empathy, shutting-off (dissociating), objectifying, and de-humanising the people one is working with, through to being snappier and having a shorter fuse. For others, connecting with vulnerability and helplessness in the people they are working with can lead to an erosion of self-esteem and a decreased sense of professional efficacy and accomplishment (Dane, 2000). Moreover, people can also develop an overwhelming sense of responsibility and accountability, which can send their rescue valency into overdrive. This can lead to the tricky tight rope between the difference between empathic care and empathetic distress and the difference between self-care and self-sacrifice.

As a result of the work, staff often experience shifts in the way they perceive themselves, others, and the world (e.g. their scripts, narratives, discourses, schemas, and core beliefs). For example, feeling 'the world is unsafe' and 'people are dangerous'. This can also contribute to more trauma, or risk attentional bias, such as seeing and noticing risk or trauma more frequently.

Staff may experience similar symptoms to the people they are working with, such as intrusive thoughts, nightmares, difficulties with regulating emotions, feeling helpless, hopeless, powerless, and vulnerable. Staff might also experience physical symptoms such as headaches, stomach aches, rashes, a compromised immune system, difficulties with sleeping and eating (McElvaney et al., 2016; Motta, 2012; Pistorius, 2006; Braley, 2010).

The above sections shine a spotlight on why reflection, supervision, containment, and emotional spaces for staff are so crucial. We need to think about how we can support staff to feel it but not become it. This is why staff wellness and wellbeing are so essential, as it is very tricky to support someone who is in emotional quicksand, if that person themselves is also in emotional quicksand; or similarly for them to be the rainbow in the storm, if they are in a storm themselves (Treisman, 2018).

Organisational protective factors

As with a person, it is important to think about an organisation's strengths, survivorship, resources, and protective factors. We need to find ways to celebrate and magnify these. Stephanie Covington (2008) discussed how a team is like a container; if cracks come in, then it is more likely that things are going to spill out. I would extend this to say it is also about how we try to create as strong a container as possible, and minimise the cracks, as well as trying to keep the cracks from shattering. Let's turn to factors from the literature base and from my work, that are likely to support an organisation to be as resilient as possible. We can compare these to factors that can make an organisation more susceptible to trauma. These are by no mean exhaustive or prescriptive but may be useful to think how we can increase the protective and resiliency factors and decrease the vulnerability and risk factors.

> - *Take some time to reflect on the above two images, which resonate? Which would you add?*
> - *What can you and the wider organisation do to boost the organisational immune system, and to reduce the fragility factors?*

Conclusion

As we have seen, a focus on adversity, culturally and trauma-informed, infused, and responsive organisational change is centred around creating environments which aim to increase feelings of safety and trust, and to decrease feelings of threat, danger, dysregulation, stress, and harm. It is about supporting trauma-reducing practice, rather than contributing to trauma-inducing practice. It is about working towards being trauma informed, infused, and responsive rather than being trauma organised and trauma soaked. This includes taking what we know about trauma, and moving from knowing to being, feeling, and doing, and responding to this knowledge by actively infusing it into daily practice.

(Continued on p68)

Factors which might make an Organisation more Susceptible to Trauma, Dysregulation, and Stress, and Weaken its Immune System

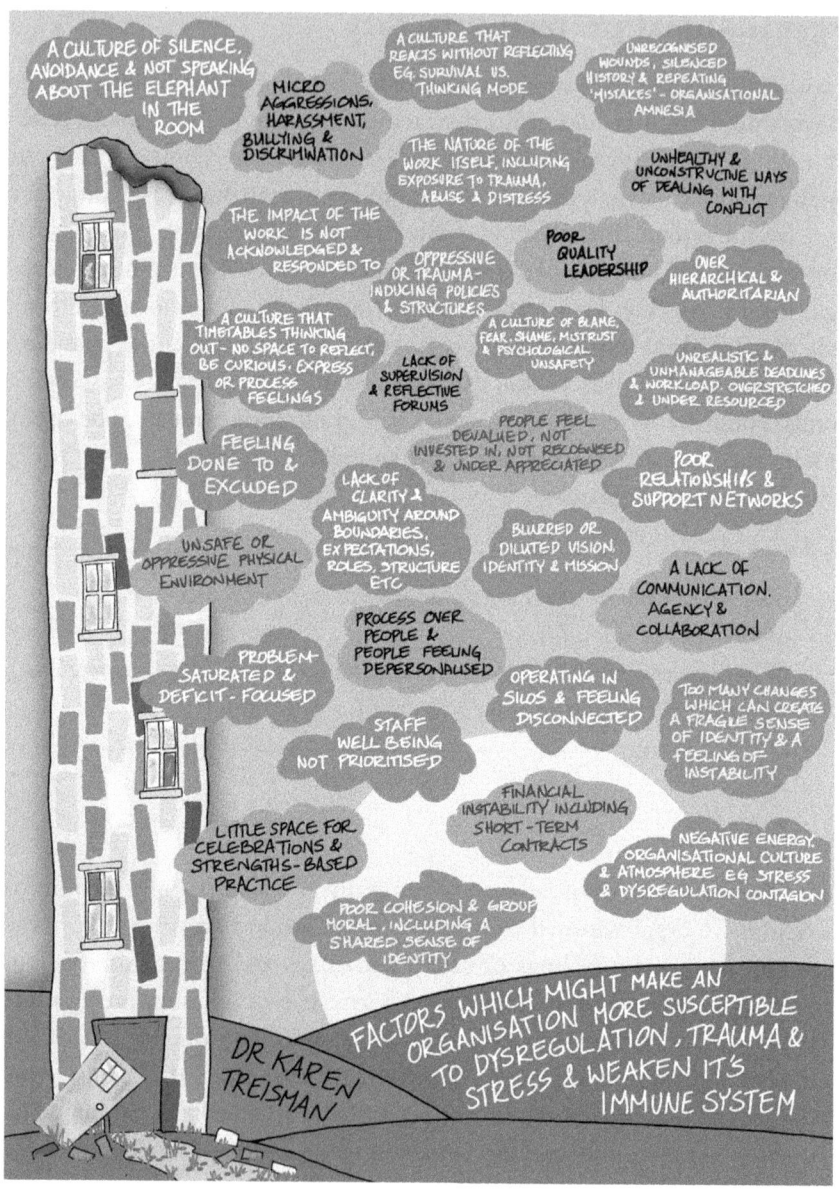

Some Protective Factors which Support Teams and Organisations to Buffer and Reduce the Impact of Organisational Trauma and Stress – Boosting the Organisation's Immune System

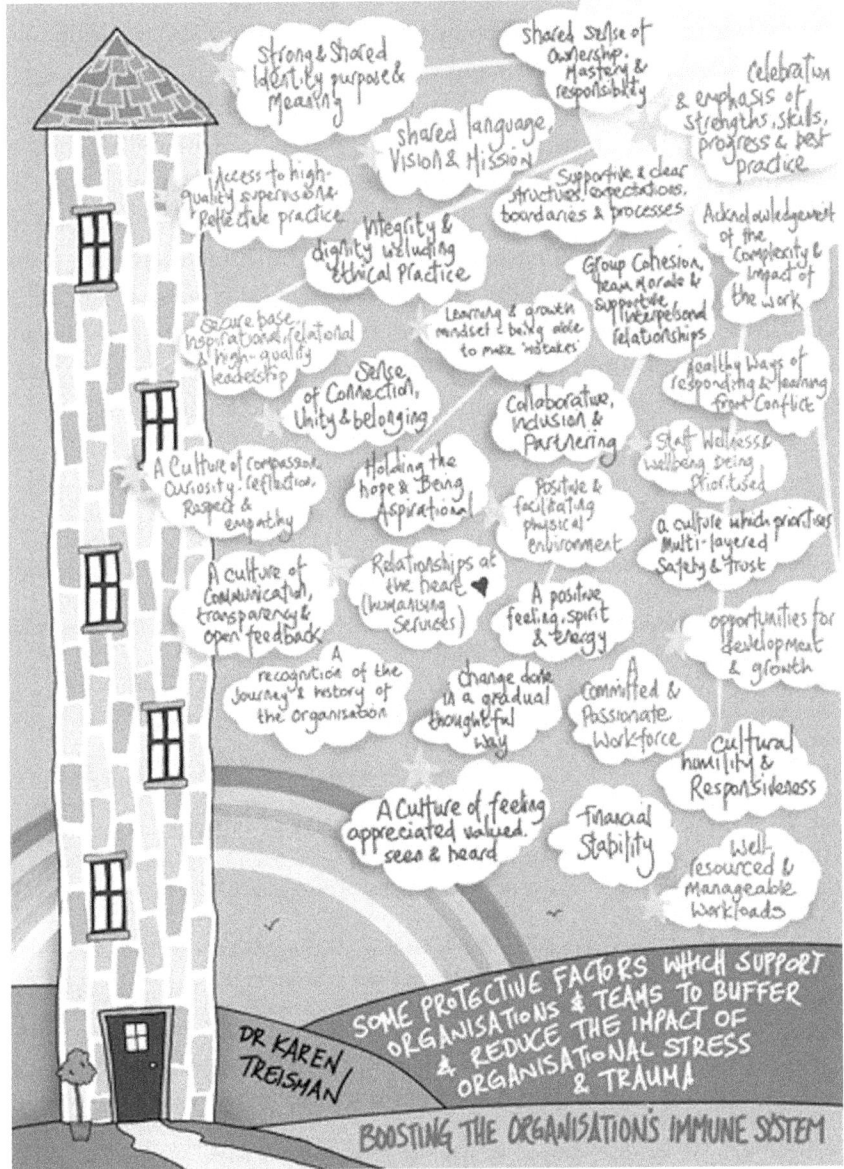

This focus is about trying to find ways to support healing, connection, belonging, relationships, recovery, and attachment to the people/organisation/community. Furthermore, it is about supporting staff and organisations to be able to breathe, reflect, communicate, feel, and think when in the presence of emotions and trauma, instead of operating in survival and reactive mode, and adding to the harm or distress. It is also about supporting healthcare staff to find ways to release, recharge, and decompress, while having the complexity of the work acknowledged, legitimised, and validated.

This involves us taking a crucial and widening lens about system, organisational, and vicarious trauma. Additionally, people understanding their own role within the work; the impact of organisational trauma; and about how systems can create, reinforce, and pass on trauma. It is also about trying to be proactive in supporting wellness, and in reducing burnout, secondary trauma, and work strain, which includes creating awareness, spaces, strategies, and mechanisms to address and further understand and reduce these dynamics and mirroring processes. This is key for both modelling the model, and for putting everyone's wellbeing, multilayered safety, and trust at its heart.

References and further reading

Baginsky, M. (2013). *Retaining Experienced Social Workers in Children's Services: The Challenge Facing Local Authorities in England.* London: Department for Education.

Bloom, S., and Farragher, B. (2010). *Destroying Sanctuary: The Crisis in Human Service Delivery Systems.* New York: Oxford University Press.

Bloom, S. L. (2011). Trauma-organized systems and parallel process. In N. Tehrani (Ed.), *Managing Trauma in the Workplace: Supporting Workers and Organizations,* 139–153. London: Routledge.

Bloom, S. L. (2013a). *Creating Sanctuary: Toward the Evolution of Sane Societies* (2nd ed.). New York: Routledge.

Bloom, S. L. (2013b). The Sanctuary Model: Changing Habits and Transforming the Organizational Operating System. In J. D. Ford, and C. A. Courtois (Eds.), *Treating Complex Traumatic Stress Disorders in Childhood and Adolescence,* 277–294. New York: Guilford Press.

Bloom, S. L. (2013c). The Sanctuary Model: Rebooting the Organizational Operating System in Group Care Setting. In R. Reece, C. Hanson, and J. Sargeant (Eds.), *Treatment of Child Abuse: Common Ground for Mental Health, Medical, and Legal Practitioners,* 109–117. Baltimore, MD: John Hopkins University Press.

Braley, R. A. (2010). Effects of Patient Trauma on Hospital Staff Functioning: An Exploratory Study of Psychological Distress Resulting from Trauma Exposure, Electronic Theses and Dissertations, Paper 767.

Bride, B. (2007). Prevalence of Secondary Traumatic Stress among Social Workers. *Social Work,* 25, 63–70.

Bride, B. E., Jones, J. L., and MacMaster, S. A. (2007). Correlates of Secondary Traumatic Stress in Child Protective Services Workers. *Journal of Evidence Based Social Work*, 4, 69–80.

Bride, B. E., Radey, M., and Figley, C. R. (2007). Measuring Compassion Fatigue. *Clinical Social Work Journal*, 35, 155–163.

Bride, B. E., Robinson, M., Yegidis, B., and Figley, C. (2003). Development and Validation of the STSS. *Research on Social Work Practice*, 13, 1–16.

Britton, R. (1994). *Re-Enactment as an Unwitting Professional Response to Family Dynamics: Crisis at Adolescence*. London: Jason Aronson Inc.

Covington, S. (2008). Women and Addiction: A Trauma-Informed Approach. *Journal of Psychoactive Drugs*, SARC Supplement 5, November 2008, 377–385.

Dane, B. (2000). Child Welfare Workers: An Innovative Approach for Interacting with Secondary Trauma. *Journal of Social Work Education*, 36, 27–38.

De Soir, E. (2012). The Management of Emotionally Disturbing Interventions in Fire and Rescue Services: Psychological Triage as a Framework for Acute Support. In R. Hughes, C. Cooper, and A. Kindler (Eds.), *International Handbook of Workplace Trauma Support*. New York: John Wiley & Sons. .

Dykes, G. (2011). The Implications of Adverse Childhood Experiences for the Professional Requirements of Social Work. *Social Work/Maatskaplike Werk*, 47, 521–533.

Emanuel, L. (2002). Deprivation X3: The Contribution of Organisational Dynamics to the 'Triple Deprivation' of Looked-After-Children. *Journal of Child Psychotherapy*, 28, 163–179.

Figley, C. (1995). *Compassion Fatigue: Coping with Secondary Traumatic Stress Disorder in Those Who Treat the Traumatized*. New York: Brunner/Mazel.

Fraiberg, S., Adelson, E., and Shapiro, V. (1975). Ghosts in the Nursery: A Psychoanalytic Approach to the Problems of Impaired Infant-Mother Relationships. *Journal of the American Academy of Child and Adolescent Psychiatry*, 14, 387–421.

Harris, M., and Fallot, R. D. (2001b). Envisioning a Trauma-Informed Service System: A Vital Paradigm Shift. *New Directions for Mental Health Services*, 89, 3–22.

Harris, M., and Fallot, R. D. (2001a). *Using Trauma Theory to Design Service Systems*. New Directions for Mental Health Services, 89. Jossey Bass.

Herman, J. L. (1992). *Trauma and Recovery*. New York: Basic Books.

Kadambi, M. A., and Truscott, D. (2003). An Investigation of Vicarious Traumatization among Therapists Working with Sex Offenders. *Traumatology*, 9, 216–230.

Lieberman, A. F., Padron, E., Van Horn, P., and Harris, W. W. (2005). Angels in the Nursery: The Intergenerational Transmission of Benevolent Influences. *Infant Mental Health Journal*, 26, 504–520.

Mason, B. (1993). Towards Positions of Safe Uncertainty. *Human Systems: The Journal of Systemic Consultation and Management*, 4, 189–200.

McCann, I. L., and Pearlman, L. A. (1990). Vicarious Traumatization: A Framework for Understanding the Psychological Effects of Working with Victims. *Journal of Traumatic Stress*, 3, 131–149.

McElvaney, R., and Tatlow-Golden, M. (2016). A Traumatised and Traumatising System: Professionals' Experience in Meeting the Mental Health Needs of Young People in the Care and Youth Justice Systems in Ireland. *Children and Youth Services Review*, 65, 62–69.

Motta, R. W. (2012). Secondary Trauma in Children and School Personnel. *Journal of Applied School Psychology*, 28, 256–269.

Perez, L., Jones, J., Englert, D., and Sachau, D. (2010). Secondary Traumatic Stress and Burnout among Law Enforcement Investigators Exposed to Disturbing Media Images. *Journal of Police and Criminal Psychology*, 25, 113–124.

Pistorius, K. D. (2006). *The Personal Impact on Female Therapists from Working with Sexually Abused Children*. All Theses and Dissertations. Paper 394.

Remen, R. N. (1996). *Kitchen Table Wisdom: Stories that Heal*. New York: Riverhead Books.

Shohet, R., and Shohet, J. (2019). *In Love with Supervision: Creating Transformative Conversations*. Manchester: PCCS.

Sprang, G., Craig, C., and Clark, J. (2011). Secondary Traumatic Stress and Burnout in Child Welfare Workers: A Comparative Analysis of Occupational Distress across Professional Groups. *Child Welfare*, 90, 149–168.

Stamm, B. H. (1999). *Secondary Traumatic Stress: Self-Care Issues for Clinicians, Researchers, and Educators*. Lutherville, MD: Sidran Press.

Thomas, J. (2016). Adverse Childhood Experiences among MSW Students. *Journal of Teaching in Social Work*, 36, 235–255.

Treisman, K. (2016). *Working with Relational and Developmental Trauma in Children and Adolescents*. London: Routledge.

Treisman, K. (2017). *A Therapeutic Treasure Box for Working with Developmental Trauma: Creative Activities and Tools*. London: Jessica Kingsley Publishers.

Treisman, K. (2021). *A Treasure Box for Creating Trauma Informed Organizations: A Ready-to-Use Resource for Trauma, Adversity, and Culturally Informed, Infused, and Responsive Systems*. London: Jessica Kingsley Publishers.

3 Setting up Systems of Staff Support using a Systemic Approach

Dr Harriet Conniff and Dr Neil Rees

> *What engages us with the Systemic approach is the emphasis on pattern and process and, hence, the recognition that the whole is much more than the sum of its parts. What we particularly appreciate is the focus on context, relationships, communication, and interaction: that is, what is happening between people rather than within people.*
> – FREDMAN, 2010, P. 26

Staff support and wellbeing in healthcare cannot occur without thinking about systems, yet what do we mean by working systemically? Working with a system, working systemically, and working as Systemic practitioners are not one and the same. The importance of thinking about systems related to staff wellbeing in healthcare is recognised internationally (Global Forum, 2019). Arguably, all staff support involves working systemically at different levels (individual, team, organisational) but this does not mean it follows a Systemic approach. Systemic thinking has been applied to the workplace since the approach first emerged (Roberts, 1996) and yet Systemic practice is not restricted to psychologists, psychotherapists, and family therapists but can be used by many professionals within healthcare. We know that psychological staff support needs to exist within a system of staff health and wellbeing (Richins et al., 2019; Macaulay & Conniff, 2020) and, crucially, in combination with decent working conditions (Daniels et al., 2021). Throughout the pandemic, healthcare organisations worldwide set up staff wellbeing programmes. In this chapter we describe how we were instrumental in developing a comprehensive system of staff health and wellbeing in our large organisation (an acute physical health NHS Trust in the UK) and how using a Systemic approach was key.

We begin this chapter by exploring what we mean by a Systemic approach and reflect on its application in healthcare contexts. Context, relationships, communication, and interaction have been fundamental to our work developing systems of staff support. Subsequently, we will present Fredman's[1] (2006) 5 'C' principles: Connections in relationships, Context, Collaboration, Circularity, and Curiosity about multiple perspectives and demonstrate how we used them to guide setting up staff support systems in an acute physical health context. In exploring these principles, particular attention will be paid to power and how this can play out in healthcare hierarchies. Related to this, we discuss how staff support can attempt to address the needs of disempowered groups such as individuals from marginalised groups or those at a lower staffing grade. This is particularly important because we work from the principles of social justice and the belief that there should be equality of opportunity for all staff. Unfortunately, there is still clear evidence of ethnic inequalities across a range of professions and settings in the NHS (NHS Health & Race Observatory, 2022). We will also present box examples of other wellbeing practitioners' work in the system of staff support exemplifying collaboration and connection.

A general introduction to the Systemic approach

A Systemic approach recognises that fundamentally people exist in relationship to others and works with these human connections. Rather than locating problems within the individual, it views them within their systems, creating a focus on interpersonal patterns and context (McNamee & Gergen, 1992). A system can be defined as a network of relationships where action in one part has an effect on all other parts. Healthcare organisations are complex human systems, made up of large numbers of people and teams (subsystems) connected to each other working towards shared goals.

To understand the nature of human systems, the machine metaphors used in early Systemic thinking are a useful but limited starting point. Human systems do, in some ways, function similarly to mechanical systems; for example, central heating systems are made up of separate but connected parts that must communicate to maintain the desired goal (of a certain temperature). The function of the system is to maintain this environment through a process of homeostasis requiring continuous adjustments and communications over time. Early Systemic practitioners described human systems as being stuck if they

---

[1] Glenda Fredman is a systemic family therapist and clinical psychologist experienced in working in medical settings who we have both been lucky to work with and be trained by.

could not change and adapt and believed they could take an 'expert' position by standing outside of the system and direct the changes they thought should be made.

Human systems are clearly more complex than central heating systems. Systemic practitioners moved on to focus less on people as objects within a stuck system, and more on processes of change in systems, viewing systems as perpetually changing and developing. Comparisons were made with ecological systems, considered more representative of the complexities of human systems (Bronfenbrenner, 1979; Bateson, 1972). Ecological systems have the same pull towards homeostasis, for instance requiring continual changes to balance population size with available resources. What examples of pulls towards homeostasis might we encounter in healthcare organisations?

The Systemic approach went on to recognise multiple perspectives within systems, instead of only the 'expert' ideas of the practitioner or those holding most power (Hedges, 2005; Jones, 1993). Systemic thinking then proposed that the practitioner cannot stand apart from the system and view it totally objectively. Instead, they inevitably look through the lenses of their own contexts (e.g. upbringing, ethnicity, culture, gender, sexuality, social class) and through the work will become part of the system. They therefore become more able to appreciate the multiple perspectives of other members of the system, requiring them to hold less of an expert position.

Systemic practice was further influenced by social constructionism particularly in its consideration of power. Those with most power in systems can determine its values and dominate the culture. Language use becomes critical here given the social constructionist view that realities are constructed in conversations between people and maintained by stories shared. Language therefore not only reflects realities or experiences but also influences and constructs them. Social constructionist theory puts forward that there are no fixed truths to be discovered within individuals because people are shaped by the relationships they are in and the contexts within which they live and work, and these can change of course.

Systemic practice also developed to see human systems as having lifecycles where adaptations are needed in response to changes in membership or the surrounding environment. This has traditionally been thought about in family systems (Carter & McGoldrick, 2005) and been applied to individuals with health conditions where family life stages may be impacted on by the 'illness lifecourse' (Rolland, 1987). Let us turn to how Systemic ideas can be thought about in health contexts.

Systemic thinking applied to healthcare organisations

Hospitals and healthcare organisations are large, complex human systems. We have discussed the Systemic ideas of interrelatedness which, when applied to organisations, mean that we cannot be removed from the work system we consult to (Oliver, 2005). We have this in mind, not only in considering our personal and professional contexts when setting up (and delivering) systems of staff support but that we too are staff who may require support!

Organisations, while they may include physical spaces, resources, and staff, also include ideas, approaches, and ways of working that cannot be touched or seen and are in continual flux: "The organisation never settles into an entity or thing that can be labelled and described, because it is constantly changing, or re-inventing itself, through the interactions going on within it" (Campbell, 2000, pp. 28). Lifecycle changes over time are relevant to healthcare systems, for instance, as hospitals go through growth and expansion. Events like critical incidents demand agile change and adaptation, and the COVID-19 pandemic is an obvious example. Redeploying staff to unfamiliar work areas on the scale that occurred during the pandemic demonstrates a pressure that moved the system away from homeostasis, unsettled it, broke down boundaries of subsystems (such as teams and services), and created understandable stress and anxiety as a result.

If we consider the social construction of reality through narrative and language, how might this apply to healthcare organisations? Using the example of a system that needs to quickly adapt in response to a pandemic, leaders, and those with most power in a hierarchical system, must give clear communications about the reasons for rapid changes (e.g. redeployment) while acknowledging the anxiety this causes. But more than clarity is needed. *How* leaders use language will set the tone and shape meaning and experience for staff. Normalising messages of expected human reactions is a clear example of using Systemic thinking to influence meaning. From the beginning of the pandemic, we encouraged and supported senior leaders to give messages such as 'you are only human and anxiety in this situation is natural' and 'make use of your tried and tested ways of coping'. This messaging gives legitimacy to how staff might feel, encourages self-care and peer support and, hopefully, reduces stigma. The message of using previous ways of coping connects with a narrative of staff as being resourceful and likely to have already developed coping skills in challenging situations. This fits with a Systemic view of individuals as the expert on themselves, and the value we place on the lived experience of those who have survived periods of psychological distress.

At times of stress in a healthcare system, narratives of staff being 'broken' can dominate and so we encouraged leaders to help staff uncover alternative narratives of resourcefulness while acknowledging the challenges and their impact. Similarly, in response to the early stages of the pandemic we tried to avoid language that placed problems in people. For example, instead of offering 'resilience training' when staff were being redeployed to COVID-19 areas we offered 'preparedness training' which primarily focused on identifying and building upon individuals' pre-established methods to manage stress and their own distress, as well as introducing some brief psychoeducation on managing anxiety. Of course, we must remain aware of the problems resulting from narratives that reflect competence alone. The narrative of the healthcare worker as 'hero', although appreciated by some as complimentary, is also experienced by many as constraining as it seems to give little permission to staff to struggle, be exhausted, and not feel heroic.

The assumption of competence and building on existing strengths and resources extended to setting up the system of staff support itself following ideas from appreciative enquiry and Solution-Focused working. Early in the process we identified what was already working well within the organisation, and where staff support was already provided. This prevented work being duplicated and also allowed us to avoid positioning ourselves (or being positioned by others) as holding the only legitimate perspective on what would be helpful to staff. We will now explore in more detail how we set up a system of staff support following Fredman's (2006) principles.

The 5 Cs model (Fredman, 2006) in setting up systems of staff support in healthcare

The 5 Cs model: Connections in relationships

We are aware of the core Systemic principle that humans are connected to each other in relationships and what one person does in a system has an effect on others in that system. To understand a system and how it functions it is useful to map the relationships between people; in healthcare, these relationships are often hierarchical. When setting up a system of staff support it was essential that we understood the landscape of relationships, where decisions are made and influence gained. This was a daunting task in our organisation which is vast (25,000 staff) and complex with many hospital and community sites, each with differing structures and professional groups. Obtaining accurate and up-to-date information was challenging as organisations constantly change, staff leave, and new posts are created. Identifying the holders of accurate organisational information was key.

We (Neil and Harriet) had prior connection, sharing principles and values from our Systemic training and experiences which were useful contexts in collaborating to develop the work. Prior to the pandemic there was limited designated psychological provision for staff support and wellbeing: a part-time post in the children's hospital (Harriet[2]), a part-time Schwartz facilitator role, and only a couple of psychologist posts (Neil, and a shared post) within occupational health for our large organisation. Many psychologists who work clinically with patients also offered staff support within their medical specialities, for example offering supervision to palliative care staff, running reflective practice groups, and facilitating psychological debriefs. Some areas had set up systems of staff support linking in with other professionals in Workforce and Organisational Development (OD) but overall, it was piecemeal.

With such a small staff wellbeing psychology resource, we needed to identify, connect, and collaborate with those individuals who were positioned in the system to have the greatest impact on it. These individuals are often, but not always, in positions of authority as leaders and managers. Individuals can also be given influence because their particular role or position within the organisation grants them usefulness or acceptability, such as union representatives and key members of staff networks (for instance, our Trust's multicultural staff network).

Building relationships is critical in commissioning and positioning of the work. Making connections with individuals in the system who hold influence is useful for multiple reasons: firstly, in developing an understanding of hopes they hold for our input, secondly to support key people to understand the role of staff support psychologists and, thirdly, crucially, to endorse staff support work itself (whether delivered by psychologists, OD, or other colleagues working in staff wellbeing). Sanctioning the work is vital and needs to go beyond lip service statements of support. The organisation and leadership need to address core working conditions first, then agree – and support – processes that release staff to join staff support sessions and/or attend to their own and team wellbeing. These key connections between people build a scaffold for the work of staff support. An example of OD in staff support and connection with OD colleagues is illustrated in Box 3.1.

---

[2] Harriet had developed a system of staff support in the children's hospital following Systemic and Solution-Focused principles (see Macaulay & Conniff, 2020).

Box 3.1: Organisational Development and Staff Support

OD is a behavioural science focusing on healthy, effective, sustainable organisations. The work of Kurt Lewin (1980–1947), a social psychologist, is at the core of OD. He was the first to study group dynamics within organisations and he developed force field analysis, action research and unfreeze–change–freeze, models which are still in use today. OD also has its roots in Gestalt, systems theory, psychodynamic theory, social discourse, appreciative inquiry, and social constructionism.

OD practitioners aim to help organisations by working with different levels of the system (from individual, teams, organisation). They collect data, collaborate, sense-make with stakeholders, advise on the people elements of change, and design and facilitate group interventions. They focus on use of self (i.e. how we consciously use our emotional, perceptual, and cognitive processes to create an impact that the system needs. This requires self-awareness, awareness of others, and self-management), to ensure ethical, quality practice which is in service of the organisation and its clients.

Within the NHS, OD practitioners may work as internal consultancy experts in relation to the human elements of change; they may be involved in leadership development, team development, and staff engagement. In the UK there is no formal route or professional development and many OD people come from training and HR functions.

By supporting individuals (e.g. through leadership development activities), teams (e.g. team development), and/or senior leaders (e.g. when there is conflict between two groups of staff or when organisational values require updating), OD practitioners are aiming to facilitate positive working relationships, harmony, compassion, diversity, inclusion, and adaptation to change. These all contribute to creating the conditions for people to thrive and support wellbeing.

For many organisations, the response to the COVID-19 pandemic resulted in very different ways of working. Guy's and St Thomas' NHS Foundation Trust recognised that staff wellbeing was critical. This brought together OD; clinical psychologists; HR; equality, diversity, and

(Continued)

inclusion (EDI); and representatives from doctors, nursing, and so on with the aim of supporting staff wellbeing. OD collaborated with clinical psychology in many ways. For example:

- designing and co-facilitating training to support staff in having conversations about wellbeing with their colleagues and signposting to sources of support
- designing and facilitating reflective sessions to assist groups of staff in processing their feelings and emotions, recognising they're not alone, supporting personal growth and self-compassion
- co-designing a range of self-help resources to support staff, managers, and teams.

OD brought skills in training/workshop design/facilitation, a consideration of the system from multiple perspectives, understanding of team dynamics, survey design, evaluation and data analysis, and the values of inclusion, collaboration, and support to the work.

Challenges in working between staff wellbeing psychologists and OD consultants included a slightly different use of language. Curiosity and time to explore different perspectives helped with clarity. Being brought together through the pandemic provided the opportunity to build relationships and deepen understanding of different approaches which then led to collaborations in addressing organisational challenges

Karen Walsh, OD consultant at GSTT, 2019–2021

Chartered psychologist. Full member of BPS Division of Occupational Psychology and committee member (appointed 2022). Member of BPS Division of Coaching Psychology. Member of ODN Europe (board member 2018–2021)

If we accept that interrelatedness is our focus, then we rely on the quality of the relationships we build in setting up new systems of support. This is the key mechanism for influence and change. In keeping with this, as the pandemic unfolded, we created further staff support psychologist posts dedicated to specific services to meet emerging need made apparent through relationships developed (e.g. dedicated to community sites, women's services, and emergency departments). The development of these posts in themselves further strengthened relationships in those areas. At the same time, we built a central team of psychologists able to respond and be present across the organisation. This gave essential agility to allow us to respond to inequalities in the system, especially inequalities of access. We also address this by making ourselves more available in place and time – physically present on-site as well as offering remote sessions and sometimes working outside of office hours to reach shift workers.

Communication is key when people are in relationship with each other. It is understood in Systemic practice that all behaviour is communication. Subsequently, even when time is limited, it is essential not to rush in but instead to try and slow down reactive approaches, allowing us to understand the communication underlying behaviour. An example of this is resisting the pressure to provide psychological support when more basic human needs have been left unattended to, such as time for breaks or quiet spaces to rest. In these instances, staff distress is often a manifestation of system pressures where working conditions are impacted. Only offering psychological wellbeing sessions in these situations is more likely to damage staff wellbeing, because colleagues can feel unheard and pathologised for voicing that their basic needs at work are not being addressed.

When entering new areas, to set up staff support, we link with those with influence such as clinical leads, ward managers, and/or those who have a wellbeing interest or role. We use relationships to help ideas (Reder & Fredman, 1996) to meet with key stakeholders and see how they want to use us as a resource. These ideas are based on the understanding that those giving and receiving help already have their own established beliefs about the helping process, usually based on their previous experiences of giving or receiving help. This can significantly influence the outcome of staff support or 'help'. We think carefully with stakeholders about the best time for sessions, frequency, and where they occur (on the ward, off ward, virtual).

This setting up of the work and connecting with staff does not stop once the work has been commissioned. We always begin team and individual sessions asking what would be useful to cover in the session, and gain feedback about the work while in-session, for instance, by asking 'are we talking about the right things?'. Following the work we evaluate it using surveys and seek staff views on additional staff wellbeing practices that could be developed.

> **Box 3.2: Practices that enable connection in setting up systems of staff support**
>
> - Map the system and relationships
> - Link with those with influence
> - Build allies with others with an interest in staff wellbeing
> - Meet with key stakeholders
> - Find out who wants what for whom
> - Consider ways to connect with individual staff, teams, and the system, for example presence, paper, and online surveys to capture as many views as possible
> - Consider how you connect with staff; alongside, seeking their expertise.

The 5 Cs model: Context gives meaning

The systems of connected relationships provide the context for how people live their lives in and out of the work setting. Context gives meaning to our behaviour and beliefs, so in order to understand them we must shed light on the context in which they originate. Healthcare organisations are microcosms of the societies in which they operate in and often reflect the diversity of culture within the communities from which they draw their workforce. The beliefs and values of these communities are found within healthcare systems alongside the beliefs and values of specific professional groups, teams, and services. There is interplay between these, and they map onto hierarchies of power where some are privileged over others. We do not and cannot know all these belief and values systems and therefore must remain curious about the perspectives and experiences of colleagues.

An example of the role of context when considering staff support is how a healthcare professional experiences and responds to stress. These will have been shaped by the relationship contexts of their past and present, including families, schools, faith organisations, training institutions, employers and so on. Of course, the current contexts for healthcare workers are strongly shaped by professional requirements, norms, and cultures but they are also influenced by people's personal cultures, including ethnicity, spirituality, gender, age, ability, sexuality and much more. Therefore, in setting up (and continuing) the service we needed to attend to all aspects of context and the intersections between them and considered Social GRRRAAACCEEESSS (Burnham, 2012). Some staff spoke to us about feeling unable to be their authentic selves or whole selves in work because professional cultures dominate. We were therefore careful to address spiritual contexts, for example, by building in sources of spiritual support alongside psychological support. Some of the work of chaplaincy in staff support is described in Box 3.3.

> ### Box 3.3: Chaplaincy and staff support
>
> Chaplains have always been an integral part of giving support to staff working in the NHS since its inception in 1948. A fundamental principle of chaplaincy is to offer pastoral, spiritual, ethical, cultural, and religious care to people of all faiths, beliefs, or none. During the COVID-19 pandemic, greater awareness was given to the wellbeing of the staff in the NHS. Two dedicated multi-faith and belief cross-cultural chaplaincy staff support teams were formed, one for the Trust hospitals and one for the Trust community. Teams were focused on the spiritual wellbeing of staff and work closely with staff psychologist colleagues to offer psycho-spiritual care as part of the continuum of care for staff. Chaplains respect different faiths, beliefs, and cultures of all staff, offering the choice of spiritual support to all staff, exploring shared humanity, and spiritual needs such as meaning and purpose, hope, belonging, and love.
>
> The main aspects of the staff support chaplaincy teams were to work with staff psychologists to help deliver:
>
> - Regular spiritual and pastoral care
> - Offer a listening ear
> - Give one-to-one staff support (face to face, virtual, or by phone)
> - Wellbeing support for managers and team leaders
> - Bereavement support, funeral, and memorial advice for staff, especially around staff death and ceremonial events.
>
> Each team works alongside staff psychologists, offering cross referrals and sharing joint publicity events. An example would be immunity/vaccination events when staff psychologists and chaplains work together with other healthcare professionals answering questions and offering support as part of the wellbeing package. Similarly, staff chaplains and psychologists work closely together after a staff death. Staff chaplains tend to offer immediate assistance, staff psychologists offer group and individual support, and staff chaplains offer ceremonial and memorial events in the medium to longer term.
>
> *(Continued)*

A normal part of chaplaincy is using a spiritual assessment tool, when being with a patient, family member, or staff member. The teams realised the importance of creating a new tool that was specific to helping explore the psycho-social-spiritual wellbeing of the staff member that is relevant to their own individual situation and circumstances. The tool we created uses the acronym SSSEWN (see Figure 3.1).

Staff chaplains have benefited in their work with the staff psychologists – there has been mutual sharing and reflection and respectful appreciation. It has been of particular benefit when working with the highly diverse community that makes up the workforce of Guy's and St Thomas'; some cultural groups trust psychologists, whereas others trust chaplains. Seeing the two groups work together has helped build respect for both groups and increased the reach of the staff wellbeing service.

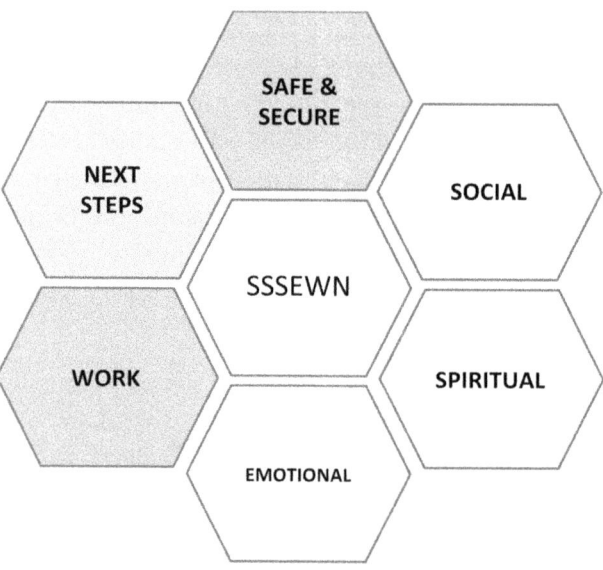

FIGURE 3.1: SSSEWN model. Authors: Mia Kyte Hilborn, William Sharpe, Tracy Morgan, Zahida Suleman, Peter Oguntimehin, Ezekiel Samuel, Josh Turner, Barth Orji, Guy's and St Thomas' NHS Foundation Trust Chaplaincy Team.

Considering diversity of personal contexts in staff support work is much more than just supporting staff to be their authentic selves; social inequalities are replicated in healthcare systems and play out in experiences of discrimination and disadvantage. Pre-pandemic, ethnically marginalised populations showed higher prevalence of mental health difficulties, linked to higher levels of comorbid risk factors such as discrimination, and social and economic inequalities. Public Health England (2020) revealed that ethnically marginalised communities are at higher risk of contracting the COVID-19 virus, increased risk of severe symptoms, and higher rates of death. A survey of over 14,000 adults by the mental health charity Mind (2020) revealed that existing inequalities in housing, employment, finances, and other issues have had a greater impact on the mental health of people from ethnically marginalised groups than White people during the pandemic. In response, we created a staff wellbeing psychologist post dedicated to supporting ethnically marginalised staff and improving access to the staff support offer by increasing the relevance and acceptability of the offer (see chapter 1).

It may seem obvious, but in physical healthcare the highest level of context is medical – staff are there to treat and care for patients who are ill, have health conditions, or have been injured. Different clinicians have different roles and tasks to perform. Changes in patient numbers, staffing levels, complexity, and acuity of patients are some of the myriad of factors that mean that a healthcare system is always in flux. We bear this in mind, remaining curious about medical contexts and the roles colleagues hold, for example, when faced with challenges such as low attendance to a group. We might consider it likely that staff are too busy to attend and think about ways around this, for example working with seniors to cover duties or changing the session time rather than be drawn to traditional psychological assumptions about ambivalence or avoidance.

Box 3.4: Consideration of context in setting up systems of staff support

- Think about what your professional and personal contexts are.
- What other contexts exist related to staff support and wellbeing in your organisation? (including history of these)
- How might the medical context vary in different areas of your healthcare organisation and impact on setting up staff support systems?
- How might Social GRRRAAACCEEESSS (Burnham, 2012) inform setting up systems of staff support and the contexts that individual staff and teams are operating in?
- How might all these contexts interrelate at different levels and change at different times?

The 5 Cs model: Collaboration across levels of the system

An emphasis on collaboration is a response to the importance of connections and context. Because of this, we actively seek people in the system to work with and alongside. This includes collaborations with other psychologists in our organisation. We have incorporated different models of psychological staff support service delivery, including psychologists embedded in medical specialties, staff support psychologists attached to medical areas and those working from within Occupational Health. We join with others from a position of cultural humility, learning what was already in place to support staff beyond psychology and co-creating further initiatives where needed. Some examples of collaborations can be found in boxes throughout this chapter. We joined with others on an individual, team/service, and organisational level.

Collaborating at the organisational level

As we joined the system and became part of it (as we cannot separate ourselves from it as we have said above), we became educated in its structures and language – we learned the 'organisational speak'. This is highlighted by the organisation's response to critical incidents when the command and control structure is established. Through the pandemic we collaborated with the strategic and tactical structure and became part of it by leading the multidisciplinary staff wellbeing subgroup of tactical command. We moved with the organisation out 'command and control' towards a restorative and recovery structure and back again. We identified allies who support the staff wellbeing agenda and collaborated closely with them to strengthen its platform. These allies include the charity[3] that funds most of the staff wellbeing programme, the Executive Board, Occupational Health, EDI, OD, Human Resources and Workforce, and the Medical Mediation Team. Box 3.5 describes the work of the Medical Mediation Team. The Psychological staff support team has been able to collaborate with their practice as an integral part of the broader system of staff health and wellbeing; we regularly liaise and occasionally do joint working.

---

[3] Guys & St Thomas Trust (GSTT) Charity.

Box 3.5: Supporting Staff to Recognise and Manage Conflict with Patients, Families, and Colleagues: The work of the Medical Mediation Foundation[a] Sarah Barclay and Dr Esse Menson

Conflict between patients, families, and health professionals is upsetting for everyone and can have a significant impact on relationships between teams and the family/patient. Health professionals join their profession to care, using their knowledge, expertise, experience, and capacity for empathy and compassion. However, when these skills fail to establish connection and trust with patients and families, the communication breakdown and conflict which may arise can lead staff to experience a range of unsettling thoughts and emotions as well as physiological stress engendered by conflict. They may be experts in their clinical field, but health professionals often report feeling out of their depth in relation to managing conflict.

The instinctive response of many health professionals when faced with conflict is to avoid it. It can be very difficult not to take things personally. It is human to want to defend yourself or your team if you're feeling attacked. Staff may have contradictory thoughts and feelings and feel unsure how best to respond. What if their input fuels the conflict and makes things worse?

Whether a conflict is short or long term, there is also a significant time cost involved in managing it.[b] Until relatively recently, there was little training available to health professionals in understanding and managing conflict between families and health professionals. MMF was established in 2010 as a not-for-profit organisation aimed at filling this gap, providing conflict management training and mediation in paediatric healthcare settings. MMF has trained more than 5,000 health professionals in multidisciplinary groups in UK NHS paediatric hospitals and internationally.

The conflict management training provided by MMF has become an important element of the staff support programme within the Evelina London Children's Hospital & Women's services.[c] Sessions include:

- Supporting staff to discuss the impact of conflict on them
- Helping staff to recognise the triggers of conflict and feel confident in acknowledging and managing, rather than avoiding them
- Practising essential mediation skills aimed at de-escalating conflict and restoring trust and empathic communication with patients and families.

(Continued)

More recently, MMF has created a structured framework for managing conflicts as a team at different levels of escalation, aiming to identify potentially painful and damaging conflict situations early and manage them proactively. Evaluation of its use found that it reduced both the time spent and the economic cost of conflict in four UK paediatric settings.[d] Ensuring that conflict is acknowledged by the multidisciplinary team (MDT) and responded to collectively and consistently is one of the key challenges involved in embedding these skills into clinical teams. For example, it is often bedside nurses who first identify and experience tensions with families while medical staff, who spend less time with them, may be less able to recognise and acknowledge the warning signs. This can delay the response time in managing it.

At Evelina London, collaboration between MMF and the staff support psychology team has been key to ensuring that if staff experience trauma or high distress as an unintended consequence of discussing a conflict they have been involved in, they can be directed to support from staff psychology. The connection between conflict management training and staff wellbeing is consistently shown in the feedback. It highlights the impact of providing staff with the resources to understand the potential triggers for conflict with families and patients and to recognise conflict at the earliest possible stage.

Making this resource available to staff reduces the time spent managing conflict and equally importantly, it increases staff confidence in approaching potentially 'difficult' conversations with families in a different way.[e] One consultant commented: "I have lots of experience in dealing with conflict but I still learned new things that I can put into practice. It made me wonder if my usual practice is always helpful." A staff nurse reported that "I now feel more confident to explore conversations with parents which may be challenging."

[a] www.medicalmediation.org.uk
[b] Forbat L, Sayer C, McNamee P, Menson E, Barclay S (2016). 'Conflict in a paediatric hospital: a prospective mixed method study'. In: Arch Dis Child 2016; pp. 23–27.
[c] Macaulay C, Conniff H. (2020) Developing a programme of staff support in a children's hospital. *Archives of Disease in Childhood British Medical Journal*. June 1–2.
[d] Lyons, O, Forbat L, Menson E, et al. (2021). 'Transforming training into practice with the conflict management framework: a mixed methods study'. In: BMJ Paediatrics Open; **5**
[e] Forbat, L, Simons J, Sayer C, Davies M, Barclay S l. (2017). 'Training paediatric healthcare staff in recognising, understanding & managing conflict with patients & families: findings from a survey on immediate & 6-month impact'. In: Arch Dis Child; pp. 250–254.

Collaborating at an individual level

We have already mentioned how crucial it is to get support from senior management to do the work – sanctioning staff members to attend. Collaborating closely with senior clinicians to appreciate the importance of staff wellbeing can aid logistical support for staff to be able to attend wellbeing sessions. For example, senior staff holding bleeps, rostering to ensure staff are released from shift, as well as people getting time back for attending wellbeing sessions from home on non-working days (should they wish to). Another valuable aspect of support from seniors is their attendance at groups run (where appropriate, for example, where positioning and power can be addressed by the facilitator). They can play an important role by modelling that it is OK to be affected by work and set an example by talking about their feelings. This is an incredibly powerful way of reducing stigma.

Collaborating at the team level

On a very practical level, it is better to offer staff support for teams in established meetings especially if there has not been anything like this before. It is useful to join healthcare staff in their language and modality, because if, as psychologists, our approach feels too alien (e.g. our language and practice) then people may not come. Sometimes it can be useful to consider offering staff support sessions in different ways, for example, a way that fits with where a staff group is at or with their professional identity. Offering a 'teaching slot' or case discussion and then encouraging reflection on the impact of scenarios or themes can feel more palatable to teams wanting something more concrete, or for those who don't want to delve into emotions during a busy shift (I, Harriet, have found reflection invariably happens even if you call it a teaching slot). Linked to this, we have found that running taster sessions can be a useful way to make explicit the kind of input that staff support practitioners can provide (e.g. wellbeing check-ins, short mindfulness sessions, and reflective practice). Holding these provides an opportunity to introduce other interventions such as debriefs, and the broader programme of staff support and wellbeing. Box 3.6 describes learning from the experiences of redeployed staff during the first wave of the pandemic to better tailor wellbeing initiatives to staff needs in subsequent waves:

Box 3.6: Setting up Psychological Staff Support Collaboratively in an NHS London Trust: Through a Systemic Lens

The following case study demonstrates how a MDT was quickly organised to support staff responding to the intense demands and pressures of the pandemic in 2020 and 2021. A small group of key individuals from across the organisation (Nursing, OD, Psychology, communications) formed a tactical group, to support staff wellbeing encompassing practical, emotional, and psychological support. As the first wave dissipated, feedback was sought from those deployed, Critical Care staff, and senior leaders to design and embed an accessible and meaningful staff wellbeing offer. The most significant and consistent points made were that staff deployed and working in critical care felt they were isolated or forgotten about and identified a lack of visibility and communication from their senior teams.

Learning from first wave

As the second wave of the pandemic took hold in December 2020, it was recognised a particular focus was again needed in supporting Critical Care staff and deployed clinical staff. Feedback from staff reflections on the first wave demonstrated the importance of feeling connected to a 'home' team during deployment. In the second wave, an experienced matron was deployed alongside the wider staff deployment with the remit of liaising and supporting this group of nurses. From there a wellbeing team evolved consisting of nursing staff from areas where staff had been deployed and a clinical psychologist.

To best utilise these resources, a collective decision was made to provide a collaborative MDT response that would be able to support as many staff impacted as possible – both deployed and permanent Critical Care staff of all disciplines. With ongoing communication with the wider wellbeing tactical team, this approach ensured shared expertise, coordination, staff familiarity, and allowed a much more holistic approach to staff wellbeing.

The wellbeing offer was focused on being responsive and adaptive to ensure it met the needs of approximately 500 deployed surge and

(Continued)

permanent Critical Care staff. While focus remained on the emotional and psychological impact on staff, it was quickly recognised that this would benefit from a broader approach linked to practical concerns of rosters, break rooms, access to food and water, and so on that were impacting the exhausted and distressed staff.

To unify diverse teams with deployed staff who had never worked together before, a structured approach to communication was implemented. This consisted of daily huddles, confidence checks for staff, virtual communication tools, wellbeing walks providing visible leadership and responding to needs as they arose, and links with the wider organisation. A weekly reflective space was introduced for the Wellbeing Team to share and discuss their experiences. This was integral to ensuring the Wellbeing Team maintained resilience, offering a safe space to openly discuss their own experiences.

Impact

It is reasonable to assume from feedback and observation that this systemic, multidisciplinary structure and approach of the Wellbeing Team was able to initiate and provide support for hundreds of staff effectively and meaningfully. The Wellbeing Team was well placed to enable actions and escalations with other supporting teams efficiently. In addition to the initial and ongoing support during deployment, the team ensured transition plans were in place for returning deployed staff. These included reflective sessions and welcome back days, ongoing support for the Critical Care staff to provide spaces to discuss their experiences and the impact on them.

What worked and transferable applications

There were key aspects relating to how the Wellbeing Team was established, and then continued to evolve that enabled an ability to remain flexible and responsive. Although this case study describes a particular time never experienced before in the NHS, the learning about staff support can be extrapolated to other times of challenge within teams

(Continued)

or an organisation such as service development, reconfiguration of teams, moving departments, or renovations. We have put these key aspects are summarised below.

Preparation – This enables an opportunity to listen to concerns and collaborate on ways to manage expectations, empowering individuals to identify what they can do to support themselves and each other during times of challenge. Ensuring an effective and sustainable structure is established and understood for varying roles and contexts.

Continued support/communication – During periods of challenge, checking in with a home team reduces the feeling of isolation and helps individuals to feel connected. Being kept informed of any changes helps individuals feel valued, transparent, and consistent communication is key. This was represented successfully in the approach our Wellbeing Team was based on, enhancing understanding, expertise, and what can be offered by bringing coordination and a multidisciplinary approach with clear and regular communication.

Realignment – At the end of the period of change, facilitating a space for reflection enables individuals to process what they have experienced, achieve closure, and ready themselves for a return to their previous role/home team. For many a change is a period of growth and learning may give opportunities for professional development. A period of reflection, coming together to hear each other's experiences helps to restore the team. Such space also allows staff to feel true recognition of the work they had experienced and bring a valuable perspective to what has been achieved.

Dr Shannon Cullerton, Lead Clinical Psychologist for Staff Wellbeing on COVID-19 Wards
Daniel Wicks, Nursing and Midwifery Information Officer (previously Matron Critical Care Wellbeing Team)
Róisín Fitzsimons, Head of Nursing and Midwifery Equality, Diversity, Inclusion, Wellbeing and Leadership Development

We do not expect medical systems to fit with traditional psychology norms of sessions being 1 hour in a room without interruptions. In acute settings the next thing will happen, and staff may need to be bleeped out or called to attend an emergency; an hour may be too long for staff in some areas (such as theatres or intensive care). Instead, we adapt our offer; with shorter interventions, going to where staff are and thinking through ways to manage interruptions for any group. We have found that healthcare staff in acute settings are usually used to interruptions, and they are perhaps more unsettling for the wellbeing practitioner!

The 5 Cs model: Circularity of relationship patterns

As we have seen, the Systemic approach focuses on circular patterns of relationships between people. Systemic practitioners are less interested in what causes problems or the need for change in the first place and are more interested in the circular patterns that maintain problems or inhibit change. Consequently, looking for the starting point of problems in healthcare systems is less productive than looking for the patterns of relationships and responses that maintain them. This serves to steer us away from blame and towards finding solutions by supporting changes in the responses between people. Interestingly, in acute healthcare systems, the use of human factors research from aviation disasters has been applied to incidents where harm has occurred to patients by using a systems lens to understand medical errors. This focuses on systemic, organisational, and broad human factors and the circular interplay between them rather than finding individual scapegoats.

Similarly, circularity helps us to move away from lineal understandings that may locate blame in an individual, for example for being tired and making a mistake. A circular understanding would view staff as tired due to work pressures, combined with the influence of professional cultures which make it difficult for staff to say they are struggling, or not being heard if they do speak up. Such a work culture may well increase anxiety in staff thereby impacting their sleep and making them more tired. By identifying these circular processes, changes can be made to shift a culture where breaks are properly built into scheduling, for instance, and that staff are able to say (and be heard) when they need a break.

> **Box 3.7: Using circularity in setting up systems of staff support**
>
> - Aids strategic response to planning what to offer and how that will fit with staff need
> - Supports strategic working with senior leaders and organisational communication
> - Opens up thinking
> - Simply drawing out of circular problem formation can be useful.

The 5 Cs model: Curiosity about multiple perspectives

Being curious about multiple perspectives helps us not to make assumptions about the 'right' approaches to supporting staff. In valuing different perspectives and skills, we appreciate that staff support while informed by psychological ideas does not always need to be delivered by psychologists. We aim to make psychological language and ideas accessible. As an example, we co-designed training on holding wellbeing conversations for all staff which allowed us to share psychological ideas and the task of creating and delivering wellbeing initiatives. We also value multiple psychological perspectives when working with our psychology colleagues and include the use of other evidence-based approaches such as responses to trauma in large-scale critical incidents, Solution-Focused approaches, and compassion practices.

As mentioned earlier, language does not just represent reality but also constructs reality; therefore, multiple perspectives are shared through stories told. Shared narratives about people can constrain them but also liberate them. This premise underpins narrative therapy (White & Epston, 1990) which views people as separate from their problems, situating them instead in wider social contexts. Conversely, healthcare organisations often focus on individual wellbeing, meaning that if a staff member is struggling emotionally, often the narrative is about the need for that individual to increase their resilience. This places the problem within the individual, as if resilience is something they alone have responsibility for and positions them as failing for not being resilient enough. The resilience narrative in healthcare tends towards a prescribed view of what resilience is rather than there being multiple renditions of resilience. A sole focus on individual resilience is also problematic because it ignores factors at a relational and systemic level that contribute to reduced staff wellbeing. We must necessarily focus on organisational and team resilience as well. Subsequently, staff support systems must provide interventions across all levels. Some examples are given in Box 3.8.

Box 3.8: Staff support interventions at multiple levels

- Ask about team coping and successes as well as individual coping and successes.
- During reflective practice sessions, invite multiple perspectives and bring in context.
- Focus on building shared narratives during psychological debriefs following critical incidents.
- Support a Just Culture approach to incidents that aim to encourage a restorative approach focused on fully understanding what's gone wrong and why instead of looking to allocate blame and punish employees.
- Share themes gathered through staff support work with leaders and managers. This 'soft intelligence' can help identify the organisational causes of stress and distress.
- Help with the creation of mechanisms to support departments to address these identified causes at a local level.
- Support campaigns to address these causes at an organisational level, such as campaigns to encourage staff to take breaks that focus on team level and manager level responsibility as well as individual responsibility.
- Work with Communications colleagues to guide messaging from senior leaders and feedback staff responses to highlight how it has been received.

Box 3.9: Using curiosity about multiple perspectives in setting up staff support

- Be aware of assumptions we may have or narratives that may exist around certain staff groups, medical specialities, and try to generate alternative hypotheses.
- Consider multiple perspectives on the problem or issue.
- Think about work at different levels of the system – individual, team, and organisational applications and at strategic levels.
- Unpick and open up thinking about loaded terms such as resilience and wellbeing.

Conclusion

In this chapter we hope we have shown that setting up a programme of staff support using Systemic principles can be done without specialist equipment or a particular physical space, or even fully trained Systemic practitioners. In its simplest form it is about being curious about the perspectives of others and therefore continually asking questions with a relational focus. Among these, 'who?' questions can be particularly useful (Lynggaard & Baum, 2006), such as 'who is most concerned here?', 'who is most affected?', 'who should we include?', 'whose voice needs to be heard?'.

Asking questions like this can challenge and disrupt the homeostasis and therefore occasionally make our role tricky to navigate. Such questions may be counter to an expectation of a quick fix from staff psychology and means the remit of our work can be varied and include mediation, advocacy, and speaking up as we try to hold on to our principles of social justice to challenge inequalities. We may be positioned by others into roles too, and the different roles we may take will vary depending on the context and how people respond to us. We are mindful of our changing roles as the work and staff support system develops. Throughout we try to maintain connection in relationships and be collaborative, think about context, and remain curious. Yet we recognise that we can also be affected by issues and themes of the work which can strongly resonate with us as healthcare workers ourselves. This is where purposeful disconnection, supervision, and peer support are vital.

References

Bateson, G. (1972). *Steps to an ecology of mind: Collected essays in anthropology, psychiatry, evolution, and epistemology.* Chicago, IL: University of Chicago Press.

Bronfenbrenner, U. (1979). *The ecology of human development.* Cambridge, MA: Harvard University Press.

Burnham, J. (2011). Developments in social GRRRAAACCEEESSS: Visible-invisible and voiced-unvoiced. In: Krause, I.-B. (Ed.), *Culture and reflexivity in systemic psychotherapy: Mutual perspectives*, 139–160. London: Karnac Books.

Burr, V. (1995). *An introduction to social constructionism.* London: Routledge.

Campbell, D. (2000). *The socially constructed organization.* London: Karnac Books. (The systemic thinking and practice series – work with organizations).

Carter, B., & McGoldrick, M. (Eds.). (2005). *The expanded family life cycle: Individual, family, and social perspectives* (3rd ed.). New York: Pearson.

Dallos, R., & Draper, R. (2015). *An introduction to family therapy: Systemic theory and practice* (4th ed.). London: Open University Press.

Daniels, J., Ingram, J., Pease, A., Wainwright, E., Beckett, K., Iyadurai, L., Harris, S., Donnelly, O., Roberts, T., & Carlton, E. (2021). The COVID-19 clinician cohort (CoCCo) study: Empirically grounded recommendations for forward-facing psychological care of frontline doctors. *International Journal of Environmental Research and Public Health*, 18, 9675.

Fredman, G. (2006). Working systemically with intellectual disability: Why not? In: Baum, S. & Lynggaard, H. (Eds.), *Intellectual disabilities: A systemic approach*, 1–20. London: Karnac Books.

Fredman, G. (Ed.). (2010). Introduction: Being with older people – A systemic approach. In: Fredman, G., Anderson, E., & Stott, J. (Eds.), *Being with older people: A systemic approach*, 1–29. London: Karnac Books.

Global Forum. (2019). 1.5-day workshop for global healthcare leaders called 'A systems-approach to alleviating work-induced stress and improving health, well-being, and resilience of health professionals within and beyond education'. Conference Summary Paper.

Hedges, F. (2005). *An introduction to systemic therapy with individuals: A social constructionist approach*. London: Palgrave Macmillan.

Jones, E. (1993). *Family systems therapy: Developments in the Milan-systemic therapies*. Chichester: Wiley Series in Family Psychology.

Lang, P., & McAdam, E. (1996). *Referrals, referrers and the system of concern: A chapter about good beginnings ... designed to lead to quicker endings!* Pre-Publication Manuscript available from: https://www.taosinstitute.net/files/Content/5694552/McAdam-lang-_Referrals,_Referrers_and_the_System.pdf.

Lynggaard, H., & Baum, S. (2006). So How Do I ...? In: Baum, S. & Lynggaard, H. (Eds.), *Intellectual disabilities: A systemic approach* (pp. 1–20). London: Karnac Books.

Macaulay, C., & Conniff, H. (2020). Developing a programme of staff support in a children's hospital. *Archives of Disease in Childhood British Medical Journal*, June, 1–2.

Maslow, A. H. (1943). A theory of human motivation. *Psychological Review*, 50(4), 370–396.

McNamee, S., & Gergen, K. J. (Eds.). (1992). *Therapy as social construction*. London: Sage.

Mind. (2020). *The mental health emergency: How has the coronavirus pandemic impacted our mental health?* London: Mind.

NHS Health & Race Observatory. (2022). *Ethnic inequalities in healthcare: A rapid evidence review*. London: NHS Health & Race Observatory.

Oliver, C. (2005). *Reflexive inquiry: A framework for consultancy practice*. London: Karnac Books.

Public Health England. (2020, June). *Beyond the data: Understanding the impact of COVID-19 on BAME groups*. London: PHE Publications.

Reder, P., & Fredman, G. (1996). The relationship to help: Interacting beliefs about the treatment process. *Clinical Child Psychology and Psychiatry*, 1(3), 457–467.

Richins, M. T., Gauntlett, L., Tehrani, N., Hesketh, I., Weston, D., Carter, H., & Amlôt, R. (2019). Public health England, British Psychological Society & Royal College of Policing Scoping Review: Post-trauma Interventions in Organisations Final Report. Available from: www.bps.org.uk

Roberts, V. Z. (1996). The organization of work: Contributions from open systems theory. In: Obholzer, A. & Roberts, V. Z. (Eds.), *The unconscious at work*, 28–38. London: Routledge. (The members of the Tavistock Clinic consulting to institutions workshop).

Rolland, J. S. (1987). Chronic illness & the life cycle: A conceptual framework. *Family Process*, 26, 203–221.

White, M., & Epston, D. (1990). *Narrative means to therapeutic ends*. New York: Norton.

4 Moral Injury

Why Exploring Novel Terms Makes Space for Talking in Staff Support

Dr Esther Murray

The ways people conceptualise issues such as stress, bullying, and sick leave inform organisational culture and the design of wellbeing interventions. Given the recent explosion of research into psychosocial distress experienced by healthcare professionals and the urgent need to both explore and map the extent of the problem, and to address the causes and consider the remedies, now may be the time to review and clarify some of our key terms. As a health psychologist, I was trained to use theoretical models and evidence to support the design and delivery of interventions, and in the importance of understanding stakeholder perspectives and working practice before seeking to intervene. This chapter will explore the ways in which emerging concepts such as moral injury impact shared institutional knowledge and therefore what staff support is offered.

We will pay special attention to the ways in which we as practitioners hold the concepts that we use with staff and unpick meanings of core concepts in staff wellbeing through exploring some key questions. Does it matter that the definition of, for example, moral injury is one that we all agree on and how can we manage the other interpretations which arise and make space for shared meanings? Can we appreciate and hold other interpretations while holding fast to our own definition? Do we need to arrive at a consensus with staff in order to talk about a particular concept? Are we required to be expert and simply tell people what a concept means? If so, does this type of expert model fit with our preferred ways of practicing and what can we do if it does not?

Habits and practices of intervention design

For those of us working with a focus on staff support, the culture of intervention design we were socialised into as part of our training and education will necessarily inform our practice at work. In Health Psychology, we train in a model based on the demonstration of competencies in the workplace. These are professional practice, consultancy, intervention design and delivery, research and teaching and training.[1] In terms of work delivered, of course consultancy, intervention and research can be combined, but they need not be. The time devoted to development, delivery, and evaluation of the projects will necessarily be different, but the rigour ought to be the same. The difficulty is likely to arise in balancing the tensions of various stakeholders in the workplace when intervention becomes part of the day job as in staff support. Other practitioner psychologists will come to their own accommodations with design and delivery of wellbeing interventions informed by their training. Due to the nature of healthcare working (which requires relatively rapid responses to relatively concrete demands) there isn't always the time to revisit the whys of our practice in intervention design.

Why do definitions matter? Creating legitimacy

When delivering staff support in the NHS, we are working with people who have been trained in the medical model, where the factors which make a concept legitimate have a lot to do with recognised and agreed signs and symptoms, diagnostic procedures, and subsequent treatments. Some models in clinical and health psychology might also follow this process. However, in psychology a biopsychosocial model of understanding human distress is preferred which takes account of wider contexts in which people are living, and the culture and life experiences which they bring to their workplace.

Part of the work in designing and delivering staff wellbeing interventions might then require us to agree definitions, particularly at the contracting stage. This might be a particularly important consideration when we are working with new or contested terms. The speed with which terms are adopted and shared for discussion can seriously compromise their usefulness. This has happened in the case of moral injury where it has been conflated with a range of perfectly legitimate hurts that might be better explored in other ways. Additionally, it is well known that the word resilience has become highly problematic in healthcare, largely due to the ways in which it has been experienced as a term which implies individual failure and weakness, decontextualised from the wider

---

[1] https://www.bps.org.uk/qualifications/health-psychology/outline

structural issues in the current healthcare system in the UK (for example). In fact, nuanced conversations about resilience, grounded in an understanding of the ways in which the term was first used in thinking about people as resilient, can be really useful.

The earliest research on resilience focused not just on intrapersonal qualities of the individual, such as optimism and intelligence, but also their ability to seek social support and to maintain beneficial social connections (Tussaie & Dyer, 2004). This could mean that wellbeing and staff support sessions could focus on the importance of maintaining social relationships and the skills which might be used to do that, especially when we are really stressed and exhausted.

When supporting staff, we need to be mindful of context in its very broadest sense, particularly in relation to staff wellbeing terminology. The ways the staff we support are interacting with academic journals, social media, conferences, online webinars, podcasts, newspapers, and all other forms of media will also influence what they bring to sessions and how they are involved in planning staff support programmes. We all know the power of coming across definitions which resonate with us and validate us; it would be worth highlighting those experiences in our interventions in order to be able to outline the focus of the work at any given time. I think this can be done by simply talking about how it feels to be validated. It is my sense that much of the scene setting and contracting work of the session should be given over to establishing what is the focus of our work together and what is not.

It is also worth foregrounding the ways in which information is shared and experienced. Academic publishing is a large part of the lives of many psychologists; for many of us, continual publication is necessary for career progression. What other healthcare professionals know about research methods and academic publishing is varied, for instance, that the papers which appear in journals are there, at least in part, for professional brownie points as much as a deep desire to ensure the right information is in the public domain. I include all my own work in this! I have given many, many talks on moral injury, published papers and book chapters, and recorded podcasts which are informed by my understandings of the term, a desire to be useful and to have my voice in the public domain because it is part of my job.

The nature and reputation of academic publishing can mean that papers become popular, not necessarily because of their quality but because they have been written by someone well known, or they support the worldview of the person who has some control over what interventions might get offered, or which speakers might be invited to the organisation. In our intervention design, we might be driven by theory or a particular therapeutic model, but it is imperative that we look at context, and at the drivers behind the work we are asked to include or support. It is important for us to explain that this is the way we establish legitimacy of terms in psychotherapeutic work, that while there will be clinical definitions in some cases there are also useful, commonly understood, non-clinical uses of words. Anxiety and depression are good examples here of describing day-to-day emotional experiences which are also debilitating conditions requiring multifaceted treatment. By defining terms early on in our work with staff (in this case), we can create space to explore, or at least acknowledge the 'what about' moments which we hope will arise when people feel safe enough.

Moral injury

Moral injury has been described in various ways, but there are two main schools of thought. Firstly, Jonathan Shay conceptualises it as the betrayal of what is right by someone who holds legitimate authority in a high stakes situation (Shay, 2014), whereas Litz and colleagues describe it as the result of "perpetrating, failing to prevent, bearing witness to or learning about acts that transgress deeply held moral beliefs or expectations" (Litz et al., 2009, p. 695). Litz et al.'s (2009) descriptions encompass the fact that the morally injured person may be the *perpetrator* of the act which causes injury, not just the person who has been acted against. Shay's (2014) observations were formed from work with US veterans recovering from their experiences in the theatre of war and highlighted the tenacious nature of their emotional reactions to these experiences. Shay (2014) spoke of their struggles to recover from events which had so rocked their view of themselves and the world that even though they had undergone effective, evidence-based treatments for PTSD, they struggled to return to 'normal' life. Processing of events that he came to understand as morally injurious seemed only to take place in peer groups where experiences across veterans were similar. Shay recognised his role as an outsider, conceptualising himself only as a facilitator of these discussions between people 'who know'.

At the point where Shay began writing about moral injury, he had worked with this population for over 20 years and his presentation of the concept grew out of these particular experiences. It is now generally understood that morally injurious events might take many forms, and indeed there is ongoing research to understand exactly what might constitute a morally injurious event (*Journal of Traumatic Stress* Special Issue June 2019). Certainly, the people I spoke to when

I undertook research in the area had their own ideas about what was morally injurious for them (Murray et al., 2018). What has become problematic is that the term moral injury is now being applied much more widely and possibly 'inappropriately'. When we are working in areas as sensitive as those where we explore the harms people have undergone as a result of their work, fussing over definitions can seem unnecessary and even unkind. It may be that you will decide there is enough shared understanding and enough currency in the term that it brings people to your intervention or is useful in a formulation and that is sufficient. Or you may decide you need to parse out the details of definition in order to explore attributions among staff. It may be that the need for a shared definition is related to the need for a sense of belonging in the group, enabling the members to be clear with one another that they are indeed experiencing the same thing.

It is worth considering why the term moral injury has gained so much traction with healthcare professionals both in the UK and the US. Ways of conceptualising the psychological harms of witnessing or experiencing trauma such as PTSD and burnout have not traditionally included a moral dimension (Nash, 2019). Being able to talk about moral issues at work opens up new conversations which are not about individual resilience, but much more about the circumstances in which people work. Examples would be moral distress (Jameton, 1984) which describes the experience of being unable to offer good care because of lack of resources such as understaffing. The experience of moral distress is largely the experience of not being able to act in ways which are congruent with an individual's self-concept because of circumstances beyond their control. It differs from moral injury in various ways such as the degree of transgression of the individual's moral code, the role of leaders and, arguably, the magnitude and frequency of events. Depending on how you conceptualise moral harms at work, moral distress could be seen as arising from the day-to-day grind, whereas moral injury might be more related to major events, and failures of leadership. We could also consider Litz et al.'s (2009, p. 695) point here about 'perpetrating or failing to prevent acts which deeply transgress deeply held moral beliefs or expectations'; it's not uncommon in health and social care to find that staff feel much more responsible for the mistakes that are made at work than might actually be 'reasonable', for want of a better word. The blame culture so prevalent in many healthcare organisations, which focuses on mistakes as the fault of a single individual, will only exacerbate this sense of personal failure.

Shay's (2014) definition of moral injury, with its emphasis on the role of leadership failings, allows the possibility of having much more open conversations about potentially contentious topics such as the role of leaders. Shay (2014, 1994) discusses the role of leadership, and how bad decisions by leaders leave subordinates at risk. In the COVID-19 pandemic, much has been made of war metaphors. While they have not always been terribly useful with regard to public health messaging, they have had an interesting impact on healthcare professionals' public identity. Newspaper stories reported staff as 'battling' on the 'front lines' of the pandemic, describing them as heroes and angels. The difficulty of adopting this metaphor, and the hero and angel tropes, is that it suggests that healthcare workers signed up to the risk of dying like a soldier might or sacrificing themselves wholly to the cause of saving humanity, like a hero. In fact, they simply chose to do a job. It also makes it harder for NHS staff to talk about how they really feel because opinions get polarised – are you a hero or a coward? During the pandemic, many healthcare staff reported feeling guilty for worrying about their own safety, even though this is a totally reasonable thing to do. Influxes of large numbers of patients with relatively high rates of mortality and morbidity, especially when many of them were younger, have increased the relevance of the war metaphor, since mass casualties are usually only seen in war. Maybe these things, coupled with scarcity of resources both in terms of staff and equipment, have meant that this concept, so resonant for the military, has gained traction with healthcare staff.

Feelings, cognitive dissonance, and moral injury

It may be that morally injurious events disrupt our individual worlds so that our attempts at meaning-making fail and we are unable to resolve the cognitive dissonance we experience. Of course, learning to assimilate events is part of our maturation as humans, but it seems that some events cannot be 'squared away' as easily as others. Possibly the painful realisation of the wrongness of the world, and maybe ourselves in it, is extremely isolating. Certainly, feelings of guilt and shame tend to make us close off from our feelings, numbing them with food, drugs, alcohol, or work or by intellectualising our experience to the point where emotion is no longer present, and also by blaming others and by expressing anger (in lieu of sadness). In moral injury specifically, like all conditions related to experiences of shame and guilt, there is a fear that by sharing 'the badness' with others, they will become contaminated by it. So that not only is our relationship with ourselves disrupted, but also our relationships with others. All these responses mean that we do not allow ourselves to access our individual experience of pain, sorrow, and regret, and thus do not work through it. I have found it useful in the past to remind any group of people I am working with that avoiding our difficult feelings relating to moral injury is an entirely human thing to do. Almost no one comes joyfully forward to 'do the work', and this work tends to get attention only when we are at crisis point.

Understanding the psychological harms of the workplace through a social psychological lens means that moral injury can be understood as happening to an individual but affecting the team and impacting the shared meanings in teams and work settings. It is clear from the literature that social support is extremely useful in mitigating the psychosocial impact of working in healthcare (Williams & Kemp, 2020, for example). However, it is important to remember that in many areas of medicine there is no tradition of debriefing or formal peer support, whether after major or even relatively routine incidents. Older physicians often talk to me about the erosion of safe spaces such as the doctors' mess, where cases could be discussed without fear of being overheard. Shift patterns have changed in many services now, resulting in long, 12-hour shifts with short handovers. There is increased lone working in prehospital care so that opportunities for peer support and rapid, informal, and timely debrief have been eroded.

In Shay's (2014) initial description of moral injury, he is explicit about the role of leadership, and how bad decisions by leaders leave subordinates at risk. In any organisation, the actions of leaders and management affect the staff, but as we have seen in the recent COVID-19 pandemic in the context of the UK, the actions of political leaders, especially, have left staff vulnerable to serious disease, disability, and even death. This is probably as stark an example of the role of failures in leadership as that faced by Shay's Vietnam veterans. But even on a more average day, decisions at the highest level leave healthcare professionals vulnerable because of understaffing, inadequate hospital estates, and insufficient equipment. The powerful hierarchies which exist in healthcare mean that staff often have no recourse and feel that they cannot raise concerns productively. When leaders do not protect and defend the safety of staff and patients, they leave them emotionally and physically vulnerable. Because the NHS holds a special place in the hearts of much of the UK nation, staff find themselves in a constant position of dissonance. They are called on to provide a service for all but are insufficiently equipped to do so, which results in their being unable to offer a standard of care they can feel proud of, and constantly exhausted by demands they cannot meet. This means that their sense of self is under constant threat because 'who I am' and 'who we are' is not 'who we should be', but nor is it within their gift to change that.

PTSD and moral injury

The symptoms which emerge after one or many morally injurious events tend to follow a pattern. Shay (2012) writes that 'both flavours of moral injury destroy the capacity for trust', and that symptoms revolve mostly around shame and guilt, with concomitant withdrawal from social networks and resulting isolation. Researchers agree that the world of someone morally injured shrinks and their social trust is replaced by the expectation of harm and exploitation, and behavioural strategies such as social isolation are then adopted (Shay, 2012; Nash, 2019; Farnsworth, 2017).

There are parallels with some of the aspects of guilt and disruption to world views which are now described in the latest iteration of the PTSD criterion and symptoms in the DSM-5 (2013), but in moral injury the source of this guilt and shame is different. Cognitive models of PTSD conceptualise the symptoms as the result of the interactions of the mind with extreme fear; that is, the world is seen as an unsafe place in which terrible things can happen. The concept of moral injury suggests that the mechanism might be more closely related to feelings and thoughts about shame and guilt: that is, the world is a *wrong* place, in which terrible things are *allowed* to happen (Farnsworth, 2019). A stark example here would be the ways in which patients with COVID-19 were discharged back to care homes early in the pandemic, or the proposed triaging of patients by age when there were likely to be insufficient ventilators, staff, and ICU beds. The guilt and shame felt as a result of moral injury will not automatically abate over time if emotions are not effectively processed, researchers point out (Griffin et al., 2019).

Nash (2019) suggests a stress *injury*, rather than a stress *appraisal* model, pointing out that cognitive/appraisal-based models could perpetuate stigma as they suggest that if people could appraise in a more effective way, then they would not become morally injured. In the current context of the NHS, an appraisal model would suggest that staff would need to rationalise every instance when they felt care was suboptimal because of a lack of resources as a result of structural failings which are nothing to do with them, but Nash suggests that there comes a point where this is no longer possible. Nash holds that 'people are breakable' if put under enough stress for long enough. Maybe it is distinctions like these which will be useful to you, and you will decide to explore fundamental understandings of how humans experience stress in order to inform how you think about issues such as moral injury.

In the special issue on moral injury in the *Journal of Traumatic Stress* (2019), Litz and Kerig also point out that there are cultural and individual factors to take into consideration with regard to understanding what might be morally injurious to any individual (Litz & Kerig, 2019). It is important to recognise a potentially biopsychosocial-spiritual aspect to the practice of medicine, especially when healthcare practitioners work in teams, often in under-resourced settings and with little time or space to debrief or benefit from peer support. A biopsychosocial-spiritual perspective (see, for example, Saad et al., 2017) simply means taking into account the whole person in healthcare, be they staff or patients. This perspective suggests that the staff under your care can be conceptualised as people who are constantly making sense of themselves and their working lives and should have access to a variety of resources for support, including spiritual communities and practice. Not only does this allow you to broaden the conversation to include moral issues, but it also recognises that staff bring their whole selves to work, with all their past history and learned behaviours around coping.

In Canada, at the Canadian Institute for Public Safety Research and Treatment, the term 'Post-Traumatic Stress Injury' (Canadian Institute for Public Safety Research and Treatment, 2019) is preferred to Post-Traumatic Stress Disorder. This is because it recognises that the harms resulting from exposure to traumatic events may manifest as very significant symptoms but that these might not meet the diagnostic criteria for PTSD, nor is it necessarily 'disordered' to experience strong and lasting psychological difficulty from traumatic situations. Like Nash (2019) we might espouse the view that to talk of injury rather than disorder calls to mind physical injuries, which can help remove some of the stigma which is often attached to mental health conditions. It is not unusual for workplace injuries to occur in medicine, and models like this one suggest that psychological or psychosocial injuries are as usual as needle sticks or injuries resulting from manual handling. The importance of using the original term of 'injury' is that it reminds staff that the organisation has a duty of care to protect them from workplace harms; it may be that conceptualising the moral harms of work like this can add weight to the argument that psychological wellbeing at work should also be protected. It's also possible, that thinking of moral injury in terms of a physical injury, that a quick fix might be expected. In fact, it's more like a genuine injury which takes time, and rehabilitation, to heal.

In her article on 'Moral Injury and the Ethic of Care', Carol Gilligan (2014) states that Shay himself reminds us how important it is to listen to the stories of the people we are working with without at the same time mentally sorting them by clinical definition. Stories of moral injury are by definition confusing and painful and should be heard in their entirety rather than parsed into their component parts according to a symptom checklist. She says that by listening in a way which creates trust, a space can be created which allows the prevailing culture to be questioned and people's own moral code to be voiced. This feels particularly pertinent when we think about equality diversity and inclusion in working with healthcare staff. Some staff have raised the issue of the ways in which moral matters are discussed at work being largely secular, for example, when they come from a strong faith tradition which frames their experience in a different way.

Acknowledging the complexities of talking about human emotion and experience is a useful starting point and can come more easily to experienced practitioners than those who are at an earlier stage in their careers. When the pressure is on to 'fix it' and the constant reply has to be 'that's not what is feasible here', it takes no small amount of strength and determination to hold the line. This might mean that if the request comes through for sessions to improve staff wellbeing, which is often measured in very hard metrics like staff retention and sick leave, then the response needs to reflect the reality that staff wellbeing is more likely to be influenced by things like free parking, hot food on night shifts, the ability to control rotas, and having sufficient staff on duty. As such, any additional wellbeing sessions can only be part of a wider package. It is worth considering that staff might not be receptive to talking about moral injury, or any other psychological aspects of their wellbeing, if the fundamental issues of food, parking, and rest areas haven't been attended to by management.

Conclusion

In this chapter we have explored some of the tensions and varied perspectives on the concept of moral injury. Is it a sort of stress injury? Some failing in appraisal? Or simply a part of being human? The question for you as the reader and practitioner must always be, what do these terms really mean in the context of staff support and wellbeing and how can I communicate that to the people I am working with? It is useful also to reflect on whether we all need to agree on a definition or a world view for any concepts used in the field of staff support in healthcare? Is it enough to propose in sessions such as these 'what if, for this session, we take it as given that…' Or do you need to present certainty as part of the work? If there is a need for you to hold the certainty in the room, it can be useful to explore where that need is coming from. There can be a narrative in the workplace that when things are hard the expert must be brought in to 'fix it'. Sometimes we are asked to come in and do work to reduce something like moral injury where our interventions are seen as the fix, which creates a pretty uncomfortable dynamic by placing us as 'experts'.

We have seen here how the term 'moral injury' can fit well in a medical context, but it does have its drawbacks. One downside to this metaphor is that it enhances the expectation of a quick fix. It is useful to remind everyone involved that mental health and wellbeing is maintained through consistent work, in exactly the same way as physical health. We know that workplace wellbeing is influenced by multiple factors and this cannot be addressed alone by psychological staff support sessions. Perhaps mulling over what staff wellbeing concepts such as moral injury might mean in healthcare settings is part of the work.

References

American Psychiatric Association. (2013). *Diagnostic and statistical manual of mental disorders: DSM-5*. Arlington, VA: American Psychiatric Association.

Gilligan, C. (2014). Moral injury and the ethic of care: Reframing the conversation about differences. *Journal of Social Philosophy, 45*(1), 89–106.

Griffin, B. J., Purcell, N., Burkman, K., Litz, B. T., Bryan, C. J., Schmitz, M., Villierme, C., Walsh, J., & Maguen, S. (2019). Moral injury: An integrative review. *Journal of Traumatic Stress, 32*(3), 350–362.

Jameton, A. (1984). *Nursing practice: The ethical issues*. Englewood Cliffs, NJ: Prentice-Hall.

Litz, B. T., & Kerig, P. K. (2019). Introduction to the special issue on moral injury: Conceptual challenges, methodological issues, and clinical applications. *Journal of Traumatic Stress, 32*(3), 341–349.

Litz, B. T., Stein, N., Delaney, E., Lebowitz, L., Nash, W. P., Silva, C., & Maguen, S. (2009). Moral injury and moral repair in war veterans: A preliminary model and intervention strategy. *Clinical Psychology Review, 29*(8), 695–706. Available at: https://www.ncbi.nlm.nih.gov/pubmed/19683376 [Accessed 16 October 2019].

Nash, W. (2019). Commentary on the special issue on moral injury: Unpacking two models for understanding moral injury. *Journal of Traumatic Stress, 32*(3). https://doi.org/10.1002/jts.22409.

Saad, M., de Medeiros, R., & Mosini, A. C. (2017). Are we ready for a true biopsychosocial-spiritual model? The many meanings of "spiritual". *Medicines (Basel, Switzerland), 4*(4), 79. https://doi.org/10.3390/medicines4040079Saad.

Shay, J. (1994). *Achilles in Vietnam: Combat trauma and the undoing of character*. New York: Scribner.

Shay, J. (2012). Moral injury. *Intertexts, 16*(1), 57–66. https://doi.org/10.1353/itx.2012.0000.

Shay, J. (2014). Moral injury. *Psychoanalytic Psychology, 31*(2), 182–191.

Tusaie, K., Dyer, J. (2004). Resilience: A historical review of the construct. *Holistic Nursing Practice, 18*(1), 3–8. https://doi.org/10.1097/00004650-200401000-00002.

Williams, R., & Kemp, V. (2020). The nature of peer support. https://doi.org/10.13140/RG.2.2.31838.25925.

www.cipsrt-icrtsp.ca. (n.d.). *CIPSRT|glossary of terms*. [online] Available at: https://www.cipsrt-icrtsp.ca/en/resources/glossary-of-terms.

5 A Relational Guide to Establish and Maintain a Psychologically Healthier Workplace

Dr Adrian Neal and Dr Julie Highfield

> *There is nothing heavier than compassion. Not even one's own pain weighs so heavy as the pain one feels for someone (else).*
>
> – (MILAN KUNDERA, 1984, P 67)

Healthcare settings globally are inherently dangerous environments where healthcare workers are exposed to a myriad of risk hazards and stressors. These include pathogen exposure, fatigue from long working hours, psychological and moral distress, as well as physical and psychological violence caused by service users and/or fellow workers, many of which have been particularly acute during the COVID-19 pandemic. The World Health Organisation (WHO, 2000) outlines that many workplace hazards and risks are avoidable, identifying inadequate staff training, poor workforce planning, inappropriate or inefficient equipment, and processes as significant contributors to the tens of thousands of healthcare workers globally who experience harm (Loeppke et al., 2016).

Aided by the now openly acknowledged negative impact of the pandemic on healthcare workers (Preti et al., 2020), organisations including the NHS (House of Commons Health and Social Care Committee, 2021) have started to promote and invest in initiatives to support the wellbeing of their workforces. An irony, however, is that in the surge to support workforce wellbeing there has been an increasingly disorganised deployment of resources, a confusion of agreed understanding as to what constitutes workforce wellbeing and what resources might be needed to make a significant positive impact. As such, we have seen a proliferation of resources supporting well-intended but often non-evidence-based initiatives, an overemphasis on mental illness and psychological treatments, as well as the inevitable push to develop interventions claiming to develop that most sought after phenomenon – 'human resilience' – all in the face of unprecedented demand in workload.

This situation necessitates that we clarify how we define workplace wellbeing, map out the established and emerging evidence base, and develop models to help us formulate what is clearly an area of complexity. All three tasks require an understanding of the psychology of both the individual and of the organisation within which they work.

What do we mean when we speak of wellbeing and psychologically healthier systems?

The concept of wellbeing is somewhat nebulous (Simons & Baldwin, 2021). Within the tightly defined parameters of the workplace, it is necessary to arrive at a more focused definition. Helpful guidance is found in the Stephenson and Farmer Report (Stephenson & Farmer, 2017) which looked specifically at healthcare. This report focuses on 'thriving at work' rather than the broader concept of *wellbeing* and health. In many ways by doing this it sidesteps the 'what is wellbeing' debate and the associated risks of falling into a binary position around health (that you are either well or ill) and therefore do or don't require a treatment.

The report acknowledges that some employees will be unwell and require treatment, but most will be struggling with different challenges (e.g. moral distress or occupational burnout, or low moral) and require very different resources to overcome. The report also highlights the fundamental point that in order to thrive an employee will need to be working in an environment that offers optimal psychosocial conditions. In short, to thrive requires a psychologically healthy working environment to mitigate the inherently hazardous nature of healthcare work. Through this lens, improved workforce wellbeing in the broadest sense (including health) and its by-product, the chance to thrive, are only possible with close attention to the systemic and often foundational biopsychosocial factors that underpin the experience of work.

To understand how to create working environments that offer opportunities for thriving, we need to explore what factors motivate the healthcare workforce to do their work, and what the work asks of them (i.e. the psychosocial demands). These issues have become increasingly relevant in the context of the pandemic and will become vital if we are to find ways to make work healthy. We know that a good experience of work is internationally recognised as a positive health outcome; conversely a poor experience of work is known to potentially harm employees (Lucian Leape Institute, 2013).

An area where healthcare is unique in its demands on the employee is the emphasis on providing the patient/client with a positive experience at a time where they are in physical pain, psychological distress, or at risk of dying. The nature of this unique dynamic is that it places added psychological demands on the worker. They are often required to be tolerant of the distress and expressed emotion of vulnerable others (psychological load), manage their own emotions (emotional labour), multitasking/holding complex information (cognitive load), all while attempting to quickly engage in a compassionate relationship. It is not until you start to break down the psychosocial demands of healthcare work that you can start to understand why it so often fails to deliver a positive experience for both worker and recipient.

The challenges of delivering compassionate healthcare

Since 2010 there has been an expansion in compassion-based initiatives within healthcare (Gilbert, 2017). The ambition to introduce truly compassionate culture into healthcare is both noble and anchored in credible evidence. It is no longer a 'nice' thing to do, it makes sound business sense, and it can positively impact the quality of healthcare (Trzeciak & Mazzarelli, 2019) and the experience of the employee. There is, however, a central problem: it is an incredibly difficult ambition to realise in modern healthcare. So why is this?

Compassion is a universally recognised virtue; however, compassionate care for another human being in distress is both physically and emotionally demanding, it cannot be sustained by intention alone. Compassionate care is hard to sustain even in close familial relationships, let alone with a stranger. It is well known that caring for a loved one is often emotionally draining, physically demanding, and can also impact negatively on the carer's financial security and social connectedness (Chang et al., 2016). In short, unless carefully managed, caring can be harmful.

Likewise providing high-quality compassionate professional care can be intensely challenging and requires a hugely psychologically resourced workforce. As such, it is not surprising that in the UK, USA, Netherlands, and New Zealand to name a few countries (Dixon-Woods et al., 2013) there have been some public failures in care and compassion. In recent years, there have been several high-profile national enquiries across the UK into failures in professional care systems (Francis Report (2013), Liverpool Care Pathway (2013), the Winterbourne Report (2012), the Morecambe Bay Report (2015), and the Andrews

Report (2015)). Each public enquiry has identified, to varying degrees, a similar pattern of interrelated individual and systemic factors: including anti-therapeutic or toxic (macro and micro) cultures, financial overcontrol, rigid targets/Key Performance Indicators, staff shortages, denial, defensiveness, demoralisation, and fear. In these conditions staff often feel deeply unsafe and unable to raise concerns, leading eventually to whistleblowing.

In addition, these public enquires identify that, in each case, staff reported experiencing compassion fatigue, poor interpersonal relationships with their managers and leaders, high degrees of stress, and burnout. These organisations appear to have had workforces with poor psychosocial capacity to cope, and leaders displayed a marked poverty in their understanding of the psychosocial needs of their staff.

It may be fair to state that such failures of care are multifactorial and hindsight is indeed an invaluable tool. That said, we know both why this happens and continues to happen. Perhaps we need a new lens through which to understand and respond.

Formulating complexity

The science of understanding the psychological needs of professional health carers is in its infancy, and even though evidence-based recommendations exist in the form of National Institute of Health and Care Excellence (NICE) guidelines (NICE, 2009, 2015) and many national reports, meaningful application of the evidence has had too little impact on the workforce. The pandemic has simply amplified this gap and added to the complexity.

Traditionally workforce development and resource management are viewed largely through the prism of an industrial model. Typically, staff are seen as resources, or parts of the organisation that must be managed and manipulated according to fiscal, strategic, or structural demands, not unlike the working parts of large machines. While this metaphor holds some validity where people are employed in highly mechanised industrial processes (e.g. factory production lines in the car industry), it quickly breaks down when the work relies on nuanced human interaction and interdependence, and where physical labour is largely exchanged for psychological labour and emotional resources.

In this chapter, which is a development of Neal et al. (2019), we argue that we must first better understand the psychosocial and the relational factors that underpin wellbeing professional healthcare if we are to meaningfully support and sustain professional carers. Furthermore, this chapter argues that there is a *relational framework* underpinning the psychosocial wellbeing of staff that can act to ameliorate many of the psychological demands (Grandey, 2000) that caring places on the healthcare professional.

The relational framework concept links to a social evolutionary theory of human interaction, as well as psychological models that focus on the subtle reciprocal nature of relationships, and wider models of relationship/emotional development such as adult Attachment theory, and models from organisational psychology.

The chapter is organised into four main parts reflecting the Relational Framework (which is illustrated in Figure 5.1):

1. Intrapersonal relationships – the relationships with colleagues and peers.
2. Interpersonal relationships – the relationship with the self.

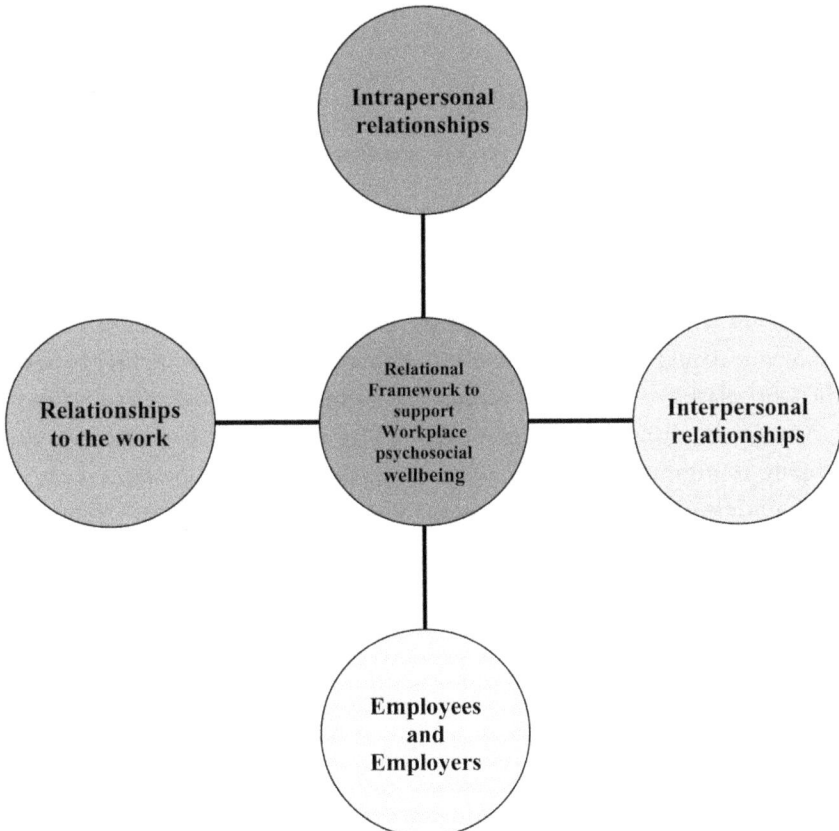

FIGURE 5.1: Relational framework to support workplace psychosocial wellbeing.

3. Relationships to the work of professional caring.
4. Relationships between employees and their employers.

The relational framework

We developed this relational framework in 2015 as a way of synthesising several theoretical models and our experience of working as part of employee wellbeing services as well as within public-facing clinical services as professional carers. As such, it is both evidenced and practice based. It offers a guide to help navigate the complex psychosocial terrain of work and has a dual purpose: firstly, to help make sense of an issue/areas of difficulty, and secondly, to help identify what intervention/resource might make the most positive impact. The factors identified in the framework should be considered important components, not solutions in themselves.

Interpersonal relationships

Relationships with others (peers and managers/leaders)

Humans are an evolved social species who rely heavily on interaction, cooperation, and interdependence. Much of what we have developed as a species relies on the passing of knowledge, the sharing of resources, and cooperation around shared goals. These factors underpin the effective functioning of virtually any human endeavours from healthcare to manufacturing. These are highly relevant in the workplace where we know relational factors such as the relationship with the manager is perhaps the biggest predictor of sickness absence and a sense of belonging to a group predictive of good psychological wellbeing. Given these factors, understanding our relationships with those we work with allows us to appreciate the wider social context that supports a psychologically healthier workplace.

Relationships with leaders

The importance of the relationship between manager and employee in workplace wellbeing is now well established (Black & Frost, 2011; NICE, 2015), the interesting question is why? Managers who genuinely value their staff, are consistent, recognise challenges, and respect boundaries, have psychologically healthier relationships with their staff. What's more, managers who help create working environments high in psychological safety (Edmondson, 1999) are more likely to have staff who feel safe and included. This specific relationship acts as an important factor in the promotion of staff wellbeing as well the psychological milieu of the workplaces. In our experience it is highly unusual to see thriving clinical teams (i.e. with high levels of motivation and/or engagement able to sustain high quality care) where these conditions are absent. Indeed, breakdowns in manager–staff relationships are often associated with higher sickness absence, complaints, errors, and poor quality of care (West et al., 2014). Although not a directly causal relationship, the quality of these relationships is a crucial factor in the wider psychosocial health of both individuals and the teams within which they work.

Relationships with team members

Knowing how peer relationships can be harnessed as a resource to offer carers greater psychosocial protection, it is vital to consider the emotional capability and capacity of managers and supervisors. This group is centrally important and can have either a positive or negative impact on the wellbeing of both individual staff and the wider team.

The second factor is to consider the identity of the team, to determine if it is indeed a team, and if it has the identified structural features and stability to achieve its purpose. Harnessing the protective value of the team is essential given the huge number of internal and external demand the average professional carer needs to manage.

As a social species, we often rely on the cooperation of those around us to both survive and then evolve. Within the workplace, groups of people who cooperate are often called 'teams' (e.g. on a shift or within the same department or sharing a physical space). Especially in healthcare they may not meet the specific criteria needed to be a 'true team'. True teams rely on their ability to sustain relationships and cooperation to achieve their shared aims and objectives. When relationships within these teams are healthy; where rules, roles, and purposes are agreed; aims and goals clarified, teams can be powerful sources of psychosocial support and, thus, wellbeing and a protective factor of their members. Thriving teams also help support their members' purpose and sense of efficacy, both well-documented predictors of workplace wellbeing. Dysfunctional teams can have the opposite effect.

A major threat to the functioning of a team, from within a team (or peer group), comes from a cluster of self-conscious emotions such as shame, humiliation, and guilt, as can be seen after social rejection and loss of rank (Gilbert, 2005). As a social species, we, like our primate cousins, are highly tuned to fit in and connect to our peer group. What's more we can experience a range of distressing emotional reactions if this connection is threatened. Gilbert argues that from an evolutionary perspective some forms of depression have their origins in social withdrawal associated with perceived or actual loss of rank within social groups.

While highly evolved to connect and cooperate, we are also evolved to identify the potential for threat and danger. Paradoxically while offering massive potential in supporting wellbeing, teams can also pose significant psychosocial threats to individual members. It is not uncommon for a range of what Campling and Ballent (2015) described as 'perverse dynamics' to be played out within teams and for relationships to become a rich source of psychological threat. Given that the psychology of the individual is complex, team psychology can be overwhelmingly so, with the addition of powerful and unhelpful emotionally driven behaviour (e.g. abusiveness, blaming, persecution, scapegoating, out grouping). In the context of such powerful dynamics, emotions and behaviour, reciprocally defensive behaviours are often triggered in teams leading to escalation and conflict. These conflicts can become a threat to the psychosocial health of the social climate of any team or peer group if unchecked. These aspects of team behavioural dynamics corrosively undermine both individual and team wellbeing, and employee's ability to offer high-quality care to others.

In addition, when considering how to try to maintain the psychosocial health, and the potential for supporting the wellbeing of teams, it is important to highlight that many teams are not teams by the true definition (West, 2008). Groups of employees are often referred to as teams when they may not be working towards a common goal. What's more when teams are set up it is common to fail to define what kind of team they need to be (independent or interdependent, command, action, advisory, or work) (Thompson, 2008). Specific forms of teams need to meet specific criteria (i.e. having 12 or fewer members; meeting at least every three weeks), though all teams need to have shared and agreed set of aims and goals, as well as identity (Shuffler et al., 2011). Teams that are not 'teams' have been referred to as *sham* or *pseudo* teams, and they are less able to offer their members many of the protective qualities found in true teams such as consistent emotional containment. As a result, staff are likely to be exposed to the stresses generated by the emotional labour of their caring roles without the protective potential of a true team. This is commonly seen in pseudo teams where membership changes frequently, such as with shift work on busy acute wards, where there is over-reliance on agency workers or within community-based services where independent work is the norm.

Intrapersonal relationships
The self and internal psychological resources

There is an abundance of evidence suggesting our *intrapersonal* relationship impacts on our wellbeing. As such, it will no doubt play an important factor in our experience of work. Factors such as self-esteem, self-compassion, self-criticalness, emotional intelligence, distress tolerance, and self-awareness are all relevant and to varying degrees also amenable to development.

The Job Demand-Resources Model (Bakker & Demerouti, 2007) can be used to predict employee engagement and burnout. It argues that the individual's experience of work rests upon the balance between the demands of their role (and the wider experience of work) and the resources that are available to them, including those that are external (e.g. team support, quality of leadership, availability of supervision) and those that can be defined as internal (e.g. their own psychological resources).

Several factors will determine what psychological resources an individual has at their disposal, and these might include:

- Ego-protecting beliefs (e.g. self-serving biases)
- The adaptiveness of dominant coping strategies
- Their capacity for self-compassion, adaptive personality traits (e.g. optimism)
- Their emotional intelligence (to a large extent the ability to manage one's emotional world).

There are, of course, many more psychological resources. Likewise, the value of these psychological resources may be limited by other psychological factors such as an individual's self-defeating coping strategies and their self-awareness – that is, the ability to understand one's own internal or psychological world. This section explores these factors and will identify what can be done to improve our intrapersonal resources.

The promotion of greater self-awareness through reflective practice has seen a slow but progressive advance across the caring professions. Its utility as an internal resource has however yet to reach its potential (Jayatilleke & Mackie, 2012).

Greater self-awareness can offer an individual the opportunity to better understand the dynamic impact their job/role and social context have on their psychological resources. What's more it can support greater psychological adaptability, and, thus, opportunities for both personal and professional development.

Improving self-awareness relies in part upon an individual's motivation and willingness to do so, and the value the organisation places on it. As such, for many professional carers an increased motivation to develop self-awareness only comes after a challenging experience. In this context, self-examination can form an important part of both personal and professional growth (Bailey et al., 2001). Yet supporting the growth and the permissibility of self-awareness needs to be done with sensitivity and in the context of a psychologically safe environment. Deliberate system-focused interventions to promote reflection of the emotional impact of work such as Schwartz Rounds (Pepper et al., 2011) and Taking Care Giving Care Rounds (Flowers et al., 2018) can help support the growth of self-awareness and reflective working cultures; however, ultimately this investment needs to be authorised, modelled, and financed by the organisation.

Hobfoll (1989) argues that without instruction or training we are often unaware of how to manage our internal resources. Hobfoll's Conservation of Resources model states that the function of much of our behaviour is to conserve and build precious emotional resources. Thus, without adequate self-awareness, we are likely to use coping styles which only have short-term effectiveness, may be self-defeating and undermining of one's own wellbeing. Such 'maladaptive coping' can take several forms though its function is to protect the individual (by experiential or affect avoidance) from uncomfortable emotions. Given that caring can often be an intensely emotional experience, feeling threatened by strong emotions is commonplace. Evidence of affect avoidance can be found across the professional caring world, from (arguably) the poor bedside manner of an overwhelmed doctor overtly dismissing distress, to a nurse who habitually depersonalises their patients, the psychologist who minimises the severity of their own distress, inappropriate team stoicism, and the use of black humour. In the extreme, Bandura (2007) argues that professional carers may start to morally disengage, which might lead to the increased permissibility of neglectful or overtly abusive behaviour. It is important to identify that affect avoidance strategies can be useful short term but have a negative impact on wellbeing in the long term. Recent research indicates that affect avoidance-based coping styles in acute medical setting maintain distress and are linked to burnout and compassion fatigue (Iglesias et al., 2010).

Given the potential for, and negative impact of, affect avoidance coping at work (especially where cultures of self-awareness are not promoted), it is important to consider more protective alternatives.

The emotional demands posed by work require us to utilise a wide range of psychological resources. These internal resources are complex but include our ability to tolerate distress, our sense of agency, and our cognitive style and belief systems, among many others. It is however not altogether clear how we develop these resources; some have their basis in our biology, many are shaped and refined through experiences and importantly our relationships. In theory, many of these resources can be modified (e.g. tolerance of distress or locus of control), though in reality the effort and motivation required to do so is huge, making change unrealistic for most. Psychological therapy research has shown that learning a disciplined application of new skills, for example, Mindfulness, can help some individuals improve their psychological adaptability (Brown et al., 2007), but this has limited impact on wider groups and is often idiosyncratic.

Alternatively, Ballatt and Campling (2011) detail a model of psychological resource management coined: Intelligent Kindness. This relies on the individual being self-aware enough to appreciate the unsustainability of being emotionally connected all the time and encourages them to actively learn how to manage their level of emotional connection (kindness/compassion) at work. This model frames emotional resources as precious and finite, in an environment that will always make demands of them. This model simply draws attention to the need to actively manage one's internal resources such as empathy, kindness, and compassion in a proactive way to prevent burnout or depletion of psychological resources.

SC can be viewed as a primary psychological resource; however, it is often overshadowed by the universal call to deliver compassionate care to others. Poor SC has clear associations with poor coping, depression (Allen & Leary, 2010), maladaptive psychological adjustment to trauma, and reduced psychological adaptability and recovery (Thompson & Waltz, 2008). SC has been identified as essential to sustained wellbeing and to the quality of relationships between colleagues and with patients. Academic understanding of this psychological construct is relatively underdeveloped, what is more, it can feel incongruent within professional settings where perfectionism and performance culture are promoted as primary values. In these settings self-criticalness can be passively encouraged, and SC seen as an indulgence. SC is most likely a predictive component of our ability (and motivation) to care for ourselves, as such if it is underdeveloped, dismissed, or discouraged it would be entirely reasonable to predict a negative impact on both individual and systemic wellbeing.

It is also important to consider EIQ as a concept. EIQ is the ability to identify and understand one's own (and others) emotional states and use this information to guide behaviour. EIQ has been acknowledged as important in good physical and psychological health (Tsaousis & Nikolaou, 2005). Several models of EIQ exist; currently one of the most empirically reliable models of EIQ is a Trait Model (Petrides & Furnham, 2003) which identifies EIQ as consisting of 5 core domains and 15 independent factors. An average EIQ (around the 50th percentile) suggests the individual should largely be aware of their emotional states and be able to regulate them, and that they can recognise the emotional states of others. High EIQ (>50th percentile) has long been associated with positive outcomes at work, including adaptive leadership styles and personal wellbeing. In this context, a better understanding of the EIQ strengths and weaknesses of yourself, teams, or individuals can, one might argue, provide a powerful framework for considering how the emotional demands of work might be better supported and which internal and external resources could be helpful.

Relationship between employer and employee

The quality of the psychological contract between employee and employer is a predictor of the quality of engagement (Rayton & Yalabik, 2014), and we know positive engagement is a protective factor against burnout (Durán et al., 2004).

Organisational psychology has identified that staff form a subtle though often unacknowledged relationship with their employing organisations coined the 'psychological contract' (Rousseau, 1989). Like the unspoken contract underpinning any meaningful relationship a 'good enough' psychological contract will bolster employee motivation, their willingness and capacity to cope with the challenges they face, a poor one will have the opposite effect. Within the professional caring environment, there are many potential threats to the psychological contract, thus the all-important employee–employer relationship.

This relationship is partly governed by an employee's expectations (both implicit and explicit) of their employers and focuses on factors such as:

- Renumeration
- Agreed working conditions
- Perceived fairness, how they (the employee) expect to be treated

- The degree to which personal agency is supported
- The anticipated demands of the role.

Breaches to this relational contract can likewise negatively impact on staff morale, their motivation and productivity.

Similarly, the concept of Organisational Justice (Adams, 1963; Barsky & Kaplin, 2007) is particularly important in maintaining an intact psychological contract, as staff are very sensitive to injustices, particularly if they a have previous experience of being treated unjustly by an employer – as they would in any other human relationship. More specifically, there are three subtypes of organisational justice: *Distributive* (relating to the fair distribution of resources), *Procedural* (relating to contracts, rules, and formal procedures), and *Interpersonal* (relating to how people feel they have been unfairly treated by others).

While a large part of the psychological contract is governed by explicit factors such as beliefs, expectations, assumptions, and values, threats to the psychological contract can also have their roots in psychosocial processes beyond our awareness (Obholzer & Roberts, 1994). These factors are usually driven by an individual's efforts to avoid unacknowledged painful emotions, including anger, loss, and anxiety. In her seminal work exploring why nurses resigned from their chosen profession, Lyth (1960) identified that a major motivator was their unconscious avoidance of deep anxiety linked to the largely unacknowledged emotional challenges of the job, and perhaps an organisational failure to acknowledge or support staff in coping with their emotional experience of work.

Both individual employees and their employing organisations can be motivated by psychological processes of which neither are fully aware. It is not uncommon for people to unknowingly re-enact unhelpful past relational patterns at work, including those that were coercive, controlling, critical, or shaming. These psychological processes can underpin disproportionate emotional and/or behavioural responses from staff following ruptures to the psychological contract. Hypothetically, this may be experienced most powerfully by staff who have been drawn to caring roles, by an unaware longing to experience some form of reciprocal experience of idealised care (Ryle et al., 1990).

In addition, it is not uncommon for employees to act out long-held adult attachment patterns with their employing organisations, usually via managers or authority figures (e.g. to feel disproportionately controlled, persecuted, or dismissed). Adult patterns such as these relate closely to secure and insecure attachment styles developed in childhood (Crittenden, & Landini, 2011) but maintained long into adulthood.

A failure to appreciate the importance of the psychosocial processes that make a 'good enough' psychological contract will inevitably result in damaged employee–employer relationships (a rupture), with negative consequences for staff wellbeing and quality of care. Fortunately, it is possible both to reduce the likelihood of these ruptures occurring in the first place and to repair them thoughtfully. It is, however, important to highlight that, in some instances, repair is not realistically possible and particularly so if relationships have been abusive, chronically neglected, or deliberately avoided. Additional complications can also be seen when ruptured relationships between employer and employee become formalised and existing organisational support such as those offered by Human Resources is unable to understand the motivation and underlying psychology of the rupture and deploy 'interventions' which only serve to perpetuate or even worsen the situation.

When considering what can be done by employing organisations, it is important to point out that repairing a 'ruptured' relationship depends upon both employees and employers accepting the reality, adopting adult positions (Berne, 1964), and correctly identifying and clarifying the problematic issues, their origins, and highlighting individual responsibility. In this way, ruptures can be seen as an opportunity to strengthen an all-important relationship and bolster staff wellbeing.

Minimising unhelpful breaches to the psychological contract rests upon a broad web of factors linked to organisational strategy. They include maintaining a workplace culture with the following characteristics:

- Clear, explicit, and relevant values (and objectives) that are consistently adhered to
- Leadership integrity and non-defensiveness
- The encouragement of collaboration across the workforce
- Clear and agreed boundaries and accountability
- A responsiveness to the emotional needs of employee and organisational fairness.

All these factors can be seen in effective individual human relationships and are equally important in healthy organisational relationships. We argue that cultures that are avoiding or denying problems, in addition to blaming, are dangerous and can lead to the creation and maintenance of toxic social climates where individuals are increasingly blamed for what may be essentially systemic problems (Wilde, 2016).

Relationship to professional caring (job and role)

Relationship with your work

The depth of a professional carer's relationships with their work is often unrecognised. Most vocationally trained carers are intrinsically motivated and report better wellbeing if they can work in a way that allows them to support their values and moral framework. For many, their work, training, and professional affiliation will have a strong relationship with their identity, who they identify with (peer group), and all importantly what gives them purpose and a sense of efficacy – all of which are well documented factors of workplace wellbeing. Understanding this specific relationship and when it experiences a crisis (e.g. moral distress or burnout) can help us understand and develop ways to avoid harm and possibly even build protective factors into the workplace.

Relationship with caring

Many professional carers are intrinsically motivated by a desire to help others. The drive to reduce distress, improve quality of life, and simply be able to positively influence another 'to make a difference' are all powerful intrinsic motivators. Not surprisingly, similar motivating values have been observed in educators (Manuel & Hughes, 2006) and police officers (Gillet et al., 2013). What attracts people to the various types of professional caring is however less well known, for example which factors lead a junior doctor to specialise in Psychiatry, Surgery, or Microbiology? Likewise, knowing why a nurse chooses to work in a Critical Care Unit over Palliative Care or Rehabilitation is also poorly understood yet highly relevant when considering the individual's relationship with their work.

In addition to the usual extrinsic motivators such as specific working conditions, availability of flexible or shift work, remuneration, associated social value/status, and structure that most paid forms of work provide, one can assume that the balance of intrinsic factors that motivate individuals into chosen roles or careers includes how the work meets and interacts with their own underlying and changing psychological needs. Given these factors it seems fair to conclude that our relationship with the work we do is both dynamic and psychologically complex, and as such it is important to consider when thinking about the potential impact (demands) of work and sustaining personal and systemic wellbeing.

In considering the potential emotional impact of work, one needs to consider two key factors: psychological labour and psychological load, neither of which are commonly identified in job adverts or descriptions. *Emotional labour* is the psychological demand placed on the individual by the effort required to show the 'appropriate' emotions despite the emotions they might be experiencing. For example, the psychological labour associated with the psychotherapist, or indeed a conscientious manager, is high as they will need to attend to, and regulate their own emotional states as triggered by their role while maintaining a calm external appearance (Brotheridge & Grandey, 2002). Unsurprisingly, high emotional labour has been linked by the same authors to burnout and employee disengagement.

Psychological load is associated with the psychological effort that is generated by exposure to the pain and distress of others. At an extreme level, vicarious traumatisation in care workers has been linked to continued exposure to the distress of patients or recipients of care (Saakvitne et al., 2000).

The psychological load and labour inherent in work varies significantly across the caring professions; it is however rarely acknowledged in job design or job planning. Within the UK and NHS context, specific profession groups seem to have greater awareness of these factors (e.g. those in the Psychological and Occupational Therapy workforce) where efforts are actively made to secure external resources such as clinical supervision, peer support, limited case numbers, and means to limit exposure. Despite these efforts to provide the right resources to offset the psychological demand, a recent survey of the psychological workforce in the UK (DCP and New Savoy Staff Wellbeing Survey, 2015, 2021) suggests that up to 46% are experiencing significant symptoms of emotional distress. One can only imagine the implications this reality will have of staff retention in a post-COVID-19 world.

Considering the issues raised, the question often asked at interview 'Why have you chosen this job?' takes an even greater significance when you must consider the need to sustain wellbeing in an ever-changing, highly demanding, and politicised health system. Perhaps a way forward lies in a shared responsibility between employee and employer. In this scenario the employer will have a more psychologically informed understanding of the complex biopsychosocial demands of the roles it is trying to recruit to offers, as well as what internal and external resources employees will need to perform in a sustainable way over time. Likewise, the employee needs to show a willingness to better understand their own motivators and internal resources, as well as the unique impact the work has on them as a unique individual.

Conclusion

Creating a consistently psychologically healthy workplace in any large healthcare organisation, including the modern NHS, is complex, and one might argue an impossibility. There is however promising evidence from the Quality Improvement literature that confirms that relational or 'connectivity' factors within an organisation play a foundational role in determining both psychological safety and patient safety (Burgess, 2019). Given the psychosocial underpinnings of these factors we believe clinical psychologists can help their organisations and the teams within which they work to have a better experience of work and create and foster the conditions where healthcare staff might hope to thrive.

To be able to achieve this, regardless of the nature of the workplace, it is essential to have a broader understanding of psychosocial wellbeing, the nature of professional care, the complex and often unacknowledged demands of the work, and the psychology of the organisation.

What's more, to do this we may be required to venture away from the familiarity of our clinical models, evidence base, and our core training. This framework maps out several areas that clinical psychologists need to better understand in order to work with staff in healthcare but also where we can make meaningful and tangible changes to our working environment for ourselves, our colleagues, our organisations, and the quality of care provided.

References and suggested reading

Adams, J. S. (1963). Towards an understanding of inequity. *Journal of Abnormal and Social Psychology*, 67, 422–436.

Allen, A. B., & Leary, M. R. (2010). Self compassion, stress and coping. *Social and Personality Compass*, 4(2), 107–118.

Andrews Report. (2015). 'Trusted to care', and independent review of the Princess of Wales Hospital and Neath Porth Talbot Hospital. August 2015. Available at: www.gov.wales.uk

Bakker & Demerouti. (2007). The job demand-resources model. *Journal of Managerial Psychology*, 22, 309–328.

Ballatt, J., & Campling, P. (2011). *Intelligent kindness: Reforming the culture of healthcare*. London. RCPsych Publications.

Bailey, K. M., Curtis, A., & Numan, D. (2001). *Pursuing professional development: The self as source*. Boston, MA: Heinle & Heinle.

Barsky, A., & Kaplin, S. A. (2007). If you feel bad, it's unfair: A quantitative synthesis of affect and organizational justice perceptions. *Journal of Applied Psychology*, 92, 286–295.

Berne, E. (1964). *Games people play: The psychology of human relationships*. London: Penguin.

Black, D. C., & Frost, D. (2011). *Health at Work – An independent review of sickness absence*. UK Department of Work and Pensions. Ref: ISBN 9780101820523,245699411/11.

British Psychological Society & New Savoy Wellbeing Survey of Psychological Professionals. (2015). Leicester, BPS.

Brotheridge, C. M., & Grandey, A. (2002). Emotional labor and burnout: Comparing two perspectives of people at work. *Journal of Vocational Behaviour*, 60, 17–39.

Brown, K. W., Ryan, R. M., & Creswell, D. (2007). Mindfulness: Theoretical foundations and evidence for its salutary effects. *Psychological Inquiry*, 18(4), 211–237.

Burges, N. (2019). Improving together: Collaboration needs to start with regulators. *BMJ*, 367, 16392.

Carter, M., West, M., Dawson, J., Richardson, J., & Dunckley, M. (2008). Developing team based working in the NHS: Report Prepared for the Department of Health, Birmingham, Aston University.

Chang, S., Zhang, Y., Jeyagurunathan, A., Wen Lau, Y., Sagayadevan, V., Chong, S. A., & Subramaniam, M. (2016). Providing care to relatives with mental illness: Reactions and distress among primary informal caregivers. *BMC Psychiatry*, 16, 80.

Crittenden, P., & Landini, A. (2011). *Assessing adult attachment: A dynamic-maturational approach to discourse analysis*. New York: W.W. Norton, 250.

Department of Health (UK) . (2012). Transforming care: A national response to Winterbourne view hospital. Available at: wwww.gov.uk

Department of Health (UK) . (2013). Berwick review into patient safety. Available at: wwww.gov.uk

Durán, A., Extremera, N., & Rey, L. (2004). 'Engagement and burnout: Analysing their association patterns'. *Psychological Reports*, June 2004, 94, 1048–1050.

Edmondson, A. (1999). Psychological safety and learning behaviour in work teams. *Administrative Science Quarterly*, 44(2), 350–383.

Faculty of Intensive Care Medicine. (2016). Regional workforce engagement report: Wales. Available at: www.ficm.ac.uk

Flowers, S., Bradfield, C., Potter, R., Stott, N., Waites, B., & Neal, A. (2018) 'Taking care, giving care' rounds: An intervention to support compassionate care amongst healthcare staff. *Clinical Psychology Forum*, March. BPS, 303, 23–30.

Gilbert, P. (Eds.). (2005). *Compassion: Conceptualisations, research, and use in psychotherapy*. London: Routledge.

Gilbert, P. (2017). Compassion: Definitions and controversies. In P. Gilbert (Ed.), *Compassion: Concepts, research and applications*, 3–15. London: Routledge/Taylor & Francis Group.

Gillet, N., Huart, I., Colombat, P., & Fouquereau, E. (2013). Perceived organisational support, motivation, and engagement among police officers. *Professional Psychology: Research and Practice*, 44(1), 46–55.

Grandey, A. A. (2000). Emotional regulation in the workplace: A new way forward to conceptualize emotional labor. *Journal of Occupational Health Psychology*, 5(1), 95–110.

Hobfoll, S. E. (1989). Conservation of resources: A new attempt at conceptualising stress. *American Psychologist*, 44(3), 513–524.

House of commons health and social care committee workforce burnout and resilience in the NHS and social care second report of session 2021–22 report, together with formal minutes relating to the report ordered by the house of commons 18 May 2021. Available at: wwww.gov.uk

Iglesias, L., Vallejo, B. B., & Fuentes, S. (2010). The relationship between experiential avoidance and burnout syndrome in critical care nurses: A cross sectional questionnaire survey. *International Journal of Nursing Studies*, 47(1), 30–37.

Jayatilleke, N., & Mackie, A. (2012). Reflection as part of continuous professional development for public health professionals: A literature review. *Journal of Public Health*, October, 35, 308–312.

Kirkup, B. (2015). *The report of the Morecambe Bay Investigation*. Morecambe Bay Investigations. Available at: wwww.gov.uk

Kundera, M. (1984). The unbearable lightness of being. London, Faber and Faber.

Loeppke, R., Boldrighini, J., Bowe, J., Braun, B., Eggins, E., Eisenberg, B. S., et al. (2016). Interaction of health care worker health and safety and patient health and safety in the US health care system: Recommendations from the 2016 summit. *Journal of Occupational & Environmental Medicine*, 59, 803.

Lucian Leape Institute. (2013). *Through the eyes of the workforce: Creating joy, meaning and safer health care*. Lucian Leape Institute at the National Patient Safety Foundation.

Lyth, I. M. (1960). Social systems as a defence against anxiety. *Human Relations*, 13, 95–121.

Manuel, J., & Hughes, J. (2006). It has always been my dream: Exploring pre-service teachers' motivation for choosing to teach. *Teacher Development*, 10(1), 5–24.

Mary Dixon-Woods, M., Baker, R., Charles, K., Dawson, J., Jerzembek, G., Martin, G., McCarthy, I., McKee, L., Minion, J., Ozieranski, P., Willars, J., Wilkie, P., & West, M. (2013). Culture and behaviour in the English national health service: Overview of lessons from a large multimethod study. *BMJ Quality & Safety*, 23(2), 106–15.

Neal, Williams & Kemp. (2019). Chapter 26, caring for the carers. In *Social scaffolding: Applying the lessons of contemporary social science to health and healthcare* (Royal College of Psychiatrists) Paperback – 30 June. 2019. Edit, Williams & Kemp.

NHS England. (2013). More care, less pathway: A review of the Liverpool care pathway. Available at: wwww.gov.uk

NICE. (2009). Promoting mental wellbeing at work. Available at: www.nice.org.uk

NICE. (2015). Workplace policy and management practices to improve health and wellbeing of employees. Available at: www.nice.org.uk

Obholzer, A., & Roberts, V. Z. (1994). *The unconscious at work: A Tavistock approach to making sense of organizational life*. London: Routledge.

Pepper, J. R., Jaggar, S. I., Mason, M. J., Finney, S. J., & Dusmet, M. (2011). Schwartz rounds: Reviving compassion in modern healthcare. *Journal of the Royal Society of Medicine*, 105(3), 94–95.

Petrides, K. V., & Furnham, A. (2003). Trait emotional intelligence: Behavioural validation in two studies of emotional recognition and reactivity to mood induction. *European Journal of Personality*, 17, 39–75. http://doi.org/10.1002/per.466.

Preti, E., Di Mattei, V., Gaia Perego, G., Ferrari, F., Mazzetti, M., Taranto, P., Di Pierro, R., Madeddu, F., & Calati, R. (2020). The psychological impact of epidemic and pandemic outbreaks on healthcare workers: Rapid review of the evidence. *Current Psychiatry Reports*, 22(8), 1–22.

Rayton, B. A., & Yalabik, Z. Y. (2014). Work engagement, psychological contract breach and job satisfaction. *The International Journal of Human Resource Management*, 25(17), 2382–2400.

Rousseau, D. M. (1989). Psychological and implied contracts in organizations. *Employee Responsibilities and Rights Journal*, 2, 121–139.

Ryle, A., Poyton, A. M., and Brockman, B. J. (1990). *Cognitive-analytic therapy: Active participation in change*. Wiley Series on psychotherapy and Counselling. London: John Wiley & Sons.

Saakvitne, K. W., Gamble, S., Pearlman, L., & Lev, B. (2000). *Risking connection: A training curriculum for working with survivors of childhood abuse.* Lutherville, MD: Sidran Press.

Shuffler, M. L., DiazGranados, D., & Salas, E. (2011). There's a science for that: Team development interventions in organizations. *Current Directions in Psychological Science,* 20(6), 365–372. http://doi.org/10.1177/0963721411422054.

Simons, G., & Baldwin, D. S. (2021). A critical review of the definition of 'wellbeing' for doctors and their patients in a post Covid-19 era. *International Journal of Social Psychiatry,* 67(8), 984–991.

Stevenson, D., & Farmer, P. (2017). Thriving at work: A review of mental health and employers (2017) thriving at work: A review of mental health and employers – GOV.UK (www.gov.uk).

Thompson, B. L., & Waltz, J. (2008). Self compassion and PTSD symptom severity. *Journal of Traumatic Stress,* 21(6), 556–558.

Thompson, L. (2008). *Making the team: A guide for managers* (3rd ed.). London: Pearson/Prentice Hall.

Trzeciak, S., & Mazzarelli, A. (2019). *Compassionomics: The revolutionary scientific evidence that caring makes a difference.* Pensacola: Student Group.

Tsaousis, I., & Nikolaou, I. (2005). Exploring the relationship between emotional intelligence with physicl and psychological health functioning. *Stress & Health,* 21(2), 77–86.

West, M. A., & Lyubovnikova, J. (2012). Real teams or pseudo teams? The changing landscape needs a better map industrial and organizational psychology. https://doi.org/10.1111/j.1754-9434.2011.01397.x.

West, M. A., Lyubovnikova, J., Eckert, R., & Denis, J. L. (2014). Collective leadership for cultures of high quality health care. *Journal of Organizational Effectiveness,* 1(3), 240–260.

Wilde, J. (2016). *The social psychology of organizations diagnosing toxicity and intervening in the workplace* (1st ed.). London: Routledge.

World Health Organisation: Mental Health Policy and Service Development Department of Mental Health and Substance Dependence Noncommunicable Diseases and Mental Health. (2000). Mental health and work: Impact, issues and good practices. Mental health and work: Impact, issues and good practices (who.int).

6 Reflections on Group Interventions in Staff Health and Wellbeing

The role of psychologists

Dr Zoe Berger, Dr Joanna Farrington-Exley, Dr Harriet Conniff, and Dr Sadie Thomas-Unsworth

Over the years, we have observed the various ways we, as psychologists, have been engaged in supporting staff with the emotional impact of their day-to-day tasks. We have observed the changing requests that have come directly from staff themselves, as well as noticed the different attempts we have made to respond to the issues we see arising in clinical spaces. One such way our input has evolved is in the form of group interventions. These groups have taken a multitude of forms and have a wide range of functions.

In 'Working More Creatively with Groups', Benson (2019) draws on the work of Kohut and Foulkes whose ideas about mirroring can help us understand the key role others play in a group intervention and help us make sense of the additional benefits we observe when running these groups. Benson reminds us that in infants, mirroring happens when a caregiver displays behaviours that show the child they are heard and their emotional state is understood (Kohut, 1977). During group interventions, the facilitator can act as an empathic mirror to help staff feel validated and connected with their own value and competence. The other group members (colleagues) can also act as mirrors. It can be easier to see in others what we cannot see in ourselves, and healthcare staff, in particular, often find it easier to be compassionate to others rather than themselves. The group can help there to be a more compassionate acceptance of unwanted parts of themselves (Foulkes, 1964).

We have also observed that group interventions, in their varying guises, have the unifying aim of bringing people together around a shared experience or theme and enhancing the group's understanding of the issue at hand. Staff have fed back to us that they enable them to connect with each other and remember their joint purpose and values. They are places where staff can give each other permission to have feelings and reactions to a situation and allow people to make sense of their own perspective and opinion of a situation by hearing and witnessing the relative positions of their colleagues.

> **What are the potential benefits of a group intervention?**
> - Space to connect that is away from clinical tasks
> - Normalise own experiences and feelings by witnessing others expressing their experiences and feelings
> - Other people bear witness to each other's thoughts and feelings
> - Look closer at an event and our reactions to it giving space to organise the experience mentally
> - Develop an understanding of our relationship and reactions to an event
> - Feel more prepared to respond to situations in future, following reflection and after learning new skills to use individually from the facilitator or other group members
> - Gain new insights into the group or the relationships within it for the facilitator or the attendee
> - Reach a larger group of staff than in individual sessions
> - Reflect on the emotional impact of the work, for example, our emotional attachment to patients and families.

Perhaps these benefits are most evident to us because the groups we are referring to tend to involve healthcare providers who already know each other and would consider themselves connected through a particular ward or clinical pathway. Of course, there are occasions when group interventions can be broader reaching than this – particularly around an adverse event when multiple teams, who may not know each other, can come together (see chapter 18 on psychological debriefs).

In this chapter, we will reflect on the dilemmas we have faced in this work, such as when to offer one-off or ongoing sessions, or when to hold preventative versus responsive groups. We will also talk about the importance of assessment, how to navigate tricky boundaries, and share our reflections on the practical issues that surround the setting up and delivery of various groups in physical healthcare settings. Lastly, we comment on the role of the embedded psychologists in this work and the more broad-reaching impact we can have in this field. The authors of this chapter are embedded psychologists and staff support is all or part of our role.

Preventative versus responsive

We recognise that one of the key considerations around group interventions is whether the intervention is positioned as part of a preventative offer of support or one in response to a specific event.

In acute hospital settings, the majority of clinical staff work with what might be considered distressing events on a regular, sometimes daily, basis. Preventative group interventions allow a culture to develop within the workplace that acknowledges the collective and cumulative impact on staff of the work they do. Rather than behind closed doors in private 1:1 sessions, group interventions allow the discussion and reflection of these issues to happen in front of peers with the benefits of fostering a supportive, compassionate environment and one that humanises healthcare. Reactive groups recognise the human impact of witnessing something distressing and, potentially traumatic, and support staff to make sense of how they feel about these experiences and find ways of continuing in their work.

Tables 6.1 to 6.3 provide examples of the type of group interventions we have offered over the years. A good menu of options should include both responsive sessions after difficult events, for example, post-incident support as well as preventative interventions to help staff stay well at work by improving working conditions and give space to talk about their experiences.

Many colleagues are keen to have a focus or topic to support their clinical reflections while others prefer to have a more fluid and unstructured space. As such, groups can range from being structured and protocol driven (such as Care Spaces) to those that are more responsive to the needs identified in the session itself. Having realistic expectations as both facilitator and attendee about what the group can and cannot offer is important for the smooth and effective running of the group.

'Well begun is half done'

Over the years, we have learnt that when offering staff support sessions, it is crucial to build relationships with the clinical colleagues we serve. 'Beginning

TABLE 6.1: Examples of types of preventative group intervention offered by practitioner psychologists.

Type of intervention	Description
Teaching sessions	**Skills to enable colleagues to support each other manage the challenges of work** Examples: • Trauma awareness • Supporting colleagues after a traumatic experience at work • Compassion-focused frameworks **Skills to use individually to manage the demands of work** Examples: • Structured courses, for example ACT[a] • Looking after ourselves • Stress • Managing working with families that challenge us **Skills to be better able to deliver clinical care to patients** Examples: • Psychological factors in physical health, for example adherence, breaking bad news, end-of-life conversations, managing and responding to ICU delirium, complex decision-making, advanced communications training These sessions have a structure or topic that provides the focus but it works well to include time for reflective practice and sharing perspectives on the topic.
Reflective practice or peer support group	**Reflective practice groups (longer term)** Examples: • Junior doctors • Consultants • Senior nurses • Pharmacists **Ad hoc reflective practice or staff support groups** Examples • New starter nurses • Ad hoc drop-ins • One-off session at a team's away day • Care Spaces • Team Time

(Continued)

TABLE 6.1 (Continued): Examples of types of preventative group intervention offered by practitioner psychologists.

Type of intervention	Description
	These groups can have a focus, for example, a complex case or can be unstructured, often drawing on Kolb's (1984) experiential learning cycle. These could be closed or open groups. With open groups it will depend on who is on shift and able to get clinical cover to attend. Supporting social spaces can also be the role of psychologists alongside their MDT colleagues, for example, coffee, cake, and chat sessions.
Schwartz Rounds (The Point of Care Foundation)	A multidisciplinary forum designed for staff to come together regularly to discuss and reflect on the emotional and social challenges associated with working in healthcare. A 1-hr meeting that involves three or four members of staff on a panel who describe an experience and the other staff attending then share their reflections and experiences. Schwartz Rounds are delivered at an organisational level and themes ideally reflect pressing issues facing the workforce at the current time.
Improving staff engagement and team culture	Tasks may include supporting the team and its leaders to: • Gather data and share themes with the team • Understand the staff survey results • Reflect on their challenges and find solutions by co-leading working groups to improve team working and team culture • Have difficult conversations in a safe space at a team away day • Discuss their values and priorities for the year ahead • Engage in a journey to becoming a high performing team using tools such as Affina Team Journey (Affina Organisation Development) This may involve working alongside OD, HR, and/or Workforce colleagues.

[a]Flaxman et al. (2013).

TABLE 6.2: Examples of types of reactive group intervention offered by practitioner psychologists.

Type of intervention	Description
Post-event group intervention or psychological debriefs	A group following an acute incident or long-term patient's death (see psychological debrief chapter)

TABLE 6.3: Examples of types of group interventions that can be both reactive and preventative offered by practitioner psychologists.

Type of intervention	Description
Team check-ins	These are one-off group interventions that can be offered to teams who are looking for an opportunity to come together and take stock. They differ from a debrief in that they do not involve exploring a particular event but do encourage and support reflection and team connectivity. They take the format of a series of rounds. These rounds help to support teams to listen and connect to each other's experiences, harness existing resources individually and as a collective. However, they should not be used when teams are experiencing high levels of conflict. In these cases advice should be sought from HR/OD departments.
Pre-briefs	Please see reference to pre-briefs in our chapter on psychological debriefs Pre-briefs are groups that offer a psychological perspective about a particular patient in an ongoing situation. These sessions offer a psychological perspective to help the wider multidisciplinary team understand the patient's difficulties and presentation and as such help prepare for events that might otherwise be difficult or potentially traumatic.

well' (Palazzoli et al., 1980; Fredman, 2007), spending time building relationships particularly with the leaders of teams and understanding the request for help enhance the likelihood of the intervention being a success (Fredman and Reder, 1996).

We have learnt, through hard experience, that staff groups might request a teaching or training session which we rush in to offer, when in fact they use it as a space for personal reflection or will request a Schwartz Round when there would have been many benefits from holding a psychological debrief first. These requests give us useful information about the team's understanding of the issue, their relationship to seeking help, and their hopes for the future. Examples of reasons staff request group support can be found in Box 6.1. The information we gain provides the ground work for a robust psychological understanding of the needs and is ultimately vital in helping to deliver the appropriate form of group intervention. We go on to discuss this in more detail later.

For non-psychologists, there is often some mystery surrounding what psychologists offer and what happens in group sessions. There can be a reluctance around talking openly about the challenges experienced especially when there is a concern about feeling vulnerable or exposed. Helping staff to understand the process and what groups can and cannot offer is a useful part of creating psychological safety and encouraging colleagues to engage. Spending time doing this well can help in the long term and save time in the future when other groups may be requested. We have found that it is easy for there to be unrealistic expectations of what groups can deliver and a hope that they may bring a neat resolution to things that, in reality, are messy and emotional.

Box 6.1: Potential triggers for group interventions to be requested/offered

- A group of staff facing particular challenges, for example, new staff, multiple tricky clinical situations
- A team may want help to grieve together about a patient death
- A team may want space to support each other following an acute traumatic event
- A team may be aware of a problem that is affecting wellness, for example, disrespectful behaviours and lack of civility between staff, changes in rostering systems
- A team may know they need some time to talk about challenges they are facing and want help to think of actions
- A psychologist is aware of the challenges faced by staff and offers a particular group intervention, for example, Acceptance and Commitment Therapy (ACT) course, reflective practice group.

One-off versus ongoing groups

One of the many dilemmas we have experienced is whether we should offer one-off or ongoing group interventions.

Highfield (2019) describes how a key aspect of being compassionate to patients and families is the ability to empathise and understand their emotional states. To do this, staff need to place their own feelings 'on hold' and express them at a later point in time, otherwise they get displaced into unhelpful behaviours in the workplace such as disrespectful behaviours to colleagues or turned inwards to themselves (Highfield, 2019). Group interventions can be a safe and healthy way of processing the emotions that come with the job of caring for others. When deciding whether groups will be one off or ongoing is partly influenced by this understanding of our need to connect and disconnect with our reactions and feelings about work. We need to respect a group's way of managing the emotional burden of caring. Papadatou's (2009) work about how staff deal with grief can be extended to managing a range of difficult feelings. Papadatou (2009) states a spectrum exists concerning staff's reactions and feelings about grief, with over connection (highly vulnerable, overwhelmed) on one side, and disconnection (invulnerable, unaffected) on the other. A good enough amount of connection sits in the healthy middle ground. Feedback from staff has suggested that one-off groups fit better with their working lives and as part of this, are seen as less of a practical and emotional commitment.

We have found that one-off groups are often easier to get 'buy-in' for from staff as they are less of a time commitment (to those attending and those covering clinical shifts) as well as to the psychologist delivering the session. On a busy or big unit/ward, it is challenging to arrange closed or longer-term groups that would enable regular commitment from rostered/shift-based staff. This is largely because in acute wards with large staff teams, such as intensive care, the chances of having the same group of people working on the same day on a regular basis to attend a closed group are virtually impossible. However, there are some teams in physical health settings that are able to manage their work pattern and other commitments in order to regularly attend a closed group.

We have found that running the same session on multiple occasions to increase reach or even at the same time but across different days of the week has been received positively. Another way of reaching groups of staff is by offering support on team study days that are organised by professional group (e.g. for nurses and allied health professionals).

The ongoing concern about one-off interventions, however, is that often the issues and dilemmas staff teams bring to us are not easily resolved or tied up neatly after one meeting. The chance for a regular and protected space to reflect on difficult themes, topics, or issues is intuitively more comfortable as providers of these groups. It most closely aligns with our clinical training and delivery of clinical services. We have therefore adopted a reverent position of respecting that one-off groups have a place and value and that these work best when there are other avenues for support available to which staff can be signposted if needed.

The reduced time commitment of one-off groups is an important consideration especially for psychologists delivering staff support interventions with very large groups of staff to serve. Where psychologists are embedded or when there is more resource, there may be capacity to offer more than one group session, for example, drop in sessions, ACT courses. Contracting the number of sessions is important in a similar way to how one might do in individual therapy.

In this part of the chapter, we want to share our reflections on the practical issues and considerations around setting up and running group interventions. We don't have all the answers but offer some of our top tips for ways to help groups run successfully.

Assess the problem and needs

As we have already mentioned, when approached to help a team with a difficulty or challenge, it is important to understand more about what the team are struggling with and their potential needs. Firstly, consider who is the right person to speak to. It would usually be the person making the request and/or the team leader or a senior member of staff. The request for a group intervention may tell you something about the leader's understanding of emotions, ability to tolerate distress in their team, and the way they respond to their colleagues' distress.

We have found it invaluable to find out as much as possible about the context the team works within, their experience of group intervention before, what has been helpful and less helpful, and what they have already tried or requested around this particular issue. Understanding the problems teams face can help to better tailor the intervention offered. We are often told that staff really value the way that embedded psychologists have a good awareness of the 'emotional temperature' and key issues of the team or the ward and, therefore, have a better awareness of what staff are facing.

The team leader may be asking for an intervention based on their assessment of the problem but through a conversation focusing on the relationship to help, as outlined below, we may come to an alternative formulation about what is needed. It sometimes helps to meet with the group themselves to have an 'assessment' session together and construct a shared formulation if a longer-term group is being requested. It is also important to consider whether what a team leader wants to get out of the group is realistic. It is here that misunderstandings can be identified and some education about group interventions can be offered.

A discussion about a problem or need can lead to other suggestions of staff support interventions (signposting to Organisational Development (OD), Occupational Health, Employee Assistance Programmes, etc.).

> **Box 6.2: Questions to reflect on when setting up group interventions based on Reder and Fredman (1996)**
>
> **In relation to the group who are requesting the intervention:**
>
> *Precipitating factors*
>
> - Why is this being asked for now?
> - Whose idea was this? Who is asking for this?
> - Has a particular event(s) triggered this request?
>
> *Predisposing factors*
>
> - What is the context of this group's difficulties?
> - What made the team vulnerable in the first place to experiencing these challenges?
>
> *Perpetuating factors*
>
> - What are the factors that are contributing to this problem? What else is going on? What is happening in the 'system', for example, not enough resources/staff?
> - What does this request tell you about the needs of the person/group requesting it?
>
> *Protective factors*
>
> - What protective factors are there?
>
> *Relationship to help(ers)*
>
> - Has anything already been tried to help with this situation or other similar situations in the past? Was it effective? How did the group respond?
> - Do the staff want this intervention? Is the manager in support of this group intervention?
> - What expectations do the group or requesting person have of the group intervention?
>
> *(Continued)*

> ***Others***
> - Whose needs could this intervention meet?
> - Who can tell us more about the needs of the group?
> - Is it a group intervention that is needed or something else?
>
> **For the psychologist who is considering delivering the intervention:**
> - What is being triggered here in your models of being a helper? Are you feeling a pull to rescue, make better, chastise?
> - What is influencing your understanding of the group's issues? Are you able to stand back and be objective?

Timing and support from senior staff

We have learnt that the timing of any group intervention is key and needs to be carefully navigated around the clinical commitments of the group. Offering an intervention mid-shift, for example, is sometimes not the optimal time and can result in staff being either unable to attend or guarded about opening up too much as they need to get on with their busy days. We have heard staff express concern that group interventions may 'open a can of worms' that either they won't be able to handle or will require too much effort to be able to get back to 'work mode' afterwards. We recognise that it can be a useful defence to detach from the sensitive and distressing nature of the work enough to be able to do our jobs and be around patient's suffering. This raises important questions for us as practitioners about the considerations needed when offering spaces for feelings and reflection during the working day, such as appropriate timings and the importance of staff being aware where to get further help should they need it. Offering sessions at the start or end of shifts or around times when there is cover from others on the ward can be helpful. If groups do happen mid-shift, it is important that staff can have a few minutes to move away from connecting with their deeper emotions at the end of the group session and ways of returning to 'work mode', for example, by having a coffee before going straight back to patients or by talking about less emotive topics before they return to their clinical duties such as plans for their day off.

When multiple group sessions are being offered consecutively, each time it is offered there needs to be consideration about whether it is the right time.

Reasons to delay or rearrange may include clinical pressures, times of change, conflict within the team, and acute clinical events. Staff need to have the 'head space' to attend and the overt permission that this is part of the ethos of the team. It may be that a change of focus is needed rather than cancelling a group. Where possible, continue to keep a dialogue with leaders about what the focus of the group may be. If a group of staff does not have the band width to do lots of 'work', perhaps a focus more on acknowledging and witnessing where they are at can be more useful.

We have mentioned support from senior managers previously. When leaders model their engagement with psychology to their team, this can demonstrate buy-in, give permission to their colleagues to prioritise attending the group, and reduce any associated stigma. It also helps us to navigate the often very tricky logistics of the running of the group (e.g. time of day, ward cover, what to do if issues or difficulties arise from the group). Some interventions are more successful if staff are given the time back or offered study leave for attending. This gives a clear message that their wellbeing is important and supported in the team and organisation. We have found that having a reciprocal arrangement with other wards or clinical teams to help provide cover for times when groups run can be a good way of managing the issues around staff being released to attend.

Consider the risks, the role of contracting and ground rules

If a team is not functioning well and there is ongoing conflict, a group intervention can potentially be more harmful than helpful. It is possible that a group intervention could make staff feel worse afterwards especially if they leave feeling blamed, shamed, or if uncontained disagreements are aired in the group. In an ideal world, we would be able to predict and understand the likelihood of this happening prior to the group. However, in reality and despite knowing the context or doing the best assessment we can, these difficult issues can surface without warning. It can help to make a plan with a colleague about how to manage this scenario if it arises and what if any ongoing action is needed following the group. It is important to assess the risk of any controversial topics, for example, any decisions that were made that some people disagree with and plan how they will be managed (see chapter 18).

We have found that it can be easier to take risks with a group when you know the group or the clinical environment well. For example, the bond between group members and the safety they feel could mean that the group can meet challenges such as moving rooms at the last minute, meeting for a shorter time than planned due to practicality issues, and running the group despite the risk it could be interrupted. In an established group, it may need to be weighed up whether having a group session is better than no session at all and what is 'good enough' in terms of boundaries and group rules.

In contrast, there are also disadvantages to knowing the group or the clinical environment well. We can be too close to a team, too aware of the issues they face, and therefore as the psychologist facilitator we can find ourselves colluding with the dynamics or dominant voices of the team that we would otherwise not have insight into with a group that we know less well. In situations like this, a fresh pair of eyes can be useful. This is where having designated staff support roles can be especially useful if they exist in your organisation. Otherwise, working in pairs can be helpful, acting as an internal governance structure to apply appropriate checks and balances to what might otherwise be difficult to hold on your own.

It is not only the facilitator who, unintentionally, can collude with the group's view. There is a risk that all group members can succumb to group pressures to agree with the way the group thinks as a whole, rather than disrupt the consensus. 'Groupthink' (Janis, 1972) refers to a process whereby differences of opinion or views are not expressed or given space and the critical thinking of individual members is discouraged. It is our role as psychologist facilitators to overtly build psychological safety (see Edmondson, 2018) within the group whereby diversity is nurtured and all individual voices are encouraged to speak up, to challenge, to offer another perspective ultimately for the richness and development of the group.

In any group session, there is of course a risk that a staff member will share that they are struggling significantly with their mental health and wellbeing. When stating the boundaries of a group session at the start, you may need to cover what will happen if risk (harm to self or others or breaches of professional practice) arises. For some group interventions, for example, teaching sessions, the chance of risk of harm being disclosed is low and this will impact on whether you explicitly state, at the start of the group, the steps that would follow disclosure. We also need to be clear about the limits of what the groups can offer in the moment and afterwards, for example, we may need to refer to community mental health services or share with managers.

For some group interventions, such as Schwartz Rounds, there needs to be consideration about how 'live' and fresh the topic is. Group interventions designed primarily to support individual and collective reflection are likely to benefit from a greater gap between any trigger event and intervention. Staff may need some time to begin processing the event themselves and for the 'dust to settle' before this happens in a group setting. However, this has to be offset by the benefit of covering topics that have resonance for staff at the time. Similarly interventions like Schwartz Rounds and training sessions bring with them the benefit of greater reach as it is often possible to have very large numbers of staff in attendance. However, with this, the greater risks around confidentiality and achieving psychological safety must be considered.

Over our collective years of practice, we have developed some tips for running group interventions successfully.

Box 6.3: Tips for running group interventions

- Ensure leadership support is in place and there is overt permission to attend for staff
- Attendance is usually voluntary and so are contributions during the session
- Have more than one facilitator
- Do only use staff trained in group interventions or if staff deliver 'off-the-shelf' protocol-driven models, they are supervised and supported by a practitioner psychologist, for example Care Spaces
- It works better if the psychologist knows the medical system
- Ideally, they are not just single sessions but as part of a system of care
- Remember you will make mistakes, not always phrase things perfectly, make gaffes
- Do only use evidence-based psychological interventions
- When staff are returning to work/clinical area after a group, encourage them to take a few minutes to shift gears
- Similar considerations to psychological debriefs – see chapter 18.

Following are some tips on how to manage the group dynamics that can be present in a group intervention.

> **Box 6.4: Tips for managing group dynamics in group interventions**
>
> - Set boundaries and ground rules
> - Try not to overplan the content of your group and what you will say as this can get in the way of creativity, empathy, and connecting with staff members' feelings
> - Use active listening skills
> - Pay attention to strong feelings in the group and manage appropriately
> - Ensure the ground rules are upheld – keep the group safe by challenging or stopping blame or criticism
> - Use psychological training and knowledge to manage group dynamics
> - Offer psychologically informed reflections, for example, make links between responses and comments
> - Notice and acknowledge themes
> - Notice and name what is happening in the group session where appropriate
> - Encourage contributions from individual voices and nurture diverse perspectives in order to prevent polarising narratives, for example, all positive or all negative
> - Draw connections with individual and team values
> - Don't be too controlling of the group process – create a space where staff can express themselves, which does carry inherent risk as groups are unpredictable
> - Model fallibility and be open about mistakes if it feels useful.
> - Signpost staff for further support

Changes in practice during the COVID-19 pandemic

During the COVID-19 pandemic we have had to adapt our group interventions to work in line with infection prevention protocols and to meet the changing needs of the wards. This has meant many interventions have been run on online platforms such as MS Teams and Zoom. We thought it would be helpful to include some reflections on how to continue to offer groups through a virtual platform.

> **Box 6.5: Tips for running group interventions on online platforms (i.e. not face to face)**
>
> - Co-facilitate – have one person responsible for tech
> - To ensure group safety remotely, devise a check-in process if the internet drops/staff get upset
> - Request people to use video – useful when others are speaking too so they can get some visual feedback from what they are saying
> - Ask people to focus on the group in hand and not to do other things like email
> - Silences can seem long! Allow longer pauses
> - Consider naming at the start the challenges of reduced emotional connection (e.g. lack of non-verbal cues) and that conversation can be 'clunky' with interruptions due to internet delay
> - If there is mix of staff joining the group session face to face and some joining remotely, regularly check if anyone wants to speak in each domain
> - Ensure confidentiality – at the start of the session, ask people to be in a private room/wear headphones if they can be overheard and if someone enters the room they are in, say you will pause the meeting
> - Be realistic about how cognitively and emotionally draining groups online are to facilitate – you may need to factor in more breaks
> - Consider the use of the chat box – it may not be helpful to have another group running in the chat box that isn't being facilitated, for example, in Schwartz Rounds; however, you may value the use of the chat box to get engagement, for example, in teaching sessions.

In the final section of this chapter, we are keen to consider the role of the embedded psychologist in the work of group intervention and staff support. For readers who offer staff support from an embedded position, we hope these reflections help to make sense of some of the challenges and opportunities you may be facing. For others who are not embedded but engaged in staff support, we hope it shines a light on the need to look after ourselves and the breadth of the role we can have in this work.

The role of the psychologist in navigating the tricky boundaries of working in staff support

There are multiple advantages of being an embedded psychologist and there are also difficult boundaries to navigate. When a psychologist knows the clinical area well because they see patients in that area or spend time in that clinical environment, they become familiar with the sights, smells, and noises of the area as well as the stories of the patients and staff. As we have seen, this can be highly valued by the staff we serve and seems to help staff feel seen and understood. We may know the colleagues they are talking about, and the themes of the difficulties staff face, especially if we offer 1:1s as well as group interventions. This can often be useful when we then occupy other professional spaces in the organisation (e.g. disseminating global themes of debriefs in Morbidity and Mortality meetings, contributing to workforce retention plans).

However, working alongside colleagues that may have, or may in the future, use our support service means that we can feel like we are always 'on duty'. We may see them in the kitchen or be side by side as colleagues in meetings. It can be hard to know how much to let our honest, messy, and vulnerable selves be present in a room with people who may need us to be in a supportive role in the future. It feels possible that staff may not come to us at a time of need for support if they are too aware of our personal lives and struggles in our own emotional life. We have found it helpful to have a physical space, for example, office that is away from the clinical area we serve, to be able to pause from always being 'on duty'. To be a safe base emotionally for others, we need a physical safe base for ourselves.

As embedded psychologists we are often asked to come in and respond to the most distressing elements of healthcare work, for example, supporting staff around a challenging crash call, death of a child, conflict with patients and families and court cases, bullying, poor working conditions, and investigations.

This invites important reflection on how we can get positioned in the work that we do and how we create our own space and structures to reflect on what we are bringing as facilitators of the intervention. We have found ourselves positioned as fixers, rescuers, advocates, and speak up guardians. We have been positioned as miracle workers with teams that want a quick fix to complex difficulties as well as wellbeing pushers. On each occasion, we navigate the delicate line of having colleagues who are 'clients' and all of this can affect our relationships with the teams we work with and our own expectations of ourselves.

> **Box 6.6: Tips for managing the challenging boundaries of staff support work**
>
> - Consider only using your work mobile phone with colleagues in the teams you serve.
> - Have a safe space where you don't have to be 'on duty' all the time, for example, a shared office with other psychologists.
> - Find a reflective practice group/space to discuss these complex boundaries and how they feel with trusted colleagues doing similar work.
> - If appropriate, adjust the boundaries with some colleagues in the teams you serve – allow yourself to be fully authentic and real with some colleagues. If these particular colleagues need 1:1 support in the future, discuss that it would not be appropriate for it to be you.
> - Pre-plan what topics you are ok to discuss in the kitchen/staff room with colleagues who may use your service in the future or have used your service in the past.

This experience of blurred boundaries was reported by Billings et al. (2021) following interviews with mental health professionals from varied professional backgrounds about their experiences supporting frontline health and social care workers during COVID-19. They reported a dilemma about whether health and social care workers were colleagues or clients. As colleagues there can be an additional emotional pull to care for them, partly because it can be easy to identify with them as a fellow healthcare worker (Billings et al., 2021). Usually there is a degree of separation with clients in other settings and we may need to work harder not to overidentify with staff we work with.

There can be additional challenges such as managing a difference of opinion about an aspect of patient care (for psychologists who also offer both staff and patient support on a ward) or differences of opinion about project work and then having to switch hats if offering a support service such as individual or group intervention. It can be an unusual position to be working alongside MDT colleagues as peers and also potentially know a lot about their personal life and struggles if they have accessed staff support. The main way we have developed to manage this is to name it and share the dilemma with staff about how to manage these tricky boundaries and ideally, allow staff to choose whether to see a psychologist from outside their clinical area or in a designated staff support role if preferred.

During the COVID-19 pandemic we have all gone through a shared experience. Supporting staff who have similar anxieties and responses to living through a pandemic has made it harder to have that more objective perspective. It became a common experience of ours to offer an individual or group session and identify with feelings shared in the group by staff.

The advantages of this identification has been more overt recognition that we too as psychologists may need spaces to reflect on the work that we do. We may want to join or be part of group interventions to reflect on issues facing the ward or be personally affected by the themes being discussed in the session. Running groups in pairs, having a robust supervision structure, and peer contact with others engaged in staff support working (for instance via national special interest groups or networks) are vital to being able to do this work well. We have often reflected on the exposing nature of facilitating group interventions and the level of responsibility we feel to be able to robustly hold the feelings and emotional experiences of our colleagues, especially when it's not always neat or easy. Our own desires to do well, for people to find it helpful and to have positive regard for our profession can all impact on how we feel about the work and the strategies we need to look after ourselves in the work.

Box 6.7: Tips for looking after ourselves

Practice what we preach:

- Reflect on your boundaries, when to stick to them and when to be flexible
- Notice if you are regularly working over your contracted hours
- Access peer support by connecting with others in a similar role locally and nationally
- Access clinical and management supervision regularly
- Enhance self-care activities
- Strive for 'good enough'
- Allow time to rest and find balance between home and work life
- Develop allies and gain leadership support where you can.

The role of the psychologist when engaging in group interventions alongside other colleagues

One challenge that requires a group intervention is supporting teams to improve staff engagement and team culture. This requires a group, rather than individual effort. As part of a preventative approach, to help staff stay well and engaged with their job role, their working conditions need to be the best they can be.

Embedded psychologists may help staff to understand how their team is functioning and offer a formulation and understanding through a systemic lens of the contributing factors rather than focussing on only the unwanted behaviours on an individual level (although these will need to be tackled too). We are only one of a range of professionals who can support the team with this. Psychologists may help to interpret staff survey results, collect data from other sources, for example, notice patterns and themes, all of which may contribute to factors influencing staff wellbeing. Psychologists can be valuable members of working groups or projects that focus on improving team culture. We have skills in bringing people together, creating safe spaces to talk about difficult topics, leadership skills to influence the system, and create behaviour change in a team, as well as being able to offer psychologically safe spaces to plan improvement projects and sometimes be in a position of not being a clinician or a manager. If we are supporting a team to improve their team culture, through leading or co-leading working groups, we can sometimes stay over the longer term, regularly review progress, and be flexible with what is offered and when. Meaningful change can be supported over time, going at the pace of the group. Multidisciplinary team colleagues are essential allies in this work who may co-lead such projects and without whom the work is unlikely to be successful.

When it comes to OD and improving working conditions such as team culture, we have learnt that it's important to be aware of our limitations and consult with the expertise of our colleagues in OD teams and Human Resources (HR). Building trust and productive working relationships with these colleagues is crucial. These teams can offer an external perspective and expertise that is very much needed.

Conclusion

In this chapter, we have shared some ideas about how to decide on the nature of group intervention to offer as well as the practical factors to consider when preparing and setting these up. We have talked about the tricky boundaries to navigate which at times can feel very uncomfortable but with good supervision and peer support can become manageable. We have found that our skills, as psychologists, of holding the group space, tolerating discomfort, and being able to respond and manage strong emotions are often used and highly valued by our colleagues. Group interventions are one of the most valuable interventions we can offer to contribute to workforce wellbeing because they involve one of our basic human needs – to be alongside others and experience social connection.

> **Key points**
>
> This chapter aims to help you choose which group interventions to offer to staff and deal with practical considerations.
>
> - We recommend using supervision and peer support to manage tricky boundaries that are inevitable when supporting staff.
> - Group interventions fulfil a basic human need to connect with others. Practitioner psychologists can hold a group space and manage strong emotions which allows groups to be run safely.

References and further reading

Affina Organisation Development, Affina Team Journey. https://www.affinaod.com/team-tools/affina-team-journey/.

Benson, J. (2019). *Working More Creatively with Groups* (4th ed.). London: Routledge.

Billings, J., Briggs, C., Ching, B. C. F., Gkofa, V., Singleton, D., Bloomfield, M., & Greene, T. (2021). Experiences of Mental Health Professionals Supporting Front-Line Health and Social Care Workers During COVID-19: Qualitative Study. *British Journal of Psychiatry Open*, 7(2), e70. https://doi.org/10.1192/bjo.2021.29.

Edmondson, A. C. (2018). *The Fearless Organisation: Creating Psychological Safety in the Workplace for Learning, Innovation and Growth*. New York: John Wiley & Sons.

Flaxman, P. E., Bond, F. W., & Livheim, F. (2013). *The Mindful and Effective Employee: An Acceptance and Commitment Therapy Training Manual for Improving Well-Being and Performance* (1st ed.). Oakland: New Harbinger Publications.

Foulkes, S. H. (1964). *Therapeutic Group Analysis*. London: Maresfield.

Fredman, G. (2007). Preparing Ourselves for the Therapeutic Relationship: Revisiting 'Hypothesizing Revisited'. *Human Systems: The Journal of Systemic Consultations and Management*, 18, 44–59.

Highfield, J. (2019). The Sustainability of the Critical Care Workforce. *British Association of Critical Care Nurses*, 24(1), 6–8.

Janis, I. L. (1972). *Victims of Groupthink: A Psychological Study of Foreign Policy Decisions and Fiascoes*. Boston, MA: Houghton Mifflin.

Kohut, H. (1977). *The Restoration of the Self*. Chicago, IL: University of Chicago Press.

Kolb, D. A. (1984). *Experiential Learning: Experience as the Source of Learning and Development*. Englewood Cliffs, NJ: Prentice-Hall.

Palazzoli, M. S., Boscolo, L., Cecchin, G., & Prata, G. (1980). The Problem of the Referring Person. *Journal of Marital and Family Therapy*, 6(1), 3–9.

Papadatou, D. (2009). *In the Face of Death: Professionals Who Care for the Dying and the Bereaved: Coping Strategies for the Helping Professional*. New York: Springer Publishing.

Reder, P., & Fredman, G. (1996). The Relationship to Help: Interacting Beliefs about the Treatment Process. *Clinical Child Psychology and Psychiatry*, 1(3), 457–467.

Schwartz Rounds, Point of Care Foundation. https://www.pointofcarefoundation.org.uk/our-programmes/staff-experience/about-schwartz-rounds/.

7 Supporting Staff and Volunteers Delivering Services to People in Crisis

Dr Sarah Davidson, Rachel Morley, Paula Aredez Arriazu, and Andrea Wood

The British Red Cross' Psychosocial and Mental Health Team provides a range of mental health and psychosocial resources and services across all its UK Services and to a range of organisations, including government departments, NHS Trusts, Fire and Rescue Services, Local Authorities and charities. In the UK, the British Red Cross is the leading third sector provider of both refugee services and crisis responses. The contexts of the work are diverse and predominantly (but not exclusively) focused on adults in community settings who have complex and diverse needs, and who experience significant health inequalities as well as a range of barriers to accessing mainstream services.

The authors of this chapter are all members of the British Red Cross' Psychosocial and Mental Health Team: Sarah Davidson is the head of Psychosocial and Mental Health for the British Red Cross. As well as leading the Psychosocial and Mental Health Team, she co-leads the Psychosocial Support Team which supports the Foreign, Commonwealth and Development Office to respond to crises around the world by having members of this team embedded in their rapid deployment teams. She also works alongside different components of the International Red Cross and Red Crescent Movement to integrate mental health and psychosocial support into all aspects of the movement's activities and resources. RM is a senior psychosocial practitioner with responsibilities for our work in Scotland and Northern Ireland, and our trauma-informed approach. Rachel Morley also co-leads our support to refugee services. Sarah and Rachel have both worked for many years as consultant clinical psychologists in the NHS. Paula Aredez Arriazu and Andrea Wood are psychosocial practitioners who deliver the resources described later. Paula is a counselling psychologist who also currently works in the NHS. Andrea is a psychotherapist and former drama therapist and international consultant for the British Council in the Middle East.

The mental health and psychosocial resources developed by the team enable staff and volunteers to support the people they are working with. This is done through a menu of offers, including workshops, reflective practice groups and one to ones, and enabling staff through a peer supporter programme. This chapter will describe the models and literature drawn on to inform the staff (and volunteer) support work carried out by the Psychosocial and Mental Health Team and will describe in detail an example of reflective practice for a staff group carried out by PAA and AW in a health service context.

The context of psychosocial support in a humanitarian organisation

'Psychosocial' refers to the interconnection between the individual (i.e. a person's internal, emotional and thought processes, feelings, and reactions) and their environment, interpersonal relationships, community, and/or culture (i.e. their social context) – 'the dynamic relationship that exists between psychological and social effects, each continually inter-acting with and influencing the other' (Save the Children, 2005)

The British Red Cross supports the psychosocial needs of people in a variety of crisis situations across the UK. These crisis situations include disasters and emergencies such as floods, fires, storms, and terrorist events. Our services also support people who have experienced cumulative crises involved in forced migration and trafficking. We also work with people who have profound health and social care needs and experiences of health inequalities.

The challenges of working in humanitarian contexts in crisis situations are considerable and the importance of effectively supporting staff and volunteers within those situations is therefore critical (Davidson, 2010a). The International Red Cross and Red Crescent Movement policy on addressing Mental Health and Psychosocial support describes the importance of protecting the mental health and psychosocial wellbeing of staff and volunteers (see Box 7.1).

The statement in box 7.1 describes the need for staff and volunteers to have the requisite training and knowledge to do the work they are doing. It highlights the need for physical and psychological safety for staff and volunteers and emphasises the need for managers to reduce work-related stressors. It also describes how staff and volunteers exposed to distressing events need to have special and additional psychosocial and mental health support. This is to promote the safety, health, and wellbeing of staff and volunteers and to ensure the quality of services offered to beneficiaries.

> **Box 7.1: International Red Cross and Red Crescent Movement policy on addressing Mental Health and Psychosocial Needs (2019)**
>
> *The mental health and psychosocial wellbeing of staff and volunteers is often affected as they work in difficult and stressful environments and are exposed to highly distressing experiences owing to the nature of mental health and psychosocial support work. The Movement exercises its duty of care and, in doing so, we not only promote the safety, health and wellbeing of staff and volunteers, but also ensure the quality of the services we provide. We will therefore:*
>
> - *Ensure that staff and volunteers have the required knowledge and psychological support skills to cope with stressful situations, look after themselves effectively, and seek support when needed.*
> - *Equip and support managers and other leaders to reduce work-related stressors for staff and volunteers.*
> - *Ensure that staff and volunteers are equipped with the required skills to support people with mental health and psychosocial needs.*
> - *We will integrate relevant mental health and psychosocial aspects into core training.*
> - *Ensure that staff, volunteers, and facilities providing mental health and psychosocial support services are protected at all times, including during armed conflicts, natural disasters, and other emergencies.*
> - *Ensure that specific and additional mental health and psychosocial support is available to individuals and teams who are exposed to distressing events owing to the nature of their work.*

This policy context informs the work of the Psychosocial and Mental Health Team in the British Red Cross. The team provide foundation courses and bespoke workshops across a range of topics (e.g. Call Handling in Crisis Situations, Dealing with Grief and Loss, Managing Anger and Aggression, Personal and Team Resilience, Supporting people who are Suicidal and/or Self Harming, Trauma-Informed Managers Training, Understanding Mental Health, and Working with Traumatised People). The team also provides written guidance for the organisation to support the workforce dealing with complex psychosocial situations (e.g. Challenging Situations, Coping with Exposure to Disturbing Imagery, Professional Boundaries, Psychosocial and Mental Health Resources Guidance, Suicide Awareness and Self Harm, Supporting Colleagues Exposed to Intense Events, and Traumatic Bereavement and Psychosocial Guidance in the Context of COVID-19).

The team provide one-to-one reflective practice sessions with managers to support them in coping with the impact of the work on them, in attending to the support needs of their staff and helping to reduce workforce stressors. The team also provides regular and ongoing reflective practice sessions for whole teams who are regularly dealing with situations involving people in crisis and doing difficult and distressing work. It provides reflective practise and diffusing sessions for groups of staff and volunteers following critical incidents and major incidents. Members of the team also offer joint consultations with a member of staff and a client together if the member of staff is particularly concerned, for example, about a client's mental health or psychosocial situation. The joint consultations offer an opportunity for the practitioners to demonstrate and consequently model their psychosocial and mental health skills, demystifying and sharing these with staff, while simultaneously supporting both staff and clients.

The CALMER framework

While awareness of psychosocial principles has been evident in the British Red Cross for many years, in December 2008 a single psychosocial framework was adopted across all services and departments. The framework, known as 'CALMER', draws on a range of ways of conceptualising and responding to the multidimensional psychosocial needs of individuals and communities. The impact of social inequalities on individuals' and communities' abilities to respond to crises and access services is acknowledged (Friedli, 2009) as is the diversity in people's experiences and backgrounds and the need to tailor responses to these (Patel et al., 2000). Coping and resilience are emphasised and fostered at individual, family, and community levels, through the provision of information, facilitation of social support, and promotion of self- and community efficacy (Cloak & Edwards, 2004; Hobfall et al., 2007). These principles are integrated into a single framework that aims to be accessible and applicable to all working with and within the British Red Cross.

Once the framework had been independently piloted with different populations in different countries (Davidson, 2010b), it was incorporated into operating manuals, policies, and procedures across the organisation. The framework was also used to develop training for staff, volunteers, and members of the public.

> **Box 7.2: The CALMER framework (Davidson, 2010a, 2010b)**
>
> CALMER first and foremost reminds staff and volunteers to be calmer and more thoughtful in their responses (particularly when crises create adrenaline rushes that work against feeling calm). CALMER is also an acronym designed to cue six sequential stages in any response:
>
> **C**onsider the situation, needs, and risks including people's experiences and wishes
> **A**cknowledge diversity, including in communication preferences and responses
> **L**isten with empathy
> **M**anage the situation to promote dignity and respect
> **E**nable contact with supportive others and people's own choices
> **R**esource through providing information and the required resources (while
> **R**emembering the responder's own needs).
>
> **C**onsider and **A**cknowledge address the importance of acknowledging diversity (in the contexts and the characteristics of those being responded to, for example the particular needs of children). Consideration is given to how responders might facilitate trust and develop rapport, through normalising and validating the individual or group's felt experience. This is further underlined within Listening skills, while Manage addresses the need to promote dignity and respect, through the management of confidentiality, for example.
>
> **E**nable and **R**esource draw from community psychology and particularly the importance of empowerment of both individuals and communities to affect not just coping, but social change and greater resilience for the future (Orford, 2008; White, 2004a, 2004b). Throughout, the needs of those responding are acknowledged in order to prevent further harm to themselves or others.

Trauma-informed approaches

The British Red Cross is on a journey to becoming a trauma-informed organisation and trauma-informed workshops are being rolled out by the

Psychosocial and Mental Health Team across the organisation to the Executive Leadership Team, Board of Trustees, and all the senior management teams. This teaching is tailored to the needs of the British Red Cross but builds on the body of evidence, experience, and frameworks from other key human service organisations. Key informants include:

- Harris and Fallot (2001) in creating cultures of trauma-informed care
- The Substance Abuse and Mental Health Services Administration (2014) in the USA
- NHS Education for Scotland (2017) and their Transforming Psychological Trauma programme
- The Mental Health Coordinating Council (MHCC) (2019) and their framework on trauma-informed leadership
- The Oregon framework for trauma-informed organisations, Trauma-Informed Oregon (2018).

The relevance of the approach is multiple: it recognises the high incidence of trauma in the populations the British Red Cross serves, it provides an understanding and acknowledgement of how trauma impacts psychosocial outcomes for clients, and of how clients can be re-traumatised even through their contacts with helping organisations. The trauma-informed work connects well with the ongoing work in the organisation to promote anti-racism, diversity, and inclusion. There is also an organisational acknowledgement of how staff and volunteers can be re-traumatised by the work they do and can experience vicarious traumatisation through hearing about and witnessing traumatic events. The metaphor of staying within the 'window of tolerance' (see The Window of Tolerance animation by Beacon House, 2018) in response to repeated stress and crises resonates at both an individual and an organisational level with managers, leaders, and practitioners being invited to consider how best to increase the windows of tolerance of those they manage and support.

The British Red Cross constantly helps people in crisis. Its staff and volunteers are often affected by the same crises affecting the populations being served, for example a significant number of staff and volunteers are from refugee backgrounds and different staff members and volunteers are variously affected by trauma experiences in their own lives not least because of their own experiences of inequality. The British Red Cross aims to step into situations where others may not, and often goes the extra mile. This means staff and volunteers are frequently exposed to very distressing and traumatic events.

The work for the British Red Cross, as for all organisations who are on a journey to become trauma informed, is to make trauma-informed principles and practices second nature. As such, its structures and processes are psychologically safe and healthy, all forms of violence and discrimination and exclusion are challenged, compassionate relationships are prioritised, and the organisation builds resilience and recovery into everything it does.

Trauma-informed principles apply equally to those delivering services as to those receiving them, so staff and volunteers also need to be treated in ways that emphasise the trauma-informed principles of safety, choice, collaboration, trustworthiness, and empowerment. For safety and support to be prioritised for staff, there needs to be attention to structural wellbeing issues which include realistic workloads and work expectations, contracts and pay, boundaries and breaks, and maintenance of appropriate skill and confidence levels including management training and support. There needs to be regular opportunities for reflecting on the work and its impact through supervision and reflective practice opportunities so that staff and volunteers can be in the best position possible to care for themselves and each other, as they care for the people they support.

Reflective practice in the British Red Cross

Reflective practice values the use of reflection to think clearly and analytically about practice (Mann, Gordon and MacLeod, 2009). In the British Red Cross, reflective practice mostly takes place in groups and draws from the models of Schön (1983), Kolb (1984), and Kurtz (2020), as well as the CALMER framework (Davidson, 2010). Both groups and one-to-one reflective practice sessions are intended to provide a reflective space for staff and volunteers to think about the emotional impacts of their work, develop competences in caring for people facing a range of crises, offer space for collaborative planning and problem-solving around areas of difficulty, support resilience in the workforce, and reinforce trauma-informed principles and the application of the CALMER framework (Davidson, 2010a, 2010b). They also aim to contribute to an organisational culture which values reflectiveness (Davidson, 2013; Wall, 2018).

Reflective practice sessions are facilitated by multiple psychosocial practitioners across a range of service and geographical locations. Therefore, there is some variation in how they are delivered and engaged with. Since they are also a product of the co-production that takes place with teams, practitioners are also led by those they work with in order to best meet those teams' needs and preferences (Wall, 2018). Features in common, as Kennard and Hartley

(2009) describe, include: time and space outside the normal work routine or environment, a focus on sharing experiences and reflecting on the work, the provision of a forum for acknowledging emotional responses associated with work, and being relatively structured by a facilitator who explicitly applies theories, evidence, and policy to the experiences of group members.

These sessions further offer an opportunity for the psychosocial practitioners to bear witness to and explore the stressful experiences staff and volunteers have and their narratives of coping. In doing this, the stigma experienced by staff and volunteers who find it difficult to cope is potentially reduced (Hartley & Kennard, 2009). The practitioners directly address phenomena related to the 'self-assigned impossible task' (Roberts, 2019) as sources of work-related distress and anxiety. Validating and normalising these experiences is often important for those who support others, in reducing distress and enabling meaningful engagement with the reflective practice sessions (Roberts, 2019). This is also the mechanism used to provide support to the team who lead the reflective practice groups. They each receive individual clinical supervision and are part of a monthly peer supervision group (together with the practitioners' managers, the senior psychosocial practitioners). In these sessions, consideration is given to the various dynamics at play, for example the impact of the team as a sponge for the distress, difficulties, and dynamics that are absorbed and, without sufficient reflection, risk being replicated (Cardona, 2020).

Evaluation of the effectiveness of the work of the Psychosocial and Mental Health Team

An external evaluation conducted over 2 ½ years and concluding in 2021 by Public Health England (now known as the UK Health and Security Agency) using structured feedback showed 'a clear and positive effect' (page 3; Public Health England, 2021) of the work of the Psychosocial and Mental Health Team which led to measurable improvements in the workforce's self-reported capacity to cope with and respond to individuals in crisis. Collating all data from September 2018 to February 2021, over 75% of those completing the measures either agreed or strongly agreed that the psychosocial practitioner sessions increased their confidence/abilities to: support and listen to clients, cope with client's distress, support others in their teams, maintain their own wellbeing and resilience, and support the resilience of others in their teams. Descriptive analyses concerning ratings across the duration also revealed a consistent picture over that time frame, namely that there had been a broad and consistent increase in the ratings of the attendees of the psychosocial practitioner sessions in relation to their confidence and abilities to both cope with intense responses and deal with the distress of others.

Supporting NHS peer supporters: A case study

The current offer of the PMHT includes funded offers to some NHS Trusts and other external organisations. While this brings a new challenge and immense learning to the psychosocial practitioners working in the PMHT, it aims to retain the essence and draws from the expertise of running reflective practice sessions offered to the British Red Cross' workforce.

One partnership was agreed with a London acute NHS Trust to support staff members who had received additional peer support training (from another agency) by offering reflective practice groups on a monthly basis. What follows is a summary of this experience, along with the learning and reflections that it brought to the practitioners involved in it since its conception, in July 2021.

The importance of coproduction

This being the first experience the two practitioners had of both working together and for an external organisation, the two spent time learning about the expectations of the project and about each other. We (Andrea Wood and Paula Aredez Arriazu) learnt that together, we encompass and share large expertise in trauma therapy, reflective practice, supervision, crisis interventions, and individual support in both NHS and charity sector settings. We share values and principles of practice, but we diverge in the ways we arrived to them, our journeys in life and our ethnic backgrounds. Consistent and continuous communication and trust between us made our own alliance flourish and, we believe, allowed for the groups to feel safe with our co-facilitating style.

While the expertise we carry from the British Red Cross is a valuable asset, we agreed from the starting point, that in order to set up a reflective practice space that would be helpful, we had to understand the needs of the people involved and engage them closely in the design and delivery of the group. We used principles of co-production (Think Local Act Personal online resources, 2021) as a loose guide for our collaboration with the hospital trust:

- *Recognising people as assets*
- *Building on people's capabilities*
- *Developing two-way, reciprocal relationships*

- *Encouraging peer support*
- *Moving away from 'delivering' services 'to' people and closer to 'co-producing' them 'with' people (i.e. drawing on participants' input, since they are 'experts by experience').*

Co-production helped create a safe space not just within the reflective practice groups but also in our communications with the Trust representatives, interactions from which we have benefited as much as they report to have from our support (see Involve: Resources on Coproduction, 2021).

Our approach

As mentioned earlier, CALMER guides and frames all the crisis and reflective practice work we do in the PMHT, and the external collaborations are no exception. While being willing to offer moments of psychoeducation where appropriate, especially around the impact on individuals and teams of working in a traumatised environment and prolonged high-level stress, and what might help to mitigate that. We both hold to a respectful 'beginner's mind' stance (seeing as if for the first time, aiming not to make too many assumptions by making as much as explicit as possible regarding perceived connections and meanings), led by acceptance and curiosity, rather than assuming 'expert' status. Respect for the diversity of views, perspectives and experiences, inclusion, transparency, and a strengths-based reflective stance which facilitates regulation of feeling states, thoughtfulness, and hope are our guiding principles. We have encountered tears and anger but also a lot of laughter.

We hold to the boundaries of safeguarding, confidentiality, and timekeeping (each online group is 1.5 hours), and work to ensure the space is welcoming, as safe as possible, respectful, and shared between the group members.

To better understand and stay connected to the needs of the groups, as well as measuring impact and success, we are in regular contact with the nominated Trust lead, we welcome informal feedback from participants, and we also ask the group to complete a short anonymised online evaluation at the end of each session. Additionally, we debrief with each other in between the monthly groups and attend both individual and group supervision to ensure and develop efficacy and take care of our own wellbeing and resilience.

Who, when, how?

The offer involves monthly, 'slow open' remote reflective practice groups for the Trust's peer supporters, conducted remotely; several staff are in their work setting, others connect from home, and both facilitators are working from home. This is a diverse staff cohort, made up of individuals from different teams with a variety of job roles (including clinical and non-clinical staff), length of experience, and sociocultural-ethnic backgrounds. It is an incredibly skilled group of people with a demonstrated psychosocially minded interest in and motivation towards supporting their colleagues through what is recognised as the largest challenge the NHS has ever faced – that of working through the COVID-19 pandemic. The group members seemed to enjoy their peer supporter training, which took place prior to the British Red Cross's involvement with the Trust, and are pleased that the Trust created that opportunity for them, as well as the ongoing British Red Cross' reflective groups.

From the conversations held with the Trust's lead for this partnership at the beginning of this collaboration, it became clear that given the acute nature of most of the participants' job roles, the offer should be both flexible and consistent to encourage and maintain attendance at its maximum, but also to secure a compassionate alternative to the fast-paced and ever-changing rhythm of their schedule.

This means that people can sign up, or even decide on the day, which of the three groups running on the same day each month they want to attend based on what best suits their very busy schedules. The consequences are cross-currents of connection between participants, on some occasions having attended a different reflective practice slot in previous months, having trained as peer supporters together in the past, or having worked together as part of the same team. Despite our initial concerns about building group identity and safety in absence of a consistent group of attendees, this method seems to suit the groups well by offering them the chance to encounter and connect to a different combination of people each time, which nurtures peer-support relationships between the peer supporters, and allows for an increased sense of control over their self-care by choosing if and when to attend the groups without feeling left out.

Themes from the sessions

Our first session began with a focus, to give everyone a task through which we could get to know each other and find commonalities and differences: that of sharing and reviewing experiences from the previous 15 months of pandemic – challenges, learning, and gains. It was quickly apparent how exhausted many people were; the camaraderie of having been through intense times together 'that no-one else would understand', with little respite and with, possibly, even greater challenges to come.

In each group different individuals quickly set a tone of emotional candour, sharing in detail some of their experiences of the pressures they have been and are under; the sheer despair at being unable to help patients, families, and colleagues as they wished; and the sense of being overwhelmed by the plethora of demands and overstretched resources.

Looking for what had had helped most the consistent themes were 'my team, my family, my friends, my pets': at a time when most of the country were locked down with immediate family or alone, NHS staff had been both exposed to the risks of being with and trying to look after many other people, as well as the benefits.

Participants are receptive to each other, mature, intelligent, thoughtful, and warm in response; on occasion perhaps responding with problem-solving, rather than acknowledging the complexity of the issue and its emotional input for the speaker; but mostly displaying understanding, empathy, practical common sense, and humour.

Subsequent groups have not had a specific topic, but rather flowed across themes surfacing from initial 'check-ins'. We support members to respond to what each shares of their working lives over the previous months. There are many crosscurrents: finding it hard to relax, feeling like 'headless chickens', not having enough time for family, witnessing and experiencing powerful feelings of grief, being worried about colleagues' mental health. We add our own responses, wonderings, offer links between participants' comments, and sometimes metaphors. Many say they appreciate this 'time out of time', to set aside the intensity of hospital life for 1.5 hours a month, to think about how they feel together.

The COVID-19 pandemic as a catalyst for past trauma

It would be unrealistic to remove the current pandemic context from the coordinates of this collaboration. As previously mentioned, the reflective practice groups started in July 2021, marking 18 months from the start of the COVID-19 pandemic. Given the global nature of this pandemic, it would be reasonable to expect any groups in any context to be impacted by it. However, when thinking about NHS staff groups, this takes a new and heightened importance.

Most of the participants of the reflective practice groups from the NHS Trust have worked face to face through the COVID-19 pandemic, in patient-facing settings and/or in acute wards. Members of staff who did not have direct clinical involvement also experienced high levels of distress since they took part in the leading, strategizing, and support for teams and services directly working with COVID-19 patients. Moreover, the non-professional impact of the pandemic should not be minimised as it added a layer of complexity to the ways that the participants managed their personal and professional routines, hygiene habits, their physical and mental health, and their self-care.

The latter seems to be an intersection of significant nuance for many: the participants have shared that they have found it (and still do at times) difficult to process and make people around them understand the importance of keeping high levels of protection for themselves and others from infection. This seems to stem from their ongoing in-person work attendance and the knowledge and/or exposure to the pain that COVID-19 continues to inflict on patients, their families, staff, and the health system as a whole. Participants have shared strong feelings about the lack of understanding from, for example 'anti-vaxxers', and anxieties about how alleged infringements of COVID-19 regulations at all levels of society, including government levels, would impact patient behaviour in already extremely fragile conditions of employment.

In addition to the complexities introduced by the COVID-19 pandemic alone, we have identified that the discussion of or exposure to pandemic-related topics can often bring up previous experiences of trauma to the surface. We have found that the groups have, on each occasion, worked well as a holding and containing space (Bion, 1961) for those who found themselves unexpectedly feeling overwhelmed by previous traumatic incidents during their practice or within the reflective practice space. An approach of support and validation was encouraged from early on from our part but seem to already be embedded in the disposition of each participant, with possible roots in their training and interest in peer support; and the invitation to reflect on how issues could signify and trigger different responses, emotions, and even physical reactions, to different people, remains open and revisited often.

What next?

The learning continues with the monthly groups. The aim to maintain these safe reflective spaces remains crucial in times when new pandemic rules are being introduced in the UK and the need for supporting people in crisis persists. With more restrictions in the opportunities healthcare staff have to access self-care due to reduced capacity, creating windows of relief or 'stopping time' can be highly impactful. Continuous monitoring is needed to understand the extent, but it is our hope that this collaboration will continue the long relationship between the NHS and the British Red Cross.

Conclusion

Staff and volunteers provide critical support to people experiencing a diversity of crises, and in doing so they require tailored interventions and responses.

Psychosocial and mental health support promotes the safety, health, and wellbeing of staff and volunteers and contributes to the quality of services offered to beneficiaries. The provision of reflective practice by psychosocial professionals has been found to increase the competence and confidence of staff and volunteers to care for their own wellbeing and resilience as well as those of their teams, and to listen to and support people in distress. This is all the more important during a period of sustained challenge as seen currently in the COVID-19 pandemic. The pandemic is increasing health inequalities and negatively impacting on people's mental health, including those delivering services (e.g. the previous case study and the report by the International Federation of Red Cross and Red Crescent Societies, 2021). It is therefore more important than ever for us to integrate appropriate mental health and psychosocial support (which is trauma informed) to ensure our responders (staff and volunteers) are able to cope and remain safe and well.

It is also important that those delivering mental health and psychosocial resources, including those which support staff and volunteers, are able to get the support that they need, and practice what they recommend. The Psychosocial and Mental Health Team value reflective spaces and trauma-informed resources and recognise the various ways that our experiences (past and present) can connect with potentially damaging consequences (Cardona, 2020; Roberts, 2019). During the pandemic the team have predominantly worked remotely, which has increased the potential for disconnection, depersonalisation, isolation, and fatigue. We have continued to meet monthly as a team for reflective practice peer supervision groups and team meetings. Our team meetings have been places for checking in, sharing our achievements and challenges, reviewing progress and learnings, and for having fun. While we have not all met in person, we have worked hard to sustain our relationships (including through regional buddy groups) and to enable our own windows of tolerance (Beacon House, 2018). In addition, the online meetings have been essential: as many of us found solo facilitation to be very challenging.

The team have extended their offer to other organisations, government departments, and charities, to provide reflective practice under contract. As an independent, impartial, and neutral organisation, we can provide spaces which enable staff and volunteers to share their challenges and dilemmas, while supporting managers and leaders to be more trauma informed. We hope that as awareness increases regarding the positive impact of providing staff and volunteers with the support that they need, more organisations will develop the resources required (using in-house and external services and materials as desired). It has never been clearer that staff and volunteers supporting others in crisis need to be supported themselves if they are to do this safely and keep well.

> **Key points**
> - Psychosocial and mental health resources can provide staff and volunteers with **training and knowledge** to do the work they are doing. Can facilitate **physical and psychological safety** for staff and volunteers and support **managers to reduce work-related stressors**. It can also deliver staff and volunteers exposed to distressing events with **special and additional psychosocial and mental health support**. This promotes **both the safety, health and wellbeing of staff and volunteers and ensures the quality of services offered to beneficiaries.**
> - CALMER is the British Red Cross' psychosocial framework. It supports staff and volunteers to be calm while guiding them through six sequential states to:
>   - **C**onsider needs and risks
>   - **A**cknowledge diversity
>   - **L**isten with empathy
>   - **M**anage the situation to promote dignity and respect
>   - **E**nable contact with supportive others and people's own choices
>   - **R**esource through providing information and the required resources (while **R**emembering the responder's own needs)
> - Reflective practice can be part of a trauma-informed approach which can enhance the perceived competence and confidence of staff and volunteers to support themselves and others (including those they are there to support and their teams) and prevent re-traumatisation.

References

Bion, W. (1961). *Experiences in Groups and Other Papers*. London: Tavistock Publications Ltd.

Cardona, F. (2020). *The Team as a Sponge: How the Nature of the Task Affects the Behaviour and Mental Life of a Team*. In Cardona, F. (2020) *Work Matters: Consulting to leaders and organisations in the Tavistock Tradition*. London, Taylor & Francis.

Cloak, N. L. & Edwards, P. (2004). Psychological First Aid: Emergency Care for Terrorism and Disaster Survivors. *Current Psychiatry*, vol. 3, 12–23.

Davidson, S. (2010a). 'Psychosocial Support within a Global Movement', *The Psychologist*, vol. 23, no. 4, 304–307.

Davidson, S. (2010b). The Development of the British Red Cross' Psychosocial Framework: Calmer. *Journal of Social Work Practice*, vol. 24, no. 1 March, 29–42. ISSN 0265-0533 print/ISSN 1465-3885.

Davidson, S. (2013). The Humanitarian and Third Sectors. In Bayne, R. & Jinks, G. (Eds.), *Applied Psychology: Training, Practice and New Directions*, 2nd ed., 278–281. New York: Sage.

Elwyn, G., Nelson, E., & Hager, A., and Price, A. (2020). Coproduction: When users Define Quality. *BMJ Quality & Safety*, vol. 29, 711–716.

Friedli, L. (2009). *Mental Health, Resilience and Inequalities.* London: WHO Europe.

Harris, M. & Fallot, R. (Eds.). (2001). *Using Trauma Theory to Design Service Systems: New Directions for Mental Health Services.* San Francisco, CA: Jossey-Bass.

Hartley, P. & Kennard, D. (Eds.). (2009). *Staff Support Groups in the Helping Professions: Principles, Practice and Pitfalls*, 11–16. Hove: Routledge.

Hobfall, S. E., Watson, P., Bell, C. C., Bryant, R. A., Brymer, M. J., Friedman, M. J., Friedman, M., Gersons, B. P. R., de Jong, J. T. V. M., Layne, C. M., Maguen, S., Neria, Y., Norwood, A. E., Pynoos, R. S., Reissman, D., Rusek, J. I., Shalev, A. Y., Solomon, Z., Steinberg, A. A. M. & Ursano, R. J. (2007). Five Essential Elements of Immediate and Mid-Term Mass Trauma Intervention: Empirical Evidence. *Psychiatry*, vol. 70, 283–315.

International Federation of Red Cross and Red Crescent Societies. (2021). Drowning Just Below the Surface: The Socioeconomic Consequences of the COVID-19 Pandemic, Geneva, 2021. Involve Resources on Coproduction accessed on 12 December 2021. https://www.involve.org.uk/resources/methods/co-production.

International Red Cross and Red Crescent Movement Policy on Addressing Mental Health and Psychosocial Needs. (2019). Document Prepared by the Working Group of the International Red Cross and Red Crescent Movement Project on Addressing Mental Health and Psychosocial Consequences of Armed Conflicts, Natural Disasters and Other Emergencies (MOMENT) and adopted by the Council of Delegates in Geneva, December 2019.

Kennard, D. & Hartley, P. (2009). What Staff Support Groups are for. In Hartley, P. & Kennard, D. (Eds.), *Staff Support Groups in the Helping Professions: Principles, Practice and Pitfalls*, 11–16. Hove: Routledge.

Kolb, D. (1984). *Experiential Learning: Experience as the Source of Learning and Development.* Englewood Cliffs, NJ: Prentice-Hall.

Kurtz, A. (2020). *How to Run Reflective Practice Groups: A Guide for Healthcare Professionals.* London: Routledge.

Mann, K., Gordon, J. & MacLeod, A. (2009). Reflection and Reflective Practice in Health Professions Education: A Systematic Review. *Advances in Health Sciences Education*, vol. 14, no. 4, 595–621.

Mental Health Coordinating Council (MHCC). (2019). Trauma-Informed Leadership for Organisational Change: A Framework, TICPOT Stage 4, MHCC, NSW, Australia, Authors: Corinne Henderson C. and Isobel S. Available: website address.

NHS Education for Scotland. (2017). Transforming Psychological Trauma. https://transformingpsychologicaltrauma.scot.

Orford, J. (2008). *Community Psychology: Challenges, Controversies and Emerging Consensus.* Chippenham, Wiltshire: Anthony Rowe Ltd.

Patel, N., Bennett, E., Dennis, M. Dosanjh, N., Mahtani, A., Miller, A. & Naidirshaw, Z. (2000). *Clinical Psychology, "Race" and Culture: A Training Manual.* Leicester: BPS Books.

Public Health England. (2021). Resilience Responders Programme Evaluation: Summative Report. Unpublished Document.

Roberts, V. Z. (2019). The Self-Assigned Impossible Task. In Obholzer, A. & Roberts, V. Z. (Eds.), *The Unconscious at Work: Individual and Organizational Stress in the Human Services*, 127–136. London: Routledge.

SAMHSA's Concept of Trauma and Guidance for a Trauma-Informed Approach. July 2014. https://ncsacw.samhsa.gov/userfiles/files/SAMHSA_Trauma.pdf.

Save the Children. (2005). Psychosocial Care and Protection and Protection of Tsunami Affected Children: Guiding Principles. https://resourcecentre.savethechildren.net/pdf/2981.pdf/ accessed 13 December 2021.

Schön, D. (1983). *The Reflective Practitioner: How Professionals Think in Action*. New York: Basic Books Inc.

The Window of Tolerance Animation by Beacon House. (2018). Last accessed 13 December 2021 https://www.youtube.com/watch?v=Wcm-1FBrDvU.

Think Local Act Personal, "Co-Production-in More Detail". Last accessed 16 December 2021. https://www.thinklocalactpersonal.org.uk/co-production-in-commissioning-tool/co-production/In-more-detail/.

Trauma Informed Oregon. (2018). Trauma Informed Care Screening Tool. https://www.traumainformedcare.chcs.org/resources-for-becoming-trauma-informed/.

Wall, A. (2018). 'A Qualitative Exploration of Reflective Practice Groups in British Red Cross Services'. Unpublished thesis for a Doctorate in Clinical Psychology at the University of East London.

White, M. (2004a). *Narrative Practice and Exotic Lives: Resurrecting Diversity in Everyday Life*. Adelaide, South Australia: Dulwich Centre Publications.

White, P. (2004b). *Working with People who are Suffering the Consequences of Multiple Trauma: A Narrative Perspective*. Adelaide, South Australia: Dulwich Centre Publications.

8 Research and Evaluation Considerations for Staff Support in Healthcare Settings

Dr Matt Hotton, Dr Louise Johnson, and Dr Anika Petrella

Research and evaluation are essential components in the field of staff wellbeing and support. As a complex and interdisciplinary field of policy and practice, staff wellbeing and support within a healthcare setting interacts with a broad spectrum of stakeholders and end users. With an increasing focus on the health and wellbeing of individuals working within healthcare, research and evaluation aid in building knowledge and understanding that directly impacts how we best support staff. It is important that such research and evaluation promote inclusivity and diversity. By ensuring cultural competency in research, the diversity of experiences within the healthcare workforce can be better understood, leading to more relevant data, which can better inform staff support practices.

The purpose of this chapter is to provide an overview of the importance of research and evaluation in the field of staff wellbeing and support and to outline ways of conducting research and evaluation within a healthcare setting. The following section considers the differences and similarities between research and evaluation, explains why research and evaluation of staff support initiatives are important, and discusses how the recent COVID-19 pandemic has led to increased awareness about the relevance of this topic. The next section discusses various research designs relevant for evaluating staff support initiatives and the final section offers some 'top tips' for putting evaluation into practice.

Research or evaluation?

Research has been defined as "the attempt to derive generalisable or transferable new knowledge to answer or refine relevant questions with scientifically sound methods". In contrast, evaluation aims to 'define or judge current care' and rather than being generalisable, is typically specific to a particular service or setting (Health Research Authority, 2017, p. 1). Audit is a further concept related to, but separate from, research and evaluation. Unlike research or evaluation, audit involves the inclusion of a standard by which outcomes are measured against (Health Research Authority, 2017). While audit plays an integral role in most aspects of service delivery, there is currently a paucity of agreed standards in the field of staff wellbeing and support against which outcomes can be compared. As such, this chapter focuses predominantly on issues related to research and evaluation, rather than audit.

Often the distinction between research and evaluation is blurred due to politics (such as funding and time constraints) and the social context (Cohen et al., 2018). There have been some important distinguishing features identified between research and evaluation (Cohen et al., 2018). However, it is also important to consider that "evaluation can be used as both a form of research as well as an evaluation procedure, and it is important to decide on which of these it is before the researcher proceeds" (Savin-Baden and Major, 2013, pp. 273–287).

Evaluation carried out in a healthcare setting has similarities and key differences when compared to research. This very distinction highlights the lack of integration between the two approaches, which have the potential to be more similar than they are different. However, in current practice, the implications of their differences should be considered to move towards pragmatic integration of evaluation and research carried out by various stakeholders.

When evaluation work is applied in a clinical setting with the same principle and rigor as academic research, the main differences left between the two are specific to the target aim which impacts practical aspects of design (e.g. methods utilised, governance) and therefore output (e.g. generalisability). For example, a hospital may be interested in understanding the feasibility, acceptability, and efficacy of a staff support programme within their unique context (i.e. one department or organisation). On the other hand, an academic conducting research may be interested in the feasibility, acceptability, and efficacy of the same staff support program, but specific to an entire population (e.g. nurses within a region or country). Therefore, there are considerations around where the work is carried out, who the intended audience or end user is, what outcomes are relevant within unique contexts, and ultimately final interpretation and generalisability.

Considering practice-based evidence

In clinical practice, evaluation, and research, both evidence-based practice and practice-based evidence are important. For example, in terms of measurement methods in psychotherapy, researchers have turned attention to the importance of practice-based evidence (Margison et al., 2000). The term 'practice-based evidence' has been defined to include "any activity in which clinicians gather scientific evidence themselves as part of routine practice" (Green and Latchford, 2012, p. 88). Practice-based evidence may include single case study designs, recording clinical activity in a database, gathering patient feedback, and incorporating session-by-session measures for each therapy session (Barkham et al., 2010, Green and Latchford, 2012, Lambert et al., 2018).

Practice-based evidence includes utilising existing outcome frameworks, as well as outcomes informed by the goals of service users (Green and Latchford, 2012). It allows for flexibility in terms of design and data collection and can lead to better therapeutic outcomes (Miller et al., 2006).

Why evaluate staff support services?

1) It can ensure that the staff support service is reaching the intended target group and provide information about uptake, effectiveness, and acceptability of staff support initiatives, which in turn can lead to important adaptations to the initiatives. It may also help identify groups of staff that may not be accessing support by collecting demographic information, for example gender, ethnicity, and job role.
2) It can provide helpful learning regarding which staff support initiatives are most effective for improving staff wellbeing and most acceptable to members of staff.
3) It can highlight the potential benefits and challenges of providing support for staff.
4) It can highlight the important role that psychologists and other healthcare professionals can play in supporting staff within their organisations.
5) It can demonstrate cost-effectiveness. This may be particularly important for stakeholders to see if a service warrants funding.

Integrating evaluation in healthcare

There are considerable challenges in integrating empirical evidence into practice within the healthcare setting. Practical limitations within the healthcare setting make it difficult to balance pragmatic approaches with evidence-based fidelity. It is important that when designing an evaluation that one carefully considers:

- The purpose or aim
- The target audience
- What outcome measures are important and feasible to consider?
- Who is best to conduct the evaluation?

There are differences in ethical and governance procedures to consider when designing research or evaluation. For example, service evaluation work may be exempt from needing research ethics approval when involving staff within a hospital. Instead, stakeholders may require approval from the site-specific head of research governance, departmental approval and/or support from the executive. Conversely, research would typically require research ethics board approval. Challenges exist with both approaches and can lead to significant time constraints when the work aims to facilitate local adaptations.

Empirical research and novel directions

Individuals working within healthcare are under immense pressure. Major incidents, such as terrorist attacks, natural disasters, and outbreaks of infectious diseases (e.g. severe acute respiratory syndrome – SARS, Ebola virus, and COVID-19), shine a light on the challenges faced by healthcare workers and provide insight into how to best support them. Prior to the COVID-19 pandemic there was a growing call for the improvement of staff health and wellbeing as well as creating healthy workplaces for healthcare workers. Research consistently highlighted high levels of sickness absence, dissatisfaction, psychological distress, and burnout when compared to other sectors. For example, research and evaluation work conducted during the SARS outbreak highlighted that high levels of persistent distress contribute to systemic burnout, poor mental health, problematic health behaviours (e.g. smoking, drinking), increased time off work, and overall reduced hours worked (Chan and Huak, 2004, Maunder, 2004, Maunder et al., 2006, Nickell et al., 2004). Following the SARs pandemic, there was an appeal for intervention and support of healthcare workers based on research and evaluation (Maunder, 2004, Maunder et al., 2006). However few changes were made. That was, until the COVID-19 pandemic struck.

The COVID-19 pandemic has played a pivotal role in highlighting the pressure healthcare workers are under, as well as the lack of systemic support and clear leadership. As the COVID-19 pandemic unfolded, healthcare services and the physical and mental health of key workers became a global focus. Rapid evaluation of staff wellbeing was commissioned at the local level (Petrella et al., 2021), national level (Barello et al., 2020, Kang et al., 2020, Xiao et al., 2020), and globally reviewed (Sheraton et al., 2020).

The collective experience of COVID-19 highlighted the current state of healthcare systems internationally and the wellbeing of those working within in healthcare settings. It also emphasised the usefulness of evaluating staff wellbeing and support interventions and sharing lessons learned broadly to appropriately respond to the evolving COVID-19 landscape. Looking beyond the pandemic, this approach will support the everyday effectiveness of the healthcare system, as well as the individual health and wellbeing of healthcare staff.

One such example of how research conducted because of the COVID-19 pandemic has led to positive changes to the field of staff wellbeing and support comes from the resilience literature. Resilience speaks to the capacity for staff to cope with a crisis and then quickly return to previous levels of functioning with as little negative impact as possible (Rosen et al., 2020). Resilience of healthcare staff is consistently highlighted as a key protective factor for wellbeing during acute stress (Rosen et al., 2020). Prior to the COVID-19 pandemic, research and evaluation had typically focused on the resilience of individual members of staff rather than occupational stresses, such as understaffing and emotional burdensome workloads. Healthcare organisations therefore place the onus on staff to achieve resilience which results in additional pressure, self-blame, and feelings of alienation and lack of support. COVID-19 brought this topic to the forefront on a global stage and a shift to considering resilience as a collective responsibility that greatly involves the healthcare organisation (Maben and Bridges, 2020). Such research also highlights how evaluation of staff support must consider the individual members of staff, as well as the responsibility of the system by which they work under unprecedented pressure. With that approach, research and evaluation will continue to play a key role in improving psychological staff support in healthcare.

Types of design

As discussed earlier, there are multiple reasons why an evaluation may be embarked on. You may be interested in monitoring the wellbeing of staff and capture use of support interventions, you may want to explore staff preferences for support interventions, or evaluate the acceptability, feasibility, and effectiveness of available interventions. This section introduces three broad approaches: monitoring staff wellbeing, evaluating staff support interventions and services, and understanding staff experiences. Throughout, we outline design considerations, methods available, and types of data that can be collected. Indeed, if the design, methodology, or data collection of a project is not suitable, there are threats to credibility, validity (i.e. bias), and overall usability of any findings.

Monitoring staff wellbeing

Monitoring staff wellbeing can provide vital information about individuals, teams, and populations of interest and allow for feedback into the team and organisation. It is important that we first consider what we know about the current climate and population of interest, as well as what outcomes we are interested in capturing (e.g. burnout, absenteeism). We then consider whether we are interested in gaining a snapshot, building insight at one specific time, or whether we are interested in detecting changes over time. The latter would involve collecting data from a cohort of staff over multiple time points (e.g. monthly). Monitoring staff wellbeing can facilitate identifying at-risk groups, impact of any changes made in response to earlier insight gained, and support the identification of individual issues among staff, group-level needs, and organisational issues. Different approaches for monitoring are outlined in Table 8.1, along with potential advantages and disadvantages of taking each approach. Indeed, given the relative merits and weaknesses of different approaches, consideration should be given to using a combination of different approaches, including mixed methodology (use of qualitative and quantitative data).

Getting the tempo right

Once you have decided upon the approach you plan to take, the next step is to consider when and how often to collect data. This can be referred to as tempo or cadence. Census data is often collected yearly given how burdensome it is to collect. This may be similar to a staff experience survey or audit of staff data (e.g. looking at absenteeism, sick leave). Cadence of cohort data varies and centres on the question of interest. Cohort data may be collected quarterly to allow for changes to be detected that occur over time, monthly to identify teething issues as changes occur, or even daily brief 'pulse' surveys to identify individual issues and at-risk groups of staff.

TABLE 8.1: Evaluation methods.

Method	What is it?	Advantage(s)	Disadvantage(s)
Census survey	Survey of a whole staff population within an organisation	Limits bias by including all members of staff	Resource intensive
Cohort survey	Survey of a subset of a population of interest that represents the whole population (sample)	Realistic, cost effective, and time efficient	Bias can occur depending on sampling strategy
Anonymous drop box	Inviting the whole population of staff to provide feedback	Anonymous feedback may reduce reporting bias by individuals	Selection bias specific to those who engage with this method
Qualitative interviews or focus groups (representative sample)	Interviewing members of staff (individual or in a group) who are part of a group of interest	Provides insight into the complex, individual experience which provides a rich narrative	Lack of generalisability and resource intensive

Usability of monitoring data

Monitoring data can be used to shed light on how staff are doing at any given time, as well as over time (trajectories and trends) at the group level. Monitoring data can facilitate crude economic analysis to assess lost productivity (absenteeism) to estimate the economic cost of illness and gain of staff support of wellness. Findings from monitoring data can identify where resources are needed (what, when, for who) and support implementation of staff support interventions. Lastly, monitoring data can impact policy at the local, regional, and national level.

Factors to consider

There are several factors to consider when monitoring staff wellbeing. Demographic differences (e.g. age, gender, ethnicity), as well as employment-specific differences (e.g. experience, seniority, role, department) may impact how you collect data, as well as how you interpret the findings. In addition, it is important to consider factors that may be interacting with data collection and outcome of interest. For example, there may be an interaction between stressors outside of the workplace, the management of a disability or illness, and ethnic or cultural differences that impact participation in an evaluation and how we may control for that interaction in our analysis of data provided.

Ethnicity and diversity are particularly relevant factors within all aspects of health research. It is essential that all ethnicities are well represented in staff wellbeing research and evaluation. However, in the United Kingdom (UK), people from Black and Minority Ethnic (BAME) groups are less likely than others to be included in health research (Farooqi et al., 2018). As of March 2020, at least 20.7% of staff working in the UK's National Health Service were from a BAME background (Government Digital Service, 2020), highlighting the importance of representation of BAME groups in research in this field and work that organisations need to do to engage this part of their workforce.

Having an impact

Feedback of evaluation results is an important design consideration. Feedback can be given to the individual members of staff as a way of validating and normalising experiences. Feedback can also be given at the team level in order to facilitate change in practice norms. To change culture, feedback at the organisational and government policy level can be made. In addition, findings can be shared within the academic field more broadly at meetings, conferences, and through peer-reviewed publications.

As an example (see Box 8.1), a mixed-methods rapid evaluation was carried out at one of London's largest university hospitals during the first year of the COVID-19 pandemic (Hughes et al., 2021, Petrella et al., 2021, Phillips et al., 2021). Results from this rapid evaluation were collated into a final report delivered to the institutions' executive and fed back to individuals who participated through Trust-wide communications. Findings presented by the evaluation team redeployed to carry out this work generated changes throughout the institution as the pandemic evolved.

Evaluation of staff support interventions and services

In addition to monitoring the wellbeing of staff groups, there are key considerations around setting up a robust evaluation to assess the feasibility, accessibility, and effectiveness of staff support interventions and services.

> **Box 8.1: Case study: COVID-19: Staff experience of health and wellbeing (Petrella et al., 2021)**
>
> *Background*
>
> Following the onset of the global pandemic (spring 2020), three hospitals in North Central London participated in a joint effort evaluating staff mental health. Healthcare workers were invited to participate in an online survey. Staff were invited to opt into a cohort study whereby follow-up data were collected every three months for the first year of the pandemic. The aims of this cohort evaluation were to:
>
> 1) Evaluate staff wellbeing during the acute phase of COVID-19 specific to moral and psychological distress, symptoms of burnout, and individual coping strategy utilisation.
> 2) Enhance our understanding of potential mechanisms of staff wellbeing and identification of at-risk populations of staff.
> 3) Monitor temporal changes in staff psychological and welfare service use, coping, and symptoms of distress and burnout among staff throughout the COVID-19 pandemic to inform emotional support needs during the recovery period.
>
> *Evaluation*
>
> The following data were collected via a bespoke survey administered using an online survey platform (Qualtrics):
>
> - Demographic information (gender, age, ethnicity)
> - Professional information (role, department, duration at the Trust, redeployment status)
> - Exposure to COVID-19 (exposure in the workplace, symptoms, positive diagnosis) (adapted from Kang et al., 2020)
> - Self-rated physical and self-rated mental health (pre-COVID-19 and currently) (Kang et al., 2020, Krause and Jay, 1994)
> - Moral distress (Corley et al., 2001)
> - Psychological distress (K10; Kessler et al., 2002)
> - Symptoms of burnout (Byrne, 1991)
> - Coping (Brief COPE; Carver, 1997)
> - Impact of Events Scale (Marmer and Weiss, 1997)
>
> *(Continued)*

> - Clinical screening questions (GAD-7 & PHQ-9; Kroenke et al., 2001; Spitzer et al., 2006)
> - Open-ended feedback regarding wellbeing needs.
>
> Dissemination is ongoing from the evaluation team (Petrella et al., 2021).
>
> ***How did the evaluation data inform practice?***
>
> Findings were fed back at the management and executive level and peer review publications were utilised to disseminate to the research field more broadly. Findings supported the justification of supporting staff during these difficult times (business cases for staff wellbeing roles) and aided in secure additional funding to support staff. These evaluative data enabled the psychology service to address areas of concern, with groups of staff identified as high risk.

What type of data to collect?

Any data collected should be recorded accurately and consistently. It can be helpful to consider the following types of data collection:

1. User data
2. Activity data
3. Feedback data
4. Outcome data

1. *User data*

User data refers to collecting information about those members of staff who are being supported. This includes collecting demographic information, such as gender, ethnicity, and religion. In addition, capturing information about job roles and teams accessing the services is important to provide context regarding who is being supported and importantly to identify groups of staff who may not be accessing support. This data should be collected routinely at the start of engagement with staff support services. When staff support services provide more informal drop-in sessions, it may still be helpful to capture this data.

2. *Activity data*

Activity data involves collecting information about the way in which staff support services are being used. This monitors whether staff support services are being delivered effectively to the intended users. The purpose of collecting such engagement data enables resources to be planned appropriately, flexibility and improvement of models of service delivery, and to understand the impact of the support service within an organisation. It is important that this information is collected consistently to provide accurate information about who is accessing the service. The amount and type of activity data collected is likely to be determined by the type of staff support service being provided and the intended use of the data collected. Thinking about how the information is going to be collected, recorded, and stored securely will help to ensure that activity data accurately reflects how the service is running and how it is being used by staff.

Those providing support to staff should strive to promote diversity and maximise access to support for people from BAME backgrounds. Certain staff groups which may have higher representation of people from BAME groups, such as cleaners and porters, may not receive information about available support or research/evaluation opportunities through traditional information cascades accessed by other members of the workforce. The routine collection of activity data can help determine whether those receiving support accurately represent the wider healthcare staff population.

Staff support initiatives may not necessarily involve face to face, video, or telephone support. It may be that resources are widely distributed online for staff to access, such as wellbeing leaflets and resources. It is important to capture this engagement, for example the use of online resources. This may include reviewing webpage traffic.

What activity data should be collected?

The following case study (Box 8.2) is an example of how a new staff support service set up in response to the first wave of the COVID-19 pandemic collected user data, activity, and feedback data (Johnson et al., 2022).

3. *Feedback data*

While the collection of user and activity data helps to provide information about which staff support services are being used, and by whom, it does not typically provide rich information about how acceptable these services are to those accessing them. It is therefore important to routinely collect direct feedback data from users of staff support services, particularly regarding how staff perceive the interventions they are receiving.

> **Box 8.2: Case study: Evaluating a COVID-19 staff support service – Department of Clinical and Health Psychology, Leeds Teaching Hospitals NHS Trust (LTHT; Johnson et al. (2022))**
>
> *Background*
>
> A new staff support service for members of staff across the Trust was set up at the beginning of April 2020 in response to the COVID-19 pandemic. Staff who worked for LTHT were able to access this support service via face-to-face drop-ins or telephone, which was initially available seven days a week, 9 am–9 pm. Qualified clinical psychologists and staff counsellors operated the service.
>
> *Evaluation*
>
> At the start of the new service, a comprehensive evaluation database and attendance log were developed to record user and activity data regarding the service. The database and survey were registered and approved as a service evaluation project by the local organisation's Research and Development department.
>
> For each staff support contact, the following data was collected:
>
> - Date and time of session
> - Job role
> - Clinical Service Unit of staff member
> - Type of support (e.g. direct or indirect support for colleague)
> - Type of session (e.g. face to face, telephone, video call, email support)
> - Reasons for accessing support (e.g. anxiety, low mood, stress, pre-existing mental health difficulties)
> - Summary of intervention delivered (e.g. psychoeducation, psychological first aid, compassion-focused therapy)
> - Issues related to risk.
>
> After each staff support session, consent was gained from the staff member being supported and clinicians would then email a summary containing the details listed above. Names of staff members were not
>
> *(Continued)*

recorded to protect confidentiality. One member of the Clinical and Health Psychology team was responsible for inputting this data into a secure database.

In addition, from joint working and sharing of resources with other healthcare organisations, a short anonymous electronic evaluation survey was developed and implemented in Leeds. With permission from the staff member, this survey was emailed to staff following support sessions.

How did the evaluation data inform practice?

The information collected was well received at a management level and was beneficial in helping to plan and adapt the service during the pandemic. For example, adjustments were made to the times and days available to access the service which was informed by the data collected. The data enabled the service to reflect on which staff groups were accessing support most frequently and which staff members were not accessing the service. Gaining insight into the difficulties that staff who accessed the service were experiencing ensured that the most appropriate support was delivered. Feedback from the staff evaluation survey helped to demonstrate the benefit and value of the service during this time and also identify areas for improvement. The evaluation data collected helped to identify a need for a business case and subsequent funding for three clinical psychology posts created specifically to work within an ongoing staff support service.

Sekhon et al. (2017) have provided a framework for different components of acceptability to collect feedback on. These different components and how they apply to evaluating staff support initiatives are summarised in Table 8.2.

Requesting staff to provide feedback, including a combination of quantitative and qualitative data, can help provide a breadth of information. An example of this is provided by Slater et al. (2018), who collected feedback on a staff wellbeing programme in paediatric oncology, haematology, and palliative care settings in Queensland, Australia. They used Likert scales to capture staff ratings of the value of specific staff support strategies, along with open-ended questions asking for suggestions about how the wellbeing initiatives might improve in the future. Such evaluation allowed the authors to produce dynamic wellbeing initiatives, in response to staff feedback.

TABLE 8.2: Components of acceptability.

Component	Description
Affective attitude	How the member of staff feels about the intervention
Burden	The amount of effort the member of staff perceives is required to participate in the intervention
Ethicality	The degree to which the intervention fits with the staff member's own value system
Intervention coherence	The degree to which the staff member understands the intervention
Opportunity costs	What is the cost (e.g. financial, time, values) to the staff member
Perceived effectiveness	The perceptions of the staff member regarding whether the intervention is likely to achieve its purpose
Self-efficacy	How confident the staff member feels that they will be able to engage in the intervention

Source: Adapted from Sekhon et al. (2017), p. 8.

It is recommended that feedback is collected for all one-to-one, group, and service-level interventions, but also that those clinicians delivering staff support interventions are mindful of keeping feedback forms brief, to not place excessive burden on staff. Online survey software can be used to aid collection of feedback, particularly following online interventions.

4. *Outcome data*

The routine collection of outcome data has become an embedded part of patient care across health settings. We argue that this should also be the case in the context of staff health and wellbeing interventions, to provide detailed information about the benefits gained from interventions. Outcome data can not only be used to determine the effectiveness of interventions, but also inform changes to interventions and service design. In addition, outcome data can help compare the effectiveness of interventions across different groups, for example different staff groups, different ethnic groups, and groups of differing years of healthcare experience. Such data can help adapt and tailor interventions, to ensure effectiveness across a range of groups.

A key aspect of collecting outcome data is selecting the right measures. A number of measures are available to monitor and measure the wellbeing of staff, and a discussion of the relative merits and disadvantages of these is beyond the scope of this chapter; however, outcomes likely to be measured include those related to stress, trauma, coping, resilience, team functioning, burnout, and psychological wellbeing. When selecting measures, researchers are advised to be mindful of the reliability and validity of measures, as well as that many measures will have been designed for a clinical population, and, as such, normative values may be less applicable for staff groups. In addition, it is important to have an awareness that certain constructs commonly investigated in the field of staff wellbeing, such as burnout, may have cultural-specific elements (Pines et al., 2002). As such, the normative values of certain outcome measures may be misleading when exploring such constructs in certain ethnic or cultural groups.

Although randomised controlled trials (RCTs; and/or systematic reviews of RCTs) provide the highest level of evidence for interventional studies (Oxford Centre for Evidence Based Medicine Levels of Evidence Working Group, 2018), in practice clinicians facilitating staff wellbeing interventions will rarely have the resources or means to conduct such studies. In addition, it may often not be ethical or feasible to conduct such a study in routine practice and currently there are very few, if any, well-conducted RCTs published in the area of staff support. Therefore, while the RCT design has considerable merit, particularly regarding controlling sources of bias, we argue that the simpler pre-post design, where measures are administered before and after an intervention (and preferably at a longer-term follow-up), has an important place in routine staff support practice.

When collecting feedback and evaluation data, it is important to ensure that samples are representative of those receiving support. There are several barriers to engaging people from BAME groups in research and evaluation, including differences in language and other sociocultural factors (Brown et al., 2014). Researchers should be mindful of these barriers and look to engage with BAME groups to identify ways of reducing them wherever possible.

Understanding staff experiences

Qualitative methods provide a systematic approach to exploring social phenomena within a natural setting. This can include the individual experiences of a specific group (e.g. nurses) or even how an organisation may function (e.g. hospital). One of the main differences between quantitative and qualitative methods is the way in which data is collected. Where quantitative methods are used to capture aspects of staff wellbeing by sampling from a specific population (e.g. nurses) and surveying global constructs (e.g. burnout), qualitative methods are used to examine the complexity of what is occurring and what that means to the specific individuals. Qualitative data is often described as providing a rich narrative to a specific phenomenon, capturing the human experience which can be absent when interpreting large numerical datasets (quantitative methods). Therefore, it is essential that the aim of an evaluation is clearly defined and the methods used to collect and analyse data are appropriately matched.

Qualitative methods or mixed methods (integration of qualitative and quantitative methods) provide powerful tools for investigating the complexity of staff wellbeing and the process of providing support. By engaging staff in individual interviews or focus groups, they are given the space to reflect and speak up about their unique experience. However, it is important to note that, like any method, there are limitations that should be considered, specifically around lack of generalisability. Although it is outside the scope of this chapter to provide insight into key principles and practices of the theoretical paradigms, methodological approaches, data collection methods, and data analysis procedures, please consult the following resources for additional guidance (Biggerstaff, 2012, Creswell et al., 2007, Fetters et al., 2013, Teherani et al., 2015).

> **Box 8.3: Case study: Virtual care and the Impact of COVID-19 on Nursing: A single centre evaluation (Hughes et al., 2021)**
>
> *Background*
>
> Following the onset of the global pandemic (spring 2020) an evaluation was carried out examining the impact of changes in nurse working practices during the COVID-19 pandemic. The focus was on how virtual care and remote working were implemented to accommodate the restrictions imposed because of the pandemic. This was a single centre evaluation that used semi-structured interviews data conducted with 48 operational leads and nurses.
>
> *Evaluation*
>
> Two overarching themes emerged relating to the patient experience and nursing experience. There were both positive and negative elements associated with virtual care and remote working related to these themes. However, the majority of nurses found that virtual clinics were useful
>
> *(Continued)*

when proper resources were provided, and managerial strategies were put in place to support them. Participants felt that virtual care could benefit many but not all patient groups moving forward, and that flexibility around working from home would be desirable in the future.

How did the evaluation data inform practice?
Telemedicine and flexible working were not common in the NHS prior to the pandemic but the current evaluation supports the role out of these as standard care with policies in place to ensure that nurses and patients are appropriately supported. It was recommended that clear policies be put in place to ensure that nurses feel supported when working remotely and there are robust assessments in place to ensure virtual care is provided to patients who have access to the necessary technology. These recommendations were taken on board by the site and in addition, educational support was developed and provided to staff.

Practice points

Conducting research or evaluation in a clinical setting does not come without challenges. The following 'Practice Points' (in Table 8.3) end our chapter and outline some of the key considerations for any clinician or researcher embarking on research or evaluation in the field of staff wellbeing and support.

Conclusions

This chapter has highlighted the critical role that research and evaluation can play in the development of staff support interventions and the delivery of effective staff support practices. We have summarised some of the key similarities and differences between research and evaluation and discussed their relative merits and challenges. There are a wide range of designs and methodologies available and we hope that this chapter has provided a helpful starting point for those looking to conduct research or evaluation in this area. Indeed, we hope to have demonstrated that even small-scale evaluation projects contribute to building the evidence base for this rapidly developing field.

TABLE 8.3: Practice points.

Build the right team	For evaluation of staff support services to be implemented effectively within an organisation, it can be helpful to identify a named individual/group of individuals who take a leading role in evaluation. It may be important to think about who within the organisation has previous experience of evaluation projects? Who may have the necessary IT skills to set up a user-friendly database? It is important to consider how you might engage staff members who are receiving support, so that evaluations are co-designed with users.
Effective collaboration	Opportunities to collaborate with others on a local, national, or even international scale. This can be facilitated by web-based communication and data collection tools (see section on maximising useful resources).
Maximise useful resources	Give consideration to the resources available to you within your organisation, for example licenses for outcome measures, computer software, and data collection tools. Electronic data collection enables multi-site access and provides reporting tools that automatically generate many standard analysis procedures, thereby saving time. There are open source programs supported by universities and hospitals, such as Research Electronic Data Capture, as well as fee for service options, such as Qualtrics or Survey Monkey. When choosing an online data collection tool it is essential that the tool is compliant with relevant regulatory standards.
The research team	It can also be useful to identify potential sources of funding, to help support your project. In terms of your workforce, your organisation may have a number of research assistants, students, assistant psychologists, or trainee clinical psychologists who could support the evaluation project. This can be a useful learning and development opportunity for more junior members of staff. It is important to ensure the necessary supervision and support is in place for assistants and trainees and any project should be supervised and overseen by a qualified member of staff.
Get buy-in from key stakeholders	Effective evaluation of staff support services is largely dependent upon on all individuals, including staff members delivering and receiving the service, to support and contribute to the evaluation initiative. Consider how a new evaluation initiative may be implemented in your organisation? What may be needed to make data collection possible? How would you ensure the data collected is reliable and valid?

(Continued)

TABLE 8.3 (Continued): Practice points.

Ethical considerations	When setting up a new evaluation project, it is recommended to discuss the idea with the organisation's local research and development department or other relevant research departments. This ensures that all the relevant research/evaluation protocols and procedures have been followed, such as consideration of ethical issues.
	Research and evaluation projects need to consider all potential ethical issues. The main ethical issues regarding staff support evaluation include: (i) Informed consent – permission for data collection, storage of confidential and possibly personal information, consent to share information, consent to be contacted for feedback regarding the service, is written consent required; (ii) Confidentiality – it is essential that any confidential and personal information collected is treated in the strictest confidence. Consideration should be given as to how data will be sufficiently anonymised as and when the data is presented to a wider audience. Accurate recording of information pertaining to risk issues is essential.
Governance issues	In recording staff support activity, it is important to consider issues related to data protection (e.g. UK General Data Protection Regulation), consent, and storage of such information on a secure database in line with local organisation governance guidance.
	Prior to collecting data, it is important that any plans for evaluation are discussed with the local organisation's relevant teams. For example, within the NHS this may include the organisation's Research and Development and Information Governance teams. Such teams can provide advice regarding local policy, particularly with regard to factors such as recording identifiable information and how best to store data securely.

References

Barello, S., Palamenghi, L. & Graffigna, G. 2020. Burnout and somatic symptoms among frontline healthcare professionals at the peak of the Italian COVID-19 pandemic. *Psychiatry Research*, 290, 113–129.

Barkham, M., Hardy, G. E. & Mellor-Clark, J. 2010. *Developing and delivering practice-based evidence: A guide for the psychological therapies.* London, John Wiley & Sons.

Biggerstaff, Deborah (2012) *Qualitative research methods in psychology.* In: Rossi, Gina, (ed.) Psychology: selected papers. Rijeka, Croatia: InTech, 175-206.

Brown, G., Marshall, M., Bower, P., Woodham, A. & Waheed, W. 2014. Barriers to recruiting ethnic minorities to mental health research: A systematic review. *International Journal of Methods in Psychiatric Research*, 23, 36–48.

Byrne, B. M. 1991. The Maslach Burnout Inventory: Validating factorial structure and invariance across intermediate, secondary, and university educators. *Multivariate Behavioral Research*, 26, 583–605.

Carver, C. S. 1997. You want to measure coping but your protocol's too long: Consider the brief cope. *International Journal of Behavioral Medicine*, 4, 92–100.

Chan, A. O. & Huak, C. Y. 2004. Psychological impact of the 2003 severe acute respiratory syndrome outbreak on health care workers in a medium size regional general hospital in Singapore. *Occupational Medicine*, 54, 190–196.

Cohen, L., Manion, L. & Morrison, K. 2018. *Evaluation and research*. Abingdon: Routledge.

Corley, M. C., Elswick, R. K., Gorman, M. & Clor, T. 2001. Development and evaluation of a moral distress scale. *Journal of Advanced Nursing*, 33, 250–256.

Creswell, J. W., Hanson, W. E., Clark Plano, V. L. & Morales, A. 2007. Qualitative research designs: Selection and implementation. *The Counseling Psychologist*, 35, 236–264.

Farooqi, A., Raghavan, R., Wison, A., Jutla, K., Patel, N., Akroyd, C., Deasi, B., Uddin, M., Kanani, R. & Campbell Morris, P. 2018. Increasing participation of Black, Asian and minority ethnic (BAME) groups in health and social care research: Toolkit. 2018.

Fetters, M. D., Curry, L. A. & Creswell, J. W. 2013. Achieving integration in mixed methods designs – Principles and practices. *Health Services Research*, 48, 2134–2156.

Government Digital Service. 2020. *Ethnicity facts and figures: NHS workforce* [Online]. Available: https://www.ethnicity-facts-figures.service.gov.uk/workforce-and-business/workforce-diversity/nhs-workforce/latest [Accessed 30 November 2021 2021].

Green, D. & Latchford, G. 2012. *Maximising the benefits of psychotherapy: A practice-based evidence approach*. London: John Wiley & Sons.

Health Research Authority. 2017. *HRA defining research table* [Online]. Available: http://www.hra-decisiontools.org.uk/research/ [Accessed 2021].

Hughes, L., Petrella, A., Phillips, N. & Taylor, R. M. 2021. Virtual care and the impact of COVID-19 on nursing: A single centre evaluation. *medRxiv*.

Johnson, L., Hardwick, K., Shand, S. & Grant, E. 2022. The development and evaluation of the Leeds clinical and health psychology department COVID-19 staff support service. *Professional Psychology: Research and Practice*, 53, 99–108.

Kang, L., Ma, S., Chen, M., Yang, J., Wang, Y., Li, R., Yao, L., Bai, H., Cai, Z. & Yang, B. X. 2020. Impact on mental health and perceptions of psychological care among medical and nursing staff in Wuhan during the 2019 novel coronavirus disease outbreak: A cross-sectional study. *Brain, Behavior, and Immunity*, 87, 11–17.

Kessler, R. C., Andrews, G., Colpe, L. J., Hiripi, E., Mroczek, D. K., Normand, S.-L., Walters, E. E. & Zaslavsky, A. M. 2002. Short screening scales to monitor population prevalences and trends in non-specific psychological distress. *Psychological Medicine*, 32, 959–976.

Krause, N. M. & Jay, G. M. 1994. What do global self-rated health items measure? *Medical Care*, 32, 930–942.

Kroenke, K., Spitzer, R. L. & Williams, J. B. 2001. The PHQ-9: Validity of a brief depression severity measure. *Journal of General Internal Medicine*, 16, 606–613.

Lambert, M. J., Whipple, J. L. & Kleinstäuber, M. 2018. Collecting and delivering progress feedback: A meta-analysis of routine outcome monitoring. *Psychotherapy*, 55, 520.

Maben, J. & Bridges, J. 2020. Covid-19: Supporting nurses' psychological and mental health. *Journal of Clinical Nursing*, Accepted Article.

Margison, F. R., Barkham, M., Evans, C., Mcgrath, G., Clark, J. M., Audin, K. & Connell, J. 2000. Measurement and psychotherapy: Evidence-based practice and practice-based evidence. *The British Journal of Psychiatry*, 177, 123–130.

Marmer, C. & Weiss, D. 1997. The impact of event scale-revised. In: Wilson, J.P. and Keane, T. M. (Eds). *Assessing psychological trauma and PTSD*. New York: Guilford, 399–411.

Maunder, R. 2004. The experience of the 2003 SARS outbreak as a traumatic stress among frontline healthcare workers in Toronto: Lessons learned. *Philosophical Transactions of the Royal Society of London. Series B: Biological Sciences,* 359, 1117–1125.

Maunder, R. G., Lancee, W. J., Balderson, K. E., Bennett, J. P., Borgundvaag, B., Evans, S., Fernandes, C. M., Goldbloom, D. S., Gupta, M. & Hunter, J. J. 2006. Long-term psychological and occupational effects of providing hospital healthcare during SARS outbreak. *Emerging Infectious Diseases,* 12, 1924.

Miller, S., Duncan, B., Sorrell, R., Brown, G. & Chalk, M. 2006. Using outcome to inform therapy practice. *Journal of Brief Therapy,* 5, 5–22.

Nickell, L. A., Crighton, E. J., Tracy, C. S., Al-Enazy, H., Bolaji, Y., Hanjrah, S., Hussain, A., Makhlouf, S. & Upshur, R. E. 2004. Psychosocial effects of SARS on hospital staff: Survey of a large tertiary care institution. *CMAJ,* 170, 793–798.

Oxford Centre For Evidence Based Medicine Levels of Evidence Working Group. 2018. Oxford centre for evidence-based medicine, 2011. Available: https://www.cebm.net/2016/05/ocebm-levels-of-evidence.

Petrella, A. R., Hughes, L., Fern, L. A., Monaghan, L., Hannon, B., Waters, A. & Taylor, R. M. 2021. Healthcare staff well-being and use of support services during COVID-19: A UK perspective. *General Psychiatry,* 34, e100458.

Phillips, N., Hughes, L., Vindrola-Padros, C., Petrella, A., Fern, L. A., Panel-Coates, F. & Taylor, R. M. 2021. The impact of leadership on the nursing workforce during the COVID-19 pandemic. *medRxiv.*

Pines, A. M., Ben-Ari, A., Utasi, A. & Larson, D. 2002. A cross-cultural investigation of social support and burnout. *European Psychologist,* 7, 256.

Rosen, B., Preisman, M., Hunter, J. & Maunder, R. 2020. Applying psychotherapeutic principles to bolster resilience among health care workers during the COVID-19 pandemic. *American Journal of Psychotherapy,* 73, 144–148.

Savin-Baden, M. & Major, C.-H. 2013. *Evaluation.* Abingdon: Routledge.

Sekhon, M., Cartwright, M. & Francis, J. J. 2017. Acceptability of healthcare interventions: An overview of reviews and development of a theoretical framework. *BMC Health Services Research,* 17, 1–13.

Sheraton, M., Deo, N., Dutt, T., Surani, S., Hall-Flavin, D. & Kashyap, R. 2020. Psychological effects of the COVID 19 pandemic on healthcare workers globally: A systematic review. *Psychiatry Research,* 292, 113360.

Slater, P. J., Edwards, R. M. & Badat, A. A. 2018. Evaluation of a staff well-being program in a pediatric oncology, hematology, and palliative care services group. *Journal of Healthcare Leadership,* 10, 67.

Spitzer, R. L., Kroenke, K., Williams, J. B. & Löwe, B. 2006. A brief measure for assessing generalized anxiety disorder: The GAD-7. *Archives of Internal Medicine,* 166, 1092–1097.

Teherani, A., Martimianakis, T., Stenfors-Hayes, T., Wadhwa, A. & Varpio, L. 2015. Choosing a qualitative research approach. *Journal of Graduate Medical Education,* 7, 669–670.

Xiao, X., Zhu, X., Fu, S., Hu, Y., Li, X. & Xiao, J. 2020. Psychological impact of healthcare workers in China during COVID-19 pneumonia epidemic: A multi-center cross-sectional survey investigation. *Journal of Affective Disorders,* 274, 405–410.

SECTION 2
PRACTICE

9 Enabling Connection and Compassion through Structured Compassion Practices

Dr Benna Waites, Dr Charlie Jones, Laura Simms, Dr Alister Scott, Andy Bradley, and Dr Rachel Potter

Compassion practices are structured dialogues designed for people working in health and social care, underpinned by key principles that support compassion through nurturing self-care and connection with others. Compassion is relational, emotional, and action oriented and seeks to alleviate suffering. Compassion practices are intended to reconnect people with their own core values and purpose, and to reconnect with each other, through group-based structured conversations. Compassion practices include Compassion Circles, Taking Care Giving Care (TCGC) rounds, and Care Spaces.

These practices are most often used in organisations with teams or with groups who may or may not know each other. The potential to use this methodology with groups of service users or within wider communities is being explored by a number of practitioners. This chapter will chart the development of the family of compassion practices, describe their background, present evaluation data, and describe a range of examples that we hope will encourage wider engagement with the practices.

History and development of compassion practices

This work started with Andy Bradley's work on compassion in the early 2000s, and his increasing sense of unease with the pervasive culture in health and social care which he found to be "dehumanising, transactional and unkind – which was leading many staff to feel burnt out, disillusioned and unable to live their values at work" (Bradley & Scott, 2021). The first formal Compassion Circle was facilitated by Andy in 2013 in the northeast of the UK in a healthcare setting and the model was rapidly adopted to support colleagues in settings such as care homes, palliative care in the Midlands (UK), and a children's hospital in Colorado (US). Bradley (2016) commented on the counter-cultural nature of the process of inviting people to think about their own and each other's compassion and self-care needs, with a starting point that compassion needs to be consciously nurtured rather than presuming its presence and persistence. Counter-cultural at that time too was the idea that in order to sustain an offering of compassionate care for patients and service users, investing time and attention in how we take care of our caregivers is required: "Why do we hear so much about compassion for patients but so little about the people who serve them?" (Bradley, 2016).

These practices were originally developed to give busy, care-focused people space to think with others who face similar challenges, and to tune into the work of maintaining and building compassion and self-care while working in tough circumstances that can erode or undermine compassion. They build on principles of dialogue: a commitment to high quality listening, listening to understand rather than to intervene, thinking and processing one's thoughts and emotions out loud, offering each other support and appreciation, avoiding rescuing. The practices deliberately disrupt the 'normal' way of having conversations in conventional society and organisations.

The assumption underpinning compassion practices is that the vast majority of people working in health and social care are drawn to the work through their own compassion and that when this reduces it is likely to relate to the system conditions in which they work. The intention is that by creating and holding the space in the context of a guided dialogue, compassion that is already there within colleagues will be 'liberated' and flow more freely.

The practices have been evaluated (Flowers et al., 2018, Jones et al., 2021, Clark et al., 2021), and there is anecdotal evidence of their use internationally in the USA, China, Canada, Australia, South Africa, Lithuania, Sweden, Denmark, France, and beyond. Clark et al. (2021) and Hewison et al. (2019) have begun to establish a literature intended to create international awareness and to share the evidence for the credibility, legitimacy, and saliency of the practices.

Background theory and research

Compassion has been defined as "a virtuous response that seeks to address the suffering and needs of a person through relational understanding and action"

(Sinclair et al., 2016, p. 195). Gilbert (2017, p. 11) defines it as "a sensitivity to suffering in self and others with a commitment to try to alleviate and prevent it". These two definitions highlight the relational, emotional, and action-oriented nature of compassion. With the advent of the COVID-19 pandemic, loss and grief have felt more omnipresent than ever and spaces where this can be held and heard compassionately feel all the more necessary.

Compassion in healthcare is commonly understood to refer to something a caregiver offers to a patient. However, Gilbert (2009) proposes that in addition to the flow of compassion from self to others, compassion also involves the flow of compassion from self to self (i.e. self-care), and the flow of compassion from others to self (i.e. what we might receive from colleagues, family, and friends). Table 9.1 outlines the flow of compassion. Evidence suggests that intentionally practising each of these can have impacts on mental states and prosocial behaviour. Hewison et al. (2019) share useful evidence to show that even those who are meant to be 'good at compassion' need nurturing; compassion and self-compassion are behaviours, skills, and habits to be learned and encouraged in self and others. The original Compassion Circle moves through each of these areas, with an inquiry into the qualities underlying care.

The invitation to appreciate colleagues during the practice in a structured way also gives the chance for people to give and receive compassion to and from each other.

Compassion practices build on the principles outlined by Nancy Kline to support optimal conditions for thinking. Kline is the author of the books *Time to Think* (2002), *More Time to Think* (2009), and more recently *The Promise That Changes Everything: I Won't Interrupt You* (2020). Kline's focus is on helping groups to think well about their shared and most complex challenges together. She has developed a 'Thinking Environment' method and a global network of trained practitioners. The method outlines a number of principles and practices that disrupt the conventional way of having discussions. These conventions can often lead to domination by a few, the ignoring of people with certain think-

TABLE 9.1: Flow of compassion.

Self to other	Visualisation of the qualities needed to give compassionate care with the 'self as patient' exercise
Self to self	Exploration of taking better care of ourselves and setting of an intention
Other to self	Exploration of the obstacles and enablers of compassion in the wider system; receiving appreciation from pairs work

ing or learning styles or those who may be quieter or more introverted, and the propagation of bad habits such as interrupting that undermine creative, original, or slower thinking.

Kline's method involves identifying the question that needs to be addressed, and then giving everyone involved several opportunities to develop their thinking on that question: time on their own, rounds where each person contributes if they wish to, thinking pairs where each individual has a chance to think out loud knowing they will not be interrupted by their listening partner, appreciations – voicing qualities that you appreciate about your thinking partner and a final thinking round where each person can share their latest thinking. Compassion practices have been inspired in part by the Thinking Environment method. Kline's method not only builds up rich layers of thought as each participant's thinking is valued, listened to, and gently challenged by the contributions of others. It also builds group cohesion, listening skills, mutual and self-awareness, and new levels of appreciation of each other through enabling a respectful, creative, and powerful mode of interacting that disrupts our normal way of talking to each other.

Groups that use the Thinking Environment method usually report lasting results in how participants relate to each other, including more attentive and respectful listening, enhanced valuing of each member's contributions and potential, and stronger bonds that emanate from voicing appreciations that many of us too often keep to ourselves. To paraphrase what the motivational speaker and author William Arthur Ward once said: "Feeling positive thoughts about someone and not expressing them, is like wrapping a present and not giving it."

The marked increase in a focus on compassion in healthcare has not always been matched by an understanding of the complex systemic conditions that might contribute to an eroding of compassion. Whitby and Gracias (2013) provide an excellent account of various compassion inhibitors and obstacles including the role of systems that reinforce the achievement of (often efficiency focused) targets over and above the human quality of care. This is explored in more depth in the aptly titled article by Steven Kerr 'On the folly of rewarding A while hoping for B' and concerns have been raised about the prevalence of system conditions that set up extrinsic motivators (targets based on external rewards and punishments, such as Critical Incident reviews that focus on documentation detail), when evidence suggests that the most effective route to supporting good performance in complex environments such as healthcare is through unleashing intrinsic motivation (IHI Psychology of Change, Hilton et al.). Kate Hilton suggests using stories to connect people with their underlying values and sense of purpose as a way of connecting people with their intrinsic motivation.

Whitby and Gracias's article also covers the challenges inherent in the provision of direct care. People working in direct caring roles are highly likely to experience powerful feelings such as disgust, hostility, and even hatred. Having these feelings is normal in the context of direct care for people who are experiencing various kinds of vulnerability, and mental and physical difficulties. Understandably, these feelings can be experienced by carers as disturbing, shameful, and at odds with a self-identity of being kind and caring.

Many of these ideas speak to the importance of the frequently unacknowledged concept of emotional labour (Brotheridge & Grandey, 2002). This psychological demand in health and care work has been recognised as sizeable by Ballat and Campling (2014) in their book *Intelligent Kindness*. Emotional labour refers to the effort required by a worker to manage emotions experienced in the line of duty. Failure to acknowledge both the extent and specifics of the psychological demands of care can negatively impact on wellbeing and the capacity of the workforce to deliver high-quality care in a sustainable way.

Indeed, a failure to meaningfully acknowledge the psychological demands of professional care work can lead to the establishment of structural characteristics (values, policies, procedures, and processes) that consistently make systems vulnerable to the undermining of compassionate care (Williams et al., 2016). Even if some people are able to care for others while not looking after themselves (so in instrumental terms 'getting the job done' for the organisation), the question arises as to the ethics of this situation.

As we have seen, both the Francis Report (2013) and the Andrews Report (2014) suggested that offering opportunities for people working in healthcare to process the emotional impact of their work is likely to improve the quality of care provided. The Francis Report specifically referenced Schwartz rounds (Point of Care Foundation) as an approach that can be used to address this. Schwartz rounds share some characteristics with compassion practices, offering a safe space for sharing experiences and reflections, and providing the opportunity to give and receive peer support (Maben et al., 2018).

There is a significant overlap between the work of compassion practices and the growing field of psychological safety (Edmondson, 1999, 2019). Psychological safety concerns the ability of team members to speak up with concerns or questions without fear of punishment, criticism, or humiliation. The structure of compassion practices, with their turn taking and consequent democratising of airtime, inherently supports the development of 'voice' across all participants. Compassion practices have been cited in work undertaken as part of the Health Foundation's Q Community Psychology for Improvement group as approaches that are likely to support the conditions that will encourage psychological safety to thrive (Health Foundation Q Community, 2022) and used as a basis for the Building Safer Spaces tool (Waites, 2022).

Case study from Wales

Compassion circles were adapted and taken up by Aneurin Bevan University Health Board (ABUHB), which is in South Wales, UK, in response to both the Francis and Andrews reports which examined systemic failings in care in the NHS (Francis, 2013; Andrews and Butler, 2014) and the subsequent need to focus on the challenge of sustaining compassion. ABUHB provides care for a population of 630,000, employing approximately 13,000 people and covering some of the most deprived areas of the UK. Both Francis and Andrews called for increased openness, candour, and support for compassionate care for patients. A key part of fostering this involves organisations creating compassionate conditions for staff that were more sustainable. A group of staff, led by staff from the psychology service, were exploring options for rising to this challenge.

Schwartz rounds have been used extensively in ABUHB and can be a powerful tool for acknowledging the emotional labour in work, and the vulnerability this can sometimes create. However Schwartz rounds have a number of drawbacks. They require preparation of panellists, and generally only involve contributions from a minority of attendees. Compassion practices also do not require any specialist facilitation training to implement, unlike Schwartz rounds, and there is no cost attached to implementation.

In ABUHB, we developed TCGC rounds as a 'sibling intervention' to Schwartz rounds. The name was drawn from a Division of Clinical Psychology conference of the same name and based on basic tenet of compassion practices – that if people are going to continue giving care, they need to be able to take care of themselves and each other. The adaptation also involved ensuring that the rounds could run as a 'one off' rather than as a regular practice and making detailed guidance notes available to ensure ease of facilitation. TCGC rounds were introduced in 2015 in ABUHB and made available to colleagues across the organisation and have now reached over 2,000 people. Over 60 colleagues have received additional training to support their delivery of TCGC rounds and although this is not deemed essential for facilitation of the rounds, our experiences suggest it supports people's confidence in facilitation. This provision was supported by a steering group (chaired by Rachel Potter) and delivered by a range of colleagues (initially mainly psychologists, supported by colleagues working in Organisational Development) working across physical and mental health services. TCGC rounds have also been used to particularly powerful effect in ABUHB in training settings as the means to introduce a cohort to each other and build connections based on values, rather than through job titles or professional groupings.

Initially, the TCGC rounds were facilitated in settings where members of the development team had connections or existing relationships, or where we had been specifically invited to support wellbeing initiatives within a team or service setting. Over time, the TCGC rounds were embedded into training programmes (e.g. the in-house leadership programme, mental health staff training days, health visitor training programme). Requests for TCGC rounds increasingly came from staff who had experienced a round in a particular setting (e.g. on a training programme) and wanted it to be facilitated within their team or service area, or a result of a colleague talking about their experience of attending a round.

The involvement of colleagues from Organisational Development meant that over time we were able to reach right across the health board, rather than just be limited to particular areas where we had connections. The TCGC rounds have also been supported by senior leaders and managers within ABUHB, which has helped raise their profile and embed them as one of a range of compassionate practices within the health board.

There have been challenges, particularly with reaching staff members who work within ward environments, where attending rounds during shifts is more problematic than community or office-based staff. COVID-19 raised some new challenges for facilitators; we had developed a protocol designed to facilitate rounds face to face, with participants sitting together in a circle, in a comfortable room, doing a mixture of group work and pairs discussions. Obviously, this was going to be difficult to facilitate in a time of social distancing, PPE, and remote working. However, we were able to adapt the rounds to be facilitated on virtual platforms such as Microsoft Teams, which enabled us to continue facilitating them during the pandemic. In this chapter we give high-level outlines of three of the Practices, starting here with TCGC rounds in Box 9.1.

This is to give the reader a sense of how they are structured and how they flow. We do this with caution because these outlines can appear dry – and as a result it can be hard to imagine how they could have the beneficial impact they so consistently do. For more details about any of the approaches visit: www.compassionpractices.net

> **Box 9.1: Sixty-minute Compassion Circle (or taking care giving care round) – general structure**
>
> - Welcome and brief introduction (*facilitator*)
> - Grounding exercise (*whole group*)
> - Round 1: Entering an Appreciative Frame of Mind (*whole group*)
> - Round 2: Uniting Values (*whole group*)
> - Round 3: Undivided listening 'Taking Care of Yourself' (*mixture of pairs work and whole group*)
> - Round 4: 'Inhibitors to Compassion' (*mixture of pairs work and whole group*)
> - Round 5: 'Enablers to Compassion' (*mixture of pairs work and whole group*)
> - Round 6: Evaluation and Appreciation (*whole group*)
> - Close (*facilitator*).

The recognition of the various factors which may contribute to both the erosion or sustenance of compassion suggests that, as leaders of systems, or as psychologists, coaches, or external consultants who can advise on the design of systems, we need to consider a range of Relational and Systemic approaches to sustaining compassion (e.g. see Neal and Highfield (chapter 5)). Within ABUHB, this has meant attending to leadership development, ensuring debriefing and counselling is available, and taking both systemic and individual, and reactive and proactive approaches.

Current practice, innovation, and evaluation

Flowers et al. (2018) reported a range of benefits to participating in a TCGC round, including a reconnection to the core values that had originally brought people into healthcare. Due to the rounds being short, fast paced, and validating, participants described feeling more comfortable and less anxious than they had expected. They also fed back that stating what they appreciated about one another was a novel but positive experience. Subsequent evaluation indicated that participants felt that the TCGC round made them more aware of compassion towards patients (82%), towards themselves (85%), and made them think about how to embed compassion more in their work (86%). In total, 89% of the respondents said that participating in the TCGC round would help them to work better with colleagues. Seventy-eight per cent of attendees agreed that they would like to attend a TCGC round again in the future and 85% said that they would recommend attending a round to their colleagues (Waites, 2020).

Attendees were also asked whether there was anything about the TCGC rounds that they found difficult; over half of the respondents did not identify any difficulties. Of those who did respond to this question, some of the attendees found it difficult to speak in a large group and to talk about themselves. Some attendees felt the round required them to 'think on the spot' and others identified that talking about themselves for 3 minutes was a challenge, though it became easier as the session went on.

Clark et al. (2021) provide a practice example of using compassion circles regularly in a Mental Health Commissioning team in the Midlands and show the value of doing this over time, building and deepening relationships with a team. In ABUHB the use of TCGC has been primarily one off, and some early evaluation reported in Flowers et al. (2018) suggested that this approach still had value. Team managers were interviewed between 12 and 18 months after a round had taken place and commented that the round had had a lasting impact. One hypothesis might be that TCGC rounds and CCs function as a catalyst to a change in relationships and thinking, supporting a shift in team climate, organisational culture, and specific behaviours.

Pandemic developments: Care Space, Pause Space, Me Space, and Team Space

Following extensive implementation and evaluation and interest from other organisations in adopting TCGC, a conference in the early stages of the pandemic (March 2020) led to the further expansion of compassion practices adapted to the COVID-19 pandemic. Conversations emerging from the conference concerned utilising the structure of the approach used in TCGC and compassion circles over a shorter time frame, to give healthcare colleagues a space to check in with each other, appreciate one another, and think about their own self-care.

Charlie Jones and Andy Bradley with additional input from Benna Waites developed a format entitled '20-Minute Care Space' for use in situations where people would not be able to commit a whole hour. This has been described in Jones et al. (2020). The process of the development of 20-Minute Care Space is described in detail in the ACP webinar (https://acpuk.org.uk/20_min_care_space/) and can be seen in Box 9.2.

> **Box 9.2: Twenty-minute Care Space**
> - Welcome and brief introduction (*facilitator*)
> - Round 1: One thing going well outside work (*whole group*)
> - Round 2: What's going on for you at the moment? (*pairs*)
> - Round 3: Appreciations (*same pairs*)
> - Round 4: How can you take more care of yourself? (*same pairs*)
> - Round 5: What one thing will you do to care for yourself (*whole group*)
> - Round 6: Grounding exercise to end.

Alongside this, Laura Simms introduced the idea of compassion practices into NHS England which was gathering resources for its NHS People app, to help frontline staff through the pandemic. Mindful of people's very real time constraints, but also the benefit of offering practices for pairs and individuals as well as groups and teams, Laura and Alister Scott developed: 10-Minute Pause Space: this is a practice for pairs, where each individual is listened to by the other, committing to some form of self-care and 5-Minute Me Space – a practice for individuals to give themselves a space to take a breather and pay attention to their own needs (see Box 9.3 for more details).

Alister Scott also developed both 20- and 60-minute Team Spaces, anticipating the need for rapid and easily accessible interventions that could support connection and care between colleagues in a team. The Team Spaces focus on 'how we are doing as a team' – an oft-neglected dimension in high-pressure environments, yet one that can make such a difference when team members connect, listen to each other, pay attention to each other as humans, celebrate the things that are going well, appreciate people for their contributions, and identify areas for improvement in a no-blame environment.

A core group of facilitators (Benna Waites, Laura Simms, Alister Scott) started meeting during the pandemic to create a free web resource providing how-to guides and detailed examples of compassion practices. In this way, an ecosystem of Compassion Practices was rapidly evolved, for groups, teams, pairs, and individuals all underpinned by key principles. All these compassion practices are freely available to view and download at https://compassionpractices.net/the-practices/ enabling and encouraging people to start using the practices in their own settings with no need for input or training from anyone else.

> **Box 9.3: Ten-minute Pause Space and its sibling, 5-min Me Space (Pause Spaces)** were designed for people who needed easy or rapid access to a shorter intervention that could also be used without a mental health practitioner facilitator.
>
> In Pause Space practices, the main inquiry is, 'what does caring for yourself mean to you?'. While this question is deeply invitational in nature, it makes no assumptions that self-compassion is familiar, or tolerable, to the individual. Rather this gentle inquiry can be used by a group, pair, or individual to explore compassion without prejudice. Pause Spaces have been described by Professor Michael West,[1] who often advises health and care services on compassion, as both 'delicate and powerful', and this non-assumptive approach also resonates with the research work of Professor Paul Gilbert on self-compassion. The main components of 10-minute Pause Spaces are as follows:
>
> - Welcome and brief introduction
> - A brief moment of stillness
> - Pairs listening: what does caring for yourself mean to you?
> - Pairs appreciations
> - Round: "To be wise, kind and compassionate towards myself I will …"
>
> Pause Spaces were developed at the start of the pandemic and informed by the research and emerging learning from other national and global events of significance. Co-designed by experts including co-founders of the Compassion Practices Collective, they also were shaped with specific mindful self-compassion and spiritual care input, ensuring a
>
> *(Continued)*

---

[1] See: https://compassionpractices.net.

'whole being' focus on the physical, emotional, psychological, spiritual, social, and professional dimensions. This approach also ensured that they were rapidly approved by the Mental Health Task Force for widespread use.

Like all the compassion practices, Pause Spaces can be used by people face to face or virtually using a variety of digital platforms. Made available freely and widely by the English National Health Service they have been taken up and embedded locally, and also promoted by other national organisations, including Mind in support of the Mental-Health-At-Work Commitment.

Designed to be fully accessible, allowing for systemic take-up and promotion, Pause Spaces can be accessed online or via App, and used immediately. Evaluation is therefore locally determined, though optionally also nationally captured. Some of the evaluation comments are publicly available and perhaps give the curious a sense of their impact. Anonymous examples include:

- "This 'pause space' or mini meditation is a powerful tool. Allowing the mind to fall still is as important as stepping away from a computer screen. I found doing both to be regenerative and probably better for me than additional caffeine."
- "The concept of the pause space is so ideal in the current climate we find ourselves. It is even more beautiful with different ones that can be adapted to suit each person."
- "I have built in pause time into my diary and mobile phone. I listen to classical music as I type/write my responses. I find that this is helping me to hone my reflective skills. I also find that taking time out for me better prepares me to be more compassionate to other people."

Pause Spaces are openly available via NHS England 'How-to Guides' and at the Compassion Practices website, which at time of writing has a global following of almost 500 people.

These open sources are particularly important in promoting equity and inclusion, ensuring people can invite themselves into working with compassion; compassion practices can be used and adapted in culturally appropriate and representative ways. As Compassion Practices evolve, liberating compassion for all will need inclusion philosophy at its heart.

Key practice points

Common underlying principles are shared by all the compassion practices:

- Making compassion a priority – holding space for each other and ourselves
- Creating a warm, welcoming, appreciative atmosphere to encourage a positive frame of mind
- Taking turns to speak and listen, in a circle if you are physically together (or creating a virtual circle with a set order if online)
- Having equal time to speak so that all are heard and no one dominates
- Offering the option not to speak – people know it's ok to pass when it's their turn
- Using respectful and non-judgmental language
- Ensuring the practices are accessible so that they can be widely used; creating inclusive spaces and using inclusive language so that all feel welcome
- Encouraging self-care – turning towards our challenges in resourceful ways, while bringing compassion to ourselves.

Compassion Habits developed by Andy Bradley:

- Listening with a Quiet Mind – ensuring that you are fully present and able to listen mindfully during the practices
- Asking questions that Matter – the practices attempt to frame concise and profound questions that will matter to all participants
- Appreciating from the Heart – giving regular opportunities to offer heartfelt, specific, and genuine appreciation.

Conclusion

A community is building around compassion practices which we hope will grow and support new ways to bring more compassion to the heart of health and social care. From the beginning, when Andy Bradley was so generous with his time and support in encouraging new developments in the practice in

ABUHB and elsewhere, the spirit of collaboration has remained strong, with practitioners sharing ideas and working together to nurture new ways of working. Compassion practices have established themselves as having a valuable role to play in supporting the work of employee wellbeing and sustaining compassion in caregivers. The principles lend themselves to adaptation in practice, and we hope that the practices continue to evolve.

References

ACP webinar. Retrieved from https://acpuk.org.uk/20_min_care_space.

Andrews, J. & Butler, M. (2014). *Trusted to care: An independent review of the Princess of Wales Hospital at Abertawe Bro Morgannwg University Health Board*. Stirling: Dementia Services Development Centre.

Ballatt, J. & Campling, P. (2014). *Intelligent kindness: Reforming the culture of healthcare*. London: RCPsych Publications.

Bradley, A. & Scott, A. (2021). *Compassion practices: Enabling us to be kinder*, 29, 12–13. Coaching Perspectives. April 21.

Brotheridge, C. M. & Grandey, A. A. (2002). Emotional labour and burnout: Comparing two perspectives of 'people work'. *Journal of Vocational Behaviour, 60*, 17–39. https://doi.org/10.1006/jvbe.2001.1815.

Clark, M., Bradley, A., Simms, L., Waites, B., Scott, A., Jones, C., Dodd, P., Howell, T. & Tinsley, G. (2021). Cultivating compassion through compassion circles: Learning from experience in mental health care in the NHS. *Journal of Mental Health Training, Education and Practice, 17*, 73–86.

Department of Health. (2012). Transforming care: A national response to Winterbourne view hospital. Available at: www.gov.uk

Edmondson, A. (2019). *The fearless organisation: Creating psychological safety in the workplace for learning, innovation and growth*. London: John Wiley and Sons.

Edmondson, A. C. (1999). Psychological safety and learning behavior in work teams. *Administrative Science Quarterly, 44*, 350–383.

Francis, R. (Chair) (2013). *Report of the Mid Staffordshire NHS foundation trust public inquiry*. London: Stationery Office. Retrieved from www.midstaffspublicinquiry.com.

Flowers, S., Bradfield, C., Potter, R., Waites, B., Neal, A., Simmons, J. & Stott, N. (2018). Taking care, giving care, rounds: An intervention to support compassionate care amongst healthcare staff. *Clinical Psychology Forum, 303*, 23–30.

Gilbert, P. (2017). Compassion: Definitions and controversies. In Gilbert, P. (Ed.), *Compassion: Concepts, research and applications*, 3–15. London: Routledge.

Health Foundation Q Community Psychology for Improvement Group. Retrieved from https://q.health.org.uk/community/groups/psychology-for-improvement/.

Hewison, A., Sawbridge, Y. & Tooley, L. (2019). Compassionate leadership in palliative and end-of-life care: A focus group study. *Journal of Leadership in Health Services, 32*(2), 264–279.

Jones, C., Waites, B. & Werrett, M. (2021). 20-minute care space: A practical intervention to support connection and compassion in NHS teams. *FPOP Bulletin, 153*, 6–9.

Kerr, S. (1975). On the folly of hoping for A while rewarding B. *Academy of Management Journal*, 18(4), 769–783.
Kline, N. (1999). *Time to think: Listening to ignite the human mind.* London: Hachette UK.
Kline, N. (2009). More time to think. Wakefield: Fisher King Publishing.
Maben, J., Taylor, C., Dawson, J., Leamy, M., McCarthy, I. & Reynolds, E., Ross, S., Shuldham, C., Bennet, L. and Foot, C.. (2018). A realist informed mixed-methods evaluation of Schwartz centre rounds in England. *Health Services and Delivery Research*, 6(37).
Scott, A. (2020). *Creating team cohesion in times of crisis.* Retrieved from https://compassionpractices.net/wp-content/uploads/2021/05/Creating-Team-Oneness-in-Times-of-Crisis-v4.pdf.
Waites, B. (2020). The implementation of taking care giving care rounds/compassion circles in ABUHB. Sustaining compassion in challenging times, Newport, Wales. Conference supported by Public Health Wales.
Whitby, P. & Gracias, S. (2013). Reflecting on the Francis report: This has happened before. *Clinical Psychology Forum*, 249, 13–17.
Williams, R., Kemp, V. & Neal, A. (2016). *Compassionate care: Leading and caring for staff of mental health services and the moral architecture of healthcare organisations.* London: RCPsych Publications.
Zimbardo, P. (2007). *The Lucifer effect: How good people turn evil.* New York: Random House; also *The psychology of evil*, TED Talk (2008).

10 Compassion-Focused Staff Support

An Antidote to Empathy Distress

Dr Kate Lucre, Catherine Lacey, and Dr Jon Taylor

Human beings are profoundly social animals. We call for another (our mother) from the moment we are born and continue to seek others throughout our lives. We play, we compete, we love, we argue, we seek support, and we seek approval. We are unique in our capacity both to consider others and to consider or reflect on ourselves. While other mammals can moderate their behaviour around members of their herd or flock, they do not have the same ability to conceptualise and empathise with others. Human beings have evolved a range of cognitive competencies and social and self-conscious emotions that promote our ability to consider how others experience their lives.

There are clear evolved advantages to these adaptations (Buss, 2009). Being aware of ourselves and others allows us to monitor our place in our social group and simultaneously enables us to experience emotions that guide our actions away from harmful consequences and towards helpful actions. Shame, when experienced proactively, can signal to us that we may experience disapproval, and that we may need to amend our actions accordingly. Pride, on the other hand, can signal approval and encourage us to engage in similar acts in the future (Beall & Tracy, 2020). The ability to mentalise also enables us to notice and respond to others – based on our experience of circumstances (Fonagy & Adshead, 2012). Again, these abilities are critical to survival. A parent needs to be able to respond to their child to feed them, warm them, and nurture them. Partners need to be able to respond to each other to meet their needs and connect. However, these abilities also expose us to the experience of the other. While we become a witness to joy, we also become witness to suffering and distress. We can be moved, angered, or saddened by others. When we work alongside people, particularly in services that draw together those who experience suffering, we can experience elevated levels of vicarious distress ourselves (Craig & Sprang, 2010; Eastwood & Ecklund, 2008). Just as the direct experience of distress can cause harm, so too can the exposure to this in others (Figley, 1982).

This chapter explores the debate around vicarious distress and the impact that this can have on staff. It considers the use of a particular staff support model, Compassion Focused Staff Support (CFSS), as an antidote to the distress that arises from the provision of care. We offer an overview of the emerging evidence of the importance of compassion in the settings where care is provided. The concept of 'compassion fatigue' is contested and replaced with empathy distress. This alternative definition is rooted in developing scientific evidence which separates these two neurobiological processes and consequent psychological and behavioural responses. CFSS will be offered as an antidote to many of the challenges of working in healthcare, including empathy distress. CFSS will be described, along with the processes involved in establishing a CFSS group. Common barriers and blocks to CFSS will also be explored.

Distressing empathy

The impact of care work, and the exposure to trauma and distress that is often a feature of such work, has received increasing attention over the last two decades (Craig & Sprang, 2010; Lucre & Taylor, 2021). Burnout has been used to describe what can occur when there is a disconnect between the employee and their work environment (Maslach & Leiter, 1997). Burnout is typically described as the result of nontraumatic but stressful work conditions and characterised by emotional exhaustion, depersonalisation, and a reduced sense of accomplishment (Kahill, 1988).

Vicarious trauma, on the other hand, describes the pervasive effects of providing trauma therapy on the identity of the therapist, which can include changes to identity alongside shifts in views of others and the world (McCann & Pearlman, 1990). This is contrasted with secondary traumatic stress which refers to a cluster of psychological symptoms that mimic post-traumatic stress reactions. However, unlike post-stress reactions, these are acquired through exposure to another who is suffering the effects of trauma. Secondary traumatic stress is considered by many to be as challenging as the experience of direct traumatic stress, with the experience of witnessing being associated with an increased sense of helplessness.

These terms, particularly the latter two, have emerged in the literature to narrate the potentially harmful impact of 'care' work. The term compassion fatigue has been used to describe the process by which the harmful effects of vicarious exposure can take hold (Figley, 1995). In that, it is suggested that 'too much compassion' could have a negative impact. The idea that compassion fatigue can be the cause of burnout, work-based stress and in some cases PTSD is so commonly accepted that it has unhelpfully prevailed within all sectors of healthcare provision for decades (Sinclair et al., 2017). Despite the term being commonly used, there has been little or no research into the validity of the concept (Lucre & Taylor, 2020). Instead, there is growing evidence that questions the concept of compassion fatigue (Sinclair et al., 2017). Sinclair et al. (2017), for example, note that "compassion fatigue has become a contemporary and iconic euphemism that should be critically re-examined". They go on to point out that compassion fatigue has been perceived as a process that occurs as a consequence of providing care rather than a consequence of work-related stress. Work-related stress refers to the broader context of employment (including opportunities for breaks, staffing levels, and supervision). The repercussion of this assumed link between providing care and compassion has been that it has been believed by many to be a finite resource which needs to be preserved and perhaps withheld by clinical staff. Clearly the impact of withholding compassion and care could be highly detrimental, particularly for patients who access services in need of receiving that compassion (Sinclair et al., 2017b).

Singer and Klimecki (2014) explored the potential for vicarious trauma while also considering the need for compassion and compassionate care delivery. Their work noted the beneficial nature of compassion, while contrasting this with the process of 'empathy distress'. Empathy distress was considered to result from the experience of sharing the distress of another, followed by difficulties in tolerating or coping with this. This resulted in the instinct to withdraw in order to protect oneself from being overwhelmed by the negative or aversive feelings of the other. Further, empathy distress was linked to the activation of the amygdala and therefore associated with threat response functions.

Compassion, on the other hand, is understood to have a very separate neurobiological pathway and, perhaps unsurprisingly, is associated with quite different emotional responses. Singer and Klimecki (2014, 2012: R875) described compassion "as a feeling of concern for another person's suffering which is accompanied by the motivation to help". Dowling (2018: 750) offers a similar distinction and explains that "compassion goes beyond feeling with the other to feeling for the other". Klimeki et al. (2013) identify that the deliberate practice of compassion activates the reward system (drive system) and also affiliative processes (soothing system), while enabling a more prosocial and positive response to potentially difficult and challenging situations (Gilbert, 2019). This differentiation is therefore the basis of the challenge to the idea that compassion is a source of fatigue, as Dowling (2018: 750) puts it, "Compassion does not fatigue – it is neurologically rejuvenating!" Therefore, compassion is a part of the solution and could be described as the antidote (Lucre & Taylor, 2020).

There is increasing evidence to support synaptic plasticity and neurogenesis, that is the brain's ability to adapt neural pathways and regenerate neural matter (Reisel, 2015). This adds weight to the notion of compassion as an antidote to distress with the potential to cultivate neurological and psychological experiences. The neuroplasticity of the human brain enables compassion not only to be trainable but also to facilitate our regulation of emotional responses (Gilbert, 2019; Hoffmeyer et al., 2019; Klemecki, 2015: Singer & Klemecki, 2014; Sinclair et al., 2017; Downing, 2018). Compassionate Mind Training (CMT) (Gilbert & Irons, 2005) embraces this capacity and combines it with psychoeducation and experiential practices. The psychoeducation component enables greater understanding about the evolutionary model of human nature and experiential exercises include self-directed breathing and imagery practices (Matos et al., 2017; Maratos et al., 2019; Beaumont et al., 2017; Irons & Heriot-Maitland, 2020; Gilbert, 2011, 2019). A number of studies have explored the impact of CMT using participants from various populations (Lucre & Corton, 2013; Lucre & Clapton, 2020; Taylor, 2021). Such studies have shown consistent and significant improvements across various outcomes, including self-report and physiological measures (Kirby et al., 2017). It is of particular note that these interventions have specifically targeted and measured all three flows of compassion (compassion for self, compassion for others, and sensitivity to the compassion from others), recognising that all three competencies are interconnected and therefore promote one another (Gilbert, 2019; Matos et al., 2017).

Despite these encouraging findings, pragmatism is important. Training our minds in compassion does not eliminate challenging emotions, but instead fosters strength, wisdom, and courage (Hoffmeyer etal., 2019). CMT facilitates a turning towards rather than a turning away from suffering, as well as the development of a buffer against the impact of empathy distress (Gilbert, 2019; Lucre & Taylor, 2020; Hoffmeyer et al., 2019). With this in mind, we can see the value of staff support as an antidote to empathy distress and we therefore now turn our attention to a particular model of support: CFSS.

Compassion-Focused Staff Support (an antidote to empathy distress)

CFSS draws on the emerging evidence for CMT, to provide a preventative rather than curative response to the needs of staff working in health and social care settings (Lucre &Taylor, 2020). The aim of CFSS is therefore to provide an ongoing experience for staff teams, rather than a crisis response. This model of staff support has been designed to promote and guide organisational change at all levels. The aim and impact of this training is to support development of those neurobiological processes that promote affiliative competencies and increased wellbeing in the workplace.

CFSS is derived from Compassion-Focused Therapy (CFT) which is an integrated and multi-modal approach that draws on evolutionary, social, and developmental psychology. A central focus in CFT is to help people access and stimulate care-orientated motives, affiliative emotions, and various competencies underpinning compassion. These all play important roles in threat regulation, wellbeing, and prosocial behaviour (Gilbert, 2014, 2015). To put this another way, CFT focuses on the importance of cultivating reciprocal relationships both intra- and interpersonally. A key part of the model is to learn to be compassionate towards others, open to receiving compassion from others, and have more self-compassion.

By building on the competencies and motivational systems associated with compassion, CFSS groups can provide a containing structure which wraps around and can influence the clinical work (see Figure 10.1).

A number of key concepts that permeate CFSS work are highlighted in Table 10.1. Briefly, CFSS continues the evolutionary understanding of our basic physiology and recognises that we are not accountable for the fundamental design of our brain, our processing architecture, nor our readiness to learn from, or adapt to, our environmental context (*not your fault*). Indeed, CFSS encourages participants to turn towards their distress (the first psychology of compassion) and strive to alleviate or prevent further suffering (the second psychology of compassion) (Gilbert & Choden, 2013).

Evolutionary influences and our need for compassion and connection merge in the three circles model of human motivational systems that is fundamental to CFT and CFSS. The model clusters human motives into three groups: those designed to monitor threat and promote safety (the threat system); those that support us to acquire key resources and achievements (the drive system); and those that enable us to rest, regenerate, and enjoy recreation (the safeness/sooth-

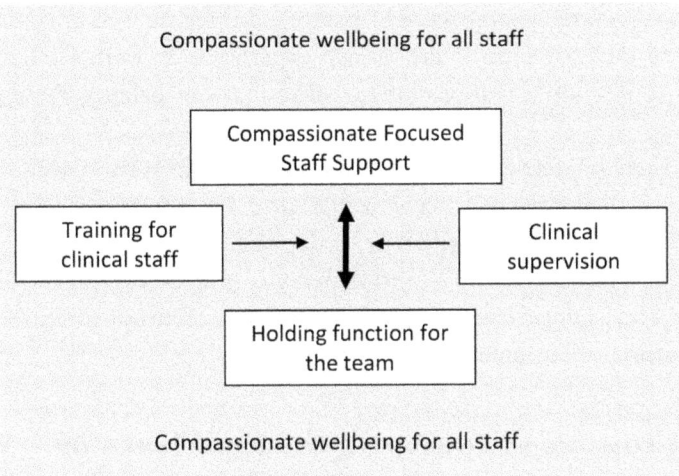

FIGURE 10.1: Compassion-focused staff support overview (Lucre &Taylor, 2020).

TABLE 10.1: Key components of Compassion-Focused Staff Support.

Not your fault, but your responsibility	Introducing the evolutionary psychology model – using key neuroscientific ideas about brain structure to support the concept of 'not your fault' (cf. Gilbert, 2011, 2017, 2019).
Compassion – what it is and what it isn't	An understanding of the two psychologies of compassion is an important component of the model of CFSS. Once staff have this understanding they can then begin to explore the core qualities of compassion and common confusions (Lucre, 2019).
Three circles	This model proposes that we have three main motivational systems that are in a constant state of interaction and interrelation. Supporting an understanding of these systems through formulation is thought to be key to developing strategies to regulate and bring balance to these internal systems (Gilbert, 2019; Lucre & Clapton, 2020 submitted).
Fears, blocks and resistances	Discussed in greater detail below
Personal practice	Personal practice is a fundamental aspect of the CFT model and as such it has been translated into the CFSS model to form the basis of the experiential work within the workshops (Gale et al., 2017; Kolts et al., 2018). Gale (2017) reported that staff who engaged in the study spoke of personal practice as becoming a 'way of life' in both personal and professional lives.

ing system). In compassion-focused practice, all three systems are considered to be central to the challenge of the human experience. In both CFT and CFSS, the aim is to develop a compassionate mind that can balance the demands of each circle.

Finally, there is a recognition that compassion, with its two psychologies, can bring its own challenges (e.g. recognising our own distress) and thus stimulate fears, blocks, and resistances (FBRs). Understanding these FBRs often forms a significant component of CFT, and experience suggests that they are equally important when considering CFSS. We therefore turn our attention to these prior to considering implementation practices.

Barriers to staff support and the experience of compassion: Fears Blocks and Resistances

CFSS operates as a reflective process; for an overview of the development and delivery of this model, see Lucre and Taylor (2020). CFSS also allows for the development of insight into the FBRs that may be encountered within, and indeed across organisations at all levels. FBRs are understood in the context of CFT as cautions and precautions rather than interference. The model recognises that people may feel reluctant to engage with distress, whether that be their own or others. FBRs are usually protective strategies that have developed in the belief that they keep us and others safe (Gilbert, 2009; Kolts et al., 2018). Therefore, these precautions have further informed the development and implementation of the model, and are worthy of particular consideration at an earlier phase.

Fears: Staff who struggle to recognise the benefits of support

In CFT, fears arise when compassion is experienced as unfamiliar, doesn't feel right, and when the person is unsure what will happen (Gilbert, 2020). In the context of care staff, a specific fear is often linked to a sense of weakness.

In these professions, staff commonly develop protective strategies as understandable mechanisms to manage the pain of working within an imperfect system and its regular reminders of human suffering. It is both understandable and expected that when asked to turn towards this suffering, particularly in a group setting, some members of the group may present with numerous fears (and indeed, blocks and resistance) to compassion. These fears can sit in any of the three flows: compassion from others, compassion for others and compassion to self (Gilbert et al., 2011, 2017; Gilbert & Mascaro, 2017). Experience would suggest that these fears may be manifest in direct comments from staff such as "it will make me weak, I don't have time, I'm not doing therapy at work, this green system won't help me when the alarms are going … I'm saying nothing" (Lucre & Taylor, 2020).

Shame and culture are common barriers to engaging staff in caring professions. Shame is known to be a threat response to a perceived social danger, linked back to our need for support from others to survive (Gilbert, 2019). Despite increasingly widespread agreement about the emotional labour involved in caring professions, a culture of concealing emotions remains. This is usually due to the misguided belief that doing so is better for ourselves and others (Davidoff, 2002; Cunningham & Wilson, 2003; Diefendorff et al., 2011; Gilbert, 2017; Kinman & Leggetter, 2016; Miles, 2020; Barton-Sweeney, 2021). As a result, being evaluated, exposed, and admitting fallibility are often experienced as shaming in this context (Gilbert, 2017; Henshall et al., 2017; Miles, 2020). The nature of some post-incident 'de-briefs', disciplinary and investigative processes, which follow this format then exacerbate these beliefs as staff can become 'second victims'. These experiences reduce confidence in professional knowledge and expertise, which can also lead to increased hypervigilance and avoidance (Wu, 2000).

It is therefore not surprising that staff are not always eager to engage in spaces designed for them to speak about the emotional impact of their work (Barton-Sweeney, 2021; Gilbert, 2017). The CFSS model and its psychologically informed language are used to gently and consistently shift away from this sense of invulnerability and infallibility and towards something that is more accepting of human frailties. Making space for naming and normalising FBRs, providing connection and commonality is a focus in both the workshops and the group setting. These elements facilitate the development of the flows of compassion, and support overall staff wellbeing (Kirby, Tellegen & Steindl, 2017; Kirby, Day & Sagar, 2019; Brown, 2021).

Blocks: Organisational culture and myopia

In CFSS, blocks are considered to flow from a misunderstanding or a different conceptualisation of compassion. They can also flow from concerns about how to experience compassion, and the level of support available if and when needed.

In care settings these blocks often manifest as a result of the fusion between outcomes or objectives and the fear of consequences when these are not demonstrable. CMT recognises that the threat and drive systems are linked in complex ways (Gilbert, 2009). In our modern environments, the distinction between these two motivational systems can become blurred as organisational drives generate threat and apprehension within the workforce. Alternatively, resource acquisition (a salary bonus or promotion for example) can only be obtained when a member of staff is considered to be 'going above and beyond'. The blurring of these systems can generate a threat-based drive rather than a resource-acquiring drive (see Figure 10.2).

In threat-based drive, internal and external dialogue often includes 'shoulds' and 'musts' which result in a motivation to avoid or to manage threat, rather than a drive towards achievement (Gilbert, 2009: p201; Palmer, 2015). In care settings, these threats can include senior leaders, regulatory boards, colleagues, and even opinions of family and friends.

Threat-based drive is not only present with patient-facing work, but is often what prompts staff support requests. Leaders perceive staff complaints, investigations, or resignations as threats and ask for an urgent response; striving to avoid, rather than driving to achieve. Given the links between threat and drive, these requests are unsurprising. However, we are best utilised by being grounded, holding boundaries, and remaining both consistent and present – in other words holding the position of the compassionate mind rather than threat or threat-based drive. This begins by holding the distress (the first psychology) without immediately problem-solving (the second psychology); 'Our job is to be the milk float and not the fire engine' (Lucre & Taylor, 2020; p?).

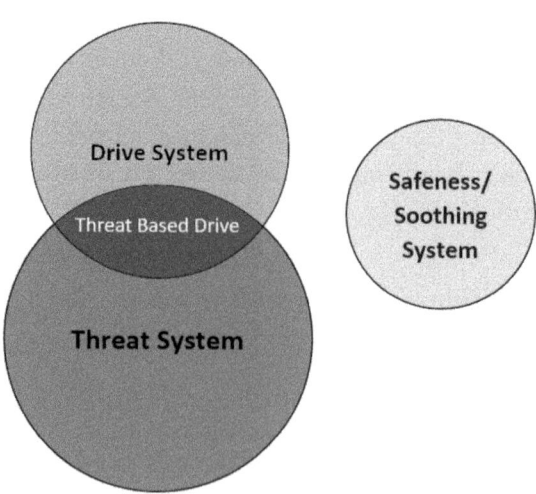

FIGURE 10.2: Threat-based drive: More striving than driving (Lucre, 2020).

Slowing the process and holding the position facilitates a sense of we-ness rather than me-ness (Feeney & Thrush, 2010). This enables time to utilise our ability to recognise what can lead to suffering before we then undertake thoughtful action. CFSS considers both short- and long-term prevention as well as alleviation. Being the milk float allows the slow considered presence required to alleviate suffering alongside prevention. This process sets the tone and is containing for the team. Together they can then think about how they can respond to one another, having taken the time to understand the nature of their distress, and subsequently cultivate compassion in their work as a group (Lucre & Taylor, 2020).

Resistance: Why us and not them – What have we done wrong (or vice versa)?

While fears represent an unfamiliarity with compassion and blocks come from concerns about the processes involved, resistance can reveal internal critical processes. Resistance is commonly associated with concerns about our worthiness or the anticipation of aversive repercussions of our compassion. Where the culture of supportive supervision and staff support is not established, there can be significant resistance. This is linked to assumptions that staff support is punitive, a response to 'problems' or indicative of deficits within the team. That the need for staff support input is a reflection of underperforming.

Kurtz (2020) identifies organisational ambivalence as another common challenge to getting regular staff support established. This is an even greater challenge when thinking about supporting staff who work in inpatient environments where they don't manage their own time or diary. There are significant challenges associated with enabling staff to access the supervision which governing bodies, and to varying degrees professional standards, require (Health and Social Care Act, 2008, Regulations, 2014). It is therefore no wonder that we often experience resistance when attempting to imbed staff group support (White et al., 1998; Brunero & Lamont, 2012). Common constraints in relation to supervision include time, money, training for supervisors, and an appreciation of how it links to patient care (White et al., 1998). Rarely is time for clinical supervision funded or even included in the overall calculation of staffing levels. It is then often when staff need this support the most that it becomes further deprioritised due to organisational change or staff pressure (Buus et al., 2018; Rothwell et al., 2021). In a system with competing demands, supervision is often the first thing to be cancelled or constricted. In some instances, this pattern has led to supervision and staff support being labelled as unhelpful and unreliable, subsequently then justifying an underinvestment at all levels of the organisation (Buus et al., 2018; Rothwell et al., 2021).

There is an additional challenge associated with the facilitation of staff support groups. The facilitation of these spaces is often expected to come from psychologists and psychotherapists who are part of the team they are being asked to support. While the organisation may prefer this for cost-saving reasons, this can complicate and undermine the message of our common humanity which underpins CFSS. If the staff support process is facilitated by a member of the team, there is a potential implication that this colleague or their discipline does not require the same support or group accountability as their peers. It also raises the question of what occurs when a conflict or difficulty worked through in the CFSS group involves the facilitator.

Given the target-driven culture, where going above and beyond has become the new normal, it is unsurprising that embedding consistent staff support in a way that truly recognises, responds to, and acts to prevent suffering is challenging (Henshall et al., 2015). The suggestion of taking staff, particularly those who don't control their diaries, away from the task at hand can be a difficult conversation with leaders. An ongoing commitment to this, even more so. Due to this, introducing the idea of compassion and how this fits in to patient, team, and individual self-care is essential. Perceived organisational compassion and self-compassion have been found to be linked to levels of compassion for others (Henshall et al., 2015). If we can embed compassion in to all levels of an organisation, it will flow on to patient care. Instead of asking the question 'what have we done wrong?', staff begin to realise that this is a core component of the work for all.

Implementing the model: Creating the flows of compassion

We have seen so far that CFSS offers an antidote to empathy distress. It also offers an opportunity for healthcare staff to continue to contribute to the experience of compassion both for themselves and for those they care for. When establishing staff support it is important to consider the key features of the model described earlier and the FBRs highlighted above. The process of implementing the model can be thought of in terms of three key areas of practice: preparation, implementation, and reflection. We will consider each of these in turn.

Preparation

The FBRs that have emerged during the implementation phase of CFSS in a number of organisations have highlighted certain areas that may benefit from attention prior to commencement. These include certain aspects of the wider organisational culture as well as establishing the pre-group workshops and their role in 'shaping the space'.

In terms of wider organisational culture, it is critical that the organisation is open to the concept of compassion and the experience of it. There seem to be two particular features of agency settings that can influence the implementation: senior level commitment and democratisation. Regarding the former, in CFSS people are seen as people. Senior managers are given the same introductory experiential sessions as those in lower banded roles. If possible, bandings are mixed to allow staff to connect with their sense of common humanity and begin to develop a shared language. Simple but meaningful rituals such as inviting all staff attending the workshops and groups to leave their name badges in a bowl by the door can support this process of flattening the hierarchy.

In relation to democratisation, CMT and the theory that sits behind it recognises the seductive nature of status, power and hierarchy, and the influence that competition or dominance can have on relationships. The CFSS group may include staff who have different personal and professional backgrounds as well as staff who have different levels of authority within the organisation. The norms that emerge in the group process can mirror existing norms in the organisation, with hierarchical and dominance-based cultures adversely affecting the group.

In this context, the pre-group workshops are critical and allow staff and the wider organisation the opportunity to 'try before you buy', experience compassion and explore concerns. The initial workshop provides an opportunity for staff to develop an understanding of the CFSS model prior to making a commitment to attend the ongoing groups. As a key part of CFSS is the voluntary nature of attendance, staff are able to use this learning opportunity as a way to meaningfully opt in to the model. As is evident in Table 10.3, the format of the workshop is variable in order to maximise attendance. The workshops can be offered in whole, half day, and shorter segments. The workshops have also been adapted to be offered in different forms using online platforms if needed.

The key concepts referred to previously (see Table 10.2) are brought to life in the pre-group workshop, aided by a playful delivery and focus on facilitating connection between participants. For example, a group-based formulation

TABLE 10.2: Elements of the preparation, implementation, and reflection phases.

Preparation		Implementation		Reflection	
Organisational culture	Accessible leadership	**CFSS group**	Group formation	Evaluate	Outcome measures
	Whole organisation commitment		Attendance		Dynamic feedback and review
Educational workshops	Clarify compassion	**FBRs**	Play and exploration	Learning and development	Supervision and CFSS group for facilitator
		Modelling	Personal practice		Personal practice

of the team using the three circles with the use of objects, scarfs, and coloured pens, enabling a light touch and play-based approach to joining up and sense making. Playfulness is an important part of social engagement systems and helps to facilitate connection between facilitator and team, as well as within the group itself (Porges, 2015). These connections are important when exploring the common FBRs that arise when thinking about compassion.

These sessions are often co-facilitated with a Lived Experience Practitioner (LEP) as well as the clinical trainer. LEP involvement in service planning and delivery has been part of NHS policy in some areas for many years. A number of studies have reported the benefits of embracing the wisdom of those with a lived experience, including collaboration and equality (Lea et al., 2016; Tate and Lester, 2018). This model of training can also offer staff a unique perspective on the experience of receiving care (Tate & Lester, 2005). As the CFSS model has evolved, a specific role for an LEP practitioner who may have graduated from their own CFT has developed (Lucre, 2022). Graduates who have considerable expertise in the lived experience of CMT and have used this as a means are able to share their learning and growth.

Anecdotal feedback from staff members (ref) who have attended these co-facilitated training agrees that they are valuable. It indicates that it is very helpful to hear about the benefits of using compassion from someone who has lived experience of using it to change their own lives. Equally the feedback from the LEP themselves supports the idea that this kind of collaboration continues to be therapeutic and provides opportunities to reinforce emotional learning.

TABLE 10.3: Workshop formats.

CFSS Programme	Timescales	Goal/aim objective
Introductory workshop "Compassion … What it is … What it isn't and Why you might need it" Facilitated by a Lived Experience Practitioner trainer and clinical trainer	2 hr/half a day/ one day	Develop understanding of and practice in self-compassion; To explore, understand, and bring compassion to the personal impact of the work undertaken within the organisation; To learn how, by understanding our own minds (i.e. our emotions, behaviours, thinking styles), we may be better placed to offer compassionate, supportive care to others in need; Explore the FBRs to compassion
CFSS group Facilitated by a psychotherapeutically trained facilitator	Ongoing twice monthly or monthly 60 or 90 min sessions depending on service need	Provision of a place of safeness to explore the impact of the work; CMT; Space to explore the unconscious communications and processes with and between group members
Booster workshop	Annually	Update and refresh skills

The workshops generally conclude with an experiential CFSS group, where participants have the opportunity to experience the structure, content, and process of the group prior to deciding to join (Lucre & Taylor, 2020).

Implementation

Once the workshop is complete, staff members are invited to join a rolling CFSS group. The purpose of these groups is the provision of a containing and supportive space. This facilitates exploration of the impact of the work, both on individuals and on the group as a whole. These groups can be team based or offered more broadly across multiple teams or service areas. This will depend on the nature of the team and the consequent capacity for releasing staff.

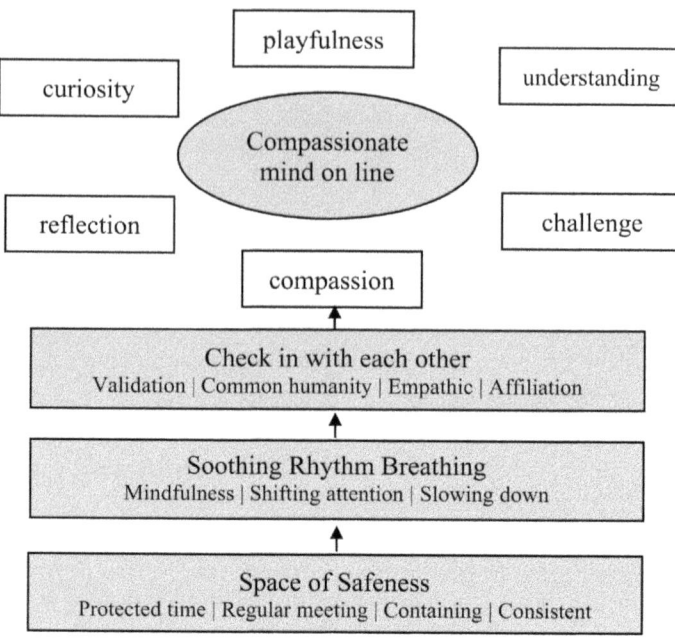

FIGURE 10.3: Group process diagram (Lucre & Taylor, 2020).

The groups are designed to enable staff involved to build on the introductory workshops. This process is facilitated by the explicit invitation to engage in CMT practices within the group setting. Figure 10.3 outlines the overall group process. The group often starts with a breathing practice to enable a transition from the work environment into a more reflective space. This is also coupled with an opportunity to embed the CMT practices and facilitate personal practice (Lucre & Taylor, 2020; Matos et al., 2017).

The structure of the group has been designed to enable members to make an attachment to the group to foster a sense of safeness within and between members (Lucre & Taylor, 2020;). A clear distinction is made between safety and safeness in the group process. The former is known to be a function of the threat and the need to run from (Gilbert, 2020). The conditions for safeness are explicitly cultivated through the open structure of the group which provides consistency, coupled with space for exploration (Gilbert, 2020; Lucre, 2022). The Soothing Breathing Rhythm practice, which is followed by a short check in from each group member, fosters a culture enquiry and a transitioning point from the workplace. SBR is a meditative breathing practice with specific attention to postural awareness, straight slightly concave back, grounded upright posture, warm friendly voice tone, and gentle facial expression, coupled with a steady diaphragmatic breathing pattern. This facilitates the activation of key physiological processes that are associated with the activation of social engagement (Geller & Porges, 2014; Porges, 2011).

As we have mentioned previously, FBRs are not uncommon and it is likely that these may manifest by some staff opting out initially (Lucre and Taylor, 2020). Instead of responding to the desire to convince those who don't attend of the validity of the model, continue the valuable work with the existing group. With time, when the CFSS language continues to grow among the team, they may see the benefits in others and want to join in. Compassion can become like a thread weaving through the team (Lucre, 2019).

Reflection

CFSS is still in the early stages of development and as such formal feedback on the model is built into both the group process and into organisational reviews, the latter of which is in progress.

The experience of being asked for feedback is linked with the nature of compassion; facilitators need to listen to the group experience and respond to the experiences that are shared. This means that feedback can be used in a responsive rather than reactive way when developing the model. It also allows for a dynamic and evolving experience of the group processes.

Reflection is similarly key for CFSS facilitators. CFSS facilitation draws on skills from CFT and from group psychotherapy. Facilitators are likely to experience projections, counter-transference invitations and to form their own impressions of group members. All of these processes are both inevitable and natural, but their form and function(s) need to be understood to prevent facilitators from acting out subtle processes in the group setting.

Finally, personal practice is vital to all compassion-focused work (Gale, Schroder & Gilbert 2017; Kolts et al., 2018; Lucre & Clapton, 2020), including the facilitation of CFSS. As we have established, the practice of compassion is beset with FBRs and therefore facilitators need frequent opportunities to reflect. An integral aspect of the CFSS model is to provide both a 'holding' and 'containing' function for the group and the work undertaken in the group process (Parry, 2010; Lucre & Taylor, 2020). In order to provide this, facilitators need the support of their own CFSS space of their own to explore the impact of the work on them, as well as regular supervision. This of course requires a significant time commitment.

Conclusion

When Charles Figley (1982) first spoke about compassion fatigue, he drew attention to an important area of research and, indeed, practice – the potential cost of caring. He recognised that those of us who work in caring professions can be touched by the distress of those around us and that, over time, the cumulative impact of this can become difficult and distressing for us. In this chapter we have offered an understanding of the process – empathy distress – that may contribute to this experience. We have then proposed a specific model for staff support that may enable care workers, therapists, and others in related fields to respond to their own distress. CFSS draws on the integrative and evolutionary model of CFT to create an opportunity for staff of all levels to turn towards their own distress and respond to that distress with compassion. The model helps us to understand organisational contexts including the human desire for power and hierarchy, the pull to threat-based drive, and the FBRs that arise when we begin to turn towards suffering with compassion. By holding these in mind and focusing on our common humanity, our need for care, and providing this containment and support, we are able to thread compassion through and influence the system.

References

Barton-Sweeney, C. (2021). *What is the lived experience for doctors when they are involved in a serious incident? A descriptive phenomenological analysis.* Doctoral Thesis. University of East London. Available at: https://repository.uel.ac.uk/download/cabb300a0083702fb54acc7344e0d8ff411d3d3219cc3164d47ae5a0ce03da82/3574147/2021_DCounPsy_BartonSweeney.pdf [Accessed 20 December 2021].

Batson, C. D. (2009). These things called empathy: Eight related but distinct phenomena. In *The social neuroscience of empathy*, 3–15. MIT Press. https://doi.org/10.7551/mitpress/9780262012973.003.0002.

Beall, A. T., & Tracy, J. L. (2020). Evolution of pride and shame. In: Workman, L. Reader, W. and Barkhow, J. H. (2020). *Cambridge handbook of evolutionary perspectives on human behavior*, Cambridge: Cambridge University Press, 179–193.

Beaumont, E., Rayner, G., Durkin, M., & Bowling, G. (2017). The effects of compassionate mind training on student psychotherapists. *The Journal of Mental Health Training, Education and Practice*, *12*(5), 300–312. https://doi.org/10.1108/JMHTEP-06-2016-0030.

Brown, B. (2012). *Daring greatly: How the courage to be vulnerable transforms the way we live, love, parent, and Llead.* New York: Gotham Books.

Brown, B. (2021). *Atlas of the heart: Mapping meaningful connection and the language of human experience.* London: Penguin.

Brunero, S., & Lamont, S. (2012). The process, logistics and challenges of implementing clinical supervision in a generalist tertiary referral hospital. *Scandinavian Journal of Caring Sciences*, *26*(1), 186–193. https://doi.org/10.1111/j.1471-6712.2011.00913.x.

Buss, D. M. (2009). The great struggles of life: Darwin and the emergence of evolutionary psychology. *American Psychologist, 64*(2), 140.

Buus, N., Delgado, C., Traynor, M., & Gonge, H. (2018). Resistance to group supervision: A semistructured interview study of non-participating mental health nursing staff members. *International Journal of Mental Health Nursing, 27*(2), 783–793. https://doi.org/10.1111/inm.12365.

Craig, C. D., & Sprang, G. (2010). Compassion satisfaction, compassion fatigue, and burnout in a national sample of trauma treatment therapists. *Anxiety, Stress, & Coping, 23*(3), 319–339.

Cunningham, W., & Wilson, H. (2013). *Being a doctor: Understanding medical practice.* Dunedin: Otago University Press.

Davidoff, F. (2002). Shame: The elephant in the room. *BMJ, 324,* 623–624. http://www.bmj.com/.

Diefendorff, J., Erickson, R., Grandey, A., & Dahling, J. (2011). Emotional display rules as work unit norms: A multilevel analysis of emotional labor among nurses. *Journal of Occupational Health Psychology, 16*(2), 170–186. https://doi.org/10.1037/a0021725.

Dowling, T. (2018). Compassion does not fatigue! *The Canadian Veterinary Journal, 59*(7), 749–750.

Eastwood, C. D., & Ecklund, K. (2008). Compassion fatigue risk and self-care practices among residential treatment center childcare workers. *Residential Treatment for Children & Youth, 25*(2), 103–122.

Feeney, B., & Thrush, R. (2010). Relationship influences on exploration of adulthood: The characteristics and function of a secure base. *Journal of Personality and Social Psychology, 98*(1), 57–76. https://doi.org/10.1037/a0016961.

Figley, C. R. (1995). Compassion fatigue: Toward a new understanding of the costs of caring. In B. H. Stamm (Ed.), *Secondary traumatic stress: Self-care issues for clinicians, researchers, and educators,* 3–28. Lutherville, The Sidran Press.

Fonagy, P., & Adshead, G. (2012). How mentalisation changes the mind. *Advances in Psychiatric Treatment, 18*(5), 353–362.

Gale, C., Schroder, T., & Gilbert, P. (2017). 'Do you practice what you preach?' A qualitative exploration of therapists' personal practice of compassion focused therapy. *Clinical Psychology & Psychotherapy, 24*(1), 171–185. https://doi.org/10.1002/cpp.1993.

Gilbert, P. (2009). Introducing compassion-focused therapy. *Advances in Psychiatric Treatment, 15*(3), 199–208. https://doi.org/10.1192/apt.bp.107.005264.

Gilbert, P. (2017). Shame and the vulnerable self in medical contexts: The compassionate solution. *Medical Humanities, 43*(4), 211–217. https://doi.org/10.1136/medhum-2016-011159.

Gilbert, P. (2019). Explorations into the nature and function of compassion. *Current Opinion in Psychology, 28,* 108–114. https://doi.org/10.1016/j.copsyc.2018.12.002.

Gilbert, P. (2020). Evolutionary psychology, compassion focused therapy & change. *The Weekend University.* [Podcast]. [Accessed 25 January 2022]. Available from https://theweekenduniversity.com/.

Gilbert, P., Catarino, F., Duarte, C., Matos, M., Kolts, R., & Stubbs, J., et al. (2017). The development of compassionate engagement and action scales for self and others. *Journal of Compassionate Health Care, 4,* 1–24. https://doi.org/10.1186/s40639-017-0033-3.

Gilbert, P., & Choden. (2013). *Mindful compassion.* London: Constable Robinson.

Gilbert, P., & Irons, C. (2005). Focused therapies and compassionate mind training for shame and self-attacking. In P. Gilbert (Ed.), *Compassion: Conceptualisations, research and use in psychotherapy,* 263–325. London, Routledge.

Gilbert, P., & Mascaro, J. (2017). Compassion: Fears, blocks, and resistances: An evolutionary investigation. In E. M. Seppälä, E. Simon-Thomas, S. L. Brown, M. C. Worline, L. Cameron, & J. R. Doty (Ed.), *The Oxford handbook of compassion science* (pp. 399–420). New York: Oxford University Press.

Gilbert, P., McEwan, K., Matos, M., & Rivis, A. (2011). Fears of compassion: Development of three self-report measures. *Psychology and Psychotherapy: Theory, Research and Practice, 84*(3), 239–255. https://doi.org/10.1348/147608310X526511.

Health and Social Care Act 2008, Regulations 2014. (2014). [Online]. [Accessed 17 February 2022]. Available from: https://www.cqc.org.uk/sites/default/files/20150510_hsca_2008 _regulated_activities_regs_2104_current.pdf.

Henshall, L. E., Alexander, T., Molyneux, P., Gardiner, E., & McLellan, A. (2017). The relationship between perceived organisational threat and compassion for others: Implications for the NHS. *Clinical Psychology & Psychotherapy, 25*(2), 231–249. https://doi.org/10.1002/cpp.2157.

Kinman, G., & Leggetter, S. (2016). Emotional labour and wellbeing: What protects nurses? *Healthcare (Basel), 4*(4), 89. https://doi.org/10.3390/healthcare4040089.

Kirby, J., Day, J., & Sagar, V. (2019). The 'flow' of compassion: A meta-analysis of the fears of compassion scales and psychological functioning. *Clinical Psychology Review, 70*, 26–39. https://doi.org/10.1016/j.cpr.2019.03.001.

Kirby, J., & Gilbert, P. (2017). The emergence of the compassion focused therapies. In P. Gilbert (Ed.), *Compassion*, 258–285. London: Routledge.

Kirby, J., Tellegen, C., & Steindl, S. (2017). A meta-analysis of compassion-based interventions: Current state of knowledge and future directions. *Behavior Therapy, 48*(6), 778–792. https://doi.org/10.1016/j.beth.2017.06.003.

Klimecki, O., & Singer, T. (2012). 'Empathic distress fatigue rather than compassion fatigue? Integrating findings from empathy research in psychology and social neuroscience'. In: B. Oakley, A. Knafo, G. Madhavan, & D. S. Wilson (Eds.), *Pathological altruism* (pp. 368–383). Oxford, Oxford University Press.

Klimecki, O. M. (2015). The plasticity of social emotions. *Social Neuroscience, 10*(5), 466–473. https://doi.org/10.1080/17470919.2015.1087427.

Klimecki, O. M., Leiberg, S., Lamm, C., & Singer, T. (2013). Functional neural plasticity and associated changes in positive affect after compassion training. *Cerebral Cortex, 23*(7), 1552–1561. https://doi.org/10.1093/cercor/bhs142.

Kolts, R., Bell, T., Bennett-Levy, J., & Irons, C. (2018). *Experiencing compassion-focused therapy from the inside out: A self-practice/self-reflection workbook for therapists.* New York: Guilford Press.

Kurtz, A. (2020). *How to run reflective practice groups: A guide for healthcare professionals.* Oxon: Routledge.

Lea, L., Holttum, S., Cooke, A., & Riley, L. (2016). Aims for service user involvement in mental health training: Staying human. *The Journal of Mental Health Training, Education and Practice, 11*(4), 208–219. https://doi.org/10.1108/JMHTEP-01-2016-0008.

Lucre, K., & Clapton, N. (2020). The compassionate kitbag: A creative and integrative approach to compassion-focused therapy. *Psychology and Psychotherapy: Theory, Research and Practice, 94*(1), 497–516. https://doi.org/10.1111/papt.12291.

Lucre, K., & Taylor, J. (2020). Compati, to suffer with: Compassion focused staff support as an antidote to the cost of caring in forensic services. In H. Swaby, B. Winder, R. Lievesley, K. Hocken, N. Blagden, & P. Banyard (Eds.), *Sexual crime and trauma: Sexual crime.* Cham: Palgrave Macmillan. https://doi.org/10.1007/978-3-030-49068-3_6n.

Maratos, F. A., Montague, J., Ashra, H., Welford, M., Wood, W., Barnes, C., Sheffield, D., & Gilbert, P. (2019). Evaluation of a compassionate mind training intervention with school teachers and support staff. *Mindfulness, 10*(11), 2245–2258. https://doi.org/10.1007/s12671-019-01185-9.

Matos, M., Duarte, C., Duarte, J., Pinto-Gouveia, J., Petrocchi, N., Basran, J., & Gilbert, P. (2017). Psychological and physiological effects of compassionate mind training: A pilot randomised controlled study. *Mindfulness, 8*(6), 1699–1712.

Parry, R. (n.d.). *A critical examination of Bion's concept of containment and Winnicott's concept of holding, and their psychotherapeutic implications.* 2. Unpublished Research Project.

Palmer, S. (2015). *The beginners guide to counselling and psychotherapy.* 2nd ed. London: SAGE Publications Ltd.

Porges, S. W. (2015). Making the world safe for our children: Down-regulating defence and up-regulating social engagement to 'optimise' the human experience. *Children Australia, 40*(2), 114–123. https://doi.org/10.1017/cha.2015.12.

Rothwell, C., Kehoe, A., Farook, S. F., & Illing, J. (2021). Enablers and barriers to effective clinical supervision in the workplace: A rapid evidence review. *BMJ Open, 11*(9). https://doi.org/10.1136/bmjopen-2021-052929.

Sinclair, S., Raffin-Bouchal, S., Venturato, L., Mijovic-Kondejewski, J., & Smith-MacDonald, L. (2017). Compassion fatigue: A meta-narrative review of the healthcare literature. *International Journal of Nursing Studies, 69*, 9–24. https://doi.org/10.1016/j.ijnurstu.2017.01.003.

Singer, T., & Klimecki, O. M. (2014). Empathy and compassion. *Current Biology, 24*(18), R875–R878.

Sinclair, S., Beamer, K., Hack, T. F., McClement, S., Raffin Bouchal, S., Chochinov, H. M., & Hagen, N. A. (2017). Sympathy, empathy, and compassion: A grounded theory study of palliative care patients' understandings, experiences, and preferences. *Palliative Medicine, 31*(5), 437–447.

Tait, L., & Lester, H. (2005). Encouraging user involvement in mental health services. *Advances in Psychiatric Treatment, 11*(3), 168–175. https://doi.org/10.1192/apt.11.3.168.

Taylor, J. (2021). Compassion in custody: Developing a trauma sensitive intervention for men with developmental disabilities who have convictions for sexual offending. *Advances in Mental Health and Intellectual Disabilities, 15*(5), 185–200.

Tuckman, B. W. (1965). Developmental sequence in small groups. *Psychological Bulletin, 63*(6), 384–399. https://doi.org/10.1037/h0022100.

Truman, C., & Raine, P. (2002). Experience and meaning of user involvement: Some explorations from a community mental health project. *Health & Social Care in the Community, 10*(3), 136–143.

White, E., Butterworth, T., Bishop, V., Jeacock, J., & Clements, A. (1998). Clinical supervision: Insider reports of a private world. *Journal of Advanced Nursing, 28*(1), 185–192. https://doi.org/10.1046/j.1365-2648.1998.00743.x.

Wu, A. W. (2000). Medical error: The second victim. The doctor who makes the mistake needs help too. *BMJ (Clinical Research ed.), 320*(7237), 726–727. https://doi.org/10.1136/bmj.320.7237.726.

11 Using the Professional Tree of Life for Staff Wellbeing and Supervision

Dr Julie Fraser and Dr Liz Matias

New beginnings, change, transformation

The lockdown, Brexit, and the murder of George Floyd in May 2020 have caused perpetual change, uncertainty, and chaos within so many of our social and professional systems. In our services, the shifting of our therapy and supervision to online platforms challenged the very basis of our thinking and forced us to find new ways to connect to families, students, supervisors, and organisations. In this maelstrom of change and increased demands on our mental and physical health, we needed to work hard to stay mindful of the values and beliefs that brought us to this kind of work and stay connected to our colleagues.

Ecotherapy and systemic practice

Watching nature flourish while we were locked down during the coronavirus pandemic inspired us to make deeper connections to the natural world and to observe nature's ability to cope with crises, by depending on the multiple relationships in our greater ecological system. Gregory Bateson (1979) was one of the first people to make the observation: "The major problems in the world are the result of the difference between how nature works and the way people think." More recently, there is rising popularity in Ecotherapy (Jordan and Hinds, 2016) which uses nature as a third party in the therapeutic process. Ecotherapy models propose that not only should we as humankind bridge the disconnection between humanity and nature and address the devastating impact the Western world has had on ecosystems. We should think more like nature as Sarah Spencer writes in her book *Think like a tree* (2019). In her book she describes natural principles to life, such as cultivating co-operative relationships, integrating and not segregating, responding creatively to change, and valuing natural resources as principles that can boost psychological and social wellbeing. Elsewhere Wohleben (2017, p. 4) describes the forest as having power as a community: "The community must remain intact no matter what. If every tree were looking out only for itself, then quite a few of them would never reach old age. Regular fatalities would result in many large gaps in the tree canopy, which would make it easier for storms to get inside the forest and uproot more trees. The heat of summer would reach the forest floor and dry out. Every tree would suffer. Every tree therefore is valuable to the community and worth keeping around for as long as possible."

The Tree and Forest of Life

Tree of Life workshops originated in Zimbabwe around 2004 as part of therapeutic work with traumatised communities (Ncube-Mlilo and Denborough, 2007). Tree of Life is a form of narrative practice that supports people to tell stories of themselves in ways that make them stronger and feel more connected to others. The metaphor of a tree is used, and each part of the tree represents different stories about our lives. The stories from the trees are shared to build a forest of stories and connections.

A professional adaptation of the Tree of Life model was developed for use with youth workers by Kis-Sines and Pluznick in Canada (date unknown). In using this model over the years in the NHS mental health trust we work in, we have adapted it to promote staff wellbeing, facilitate reflective practice, as a model for supervision and to build staff support in diverse teams and settings. In this chapter, we will introduce the Professional Tree of Life (PTOL) methodology and discuss some of its applications in our services, including as a model for supervision and to support staff teams.

Overview of the Professional Tree of Life model

The PTOL model offers us the opportunity to connect with the staff teams we work with in creative and flexible ways. We will briefly introduce the methodology here. Initially time is spent connecting to the metaphor of the tree and the forest by sharing people's favourite trees and the memories connected to them. We are then invited to draw our own tree and share our trees with others to build a forest. The forest is about strengthening connections with others, the team, and the wider organisation and a chance to reflect on the collective resources that can be accessed to help 'weather the storms'.

> **Box 11.1: Summary of meanings of parts of the tree**
>
> Roots – our training background and professional influences
> Ground – daily practices at work
> Trunk – skills and principles we bring to work
> Branches – hopes and dreams for our work, our colleagues, the team, and the people we work for
> Leaves – who supports and sustains our working lives
> Fruits/flowers – how we contribute to others at work (resources, skills, etc.) and what contributes to our working lives.

The trees are then displayed for the rest of the group to admire and stories shared among members as part of a 'Forest of Life'. The group is then invited to reflect on how the different aspects of their trees can be sustained through adversity or 'The Storms of Life'. Finally, we give 'Certificates' which facilitate the sharing and celebration of stories and ways a team can document key aspects of preferred stories of working together.

'The forest of supervision': Using the professional Tree of Life to connect and reflect in a perinatal community, Family Therapy service

I (Julie) am a clinical psychologist, systemic family therapist, and systemic supervisor in a Family Therapy clinic within a community perinatal mental health service. I supervise Family Therapy trainees from the MSc Family Therapy training for King's College. To undertake the MSc Family Therapy training the trainees have to hold a core professional qualification such as, but not exclusively, psychology, medicine, social work, or psychiatry. The purpose of the MSc training placement is to offer live supervision of the trainees in their final stage of the transition to qualified family therapist. Here I will share my experience of the PTOL as a creative model of family therapist training, support and development in our perinatal supervision group. I will link to clinical theory, and throughout we will share our reflections in action and the reflections on action (Schön, 1987) in supervision.

Reflections from our experiences of using the PTOL in our supervision group

We started by 'warming the context' and sharing our favourite, or significant trees. Using the tree metaphor, we were able to start to talk about 'self' in a safe way and bring in our Social Graces (Burnham, 2012). It helped to facilitate some cultural reflexivity (Krause, 2018) as the stories of the trees connected to our country of origins. I also used it as a way of sharing what kind of supervisor I want to be and reflecting on my differences to the group. Like the Douglas Fir: I am older than the other supervision group members; I grow well in a forest, so I am a team player; and I offer protection, so I want to look after my supervisees and nurture their development. In many respects, I have reflected on this part of the model as setting the scene for the tasks of being a supervisor. Systemic and family therapists Bertrano and Gilli (2010) describe these tasks as the focus on the therapist, the family, and the relationship between the family and therapist each with different goals; but ultimately, I wanted us to connect to the metaphor and feel like we are in a 'forest of supervision' supporting each other. The context of being online without physical connection was a fundamental driver in wanting to use a metaphor from nature to help us connect.

Some feedback from the group during this exercise: 'It felt easier to talk about myself as a tree, I wasn't sure if I would feel silly, but my supervisor going first helped ! … I was really struck by how many memories or stories this exercise reminded me of. … I felt like we got to know each other more and faster, than if we just asked each other questions about ourselves … it felt like we were saying a lot, with only a few words … so much imagery.'

We carried out this exercise over a few dedicated supervision sessions. I will run through each part of the tree illustrating our experience in more detail.

The trunk and the roots

The roots of the tree ask: what brought you to this work, or what events or people influenced you? The trunk asks: what skills and knowledge do you bring to your work/training, what values are most meaningful to you? These are narrative questions of landscape of action and landscape of identity (White, 1989). They also invite supervisees to strengthen their identities of competences (Epston, 1994). This links nicely with Paula Boston's (2010) ideas and exercise on mapping out our pre-knowledges by writing lists of strengths and resources in the categories of professional/clinical, learning styles, personal attributes, and ways of working in a group setting. In this way, Boston (2010) writes, 'the exercise aims to support the construction of a rich description of themselves as contributors to learning, rather than the thinly described version of themselves as anxious and inexperienced new students'. Seeing ourselves as learning/developing/on a journey together feels more appropriate to supervising trainees with a range of fully qualified professionals such as child psychiatrist, social worker, and psychologist.

Some of the feedback from the supervisees described this part of the model as follows: 'It felt so different to how we normally start our family therapy trainee placements. … I didn't feel like such a novice, I was reminded how much I already know … it was like being given permission to bring what we know, that we could integrate our previous working lives … it was fascinating to hear what the others have done … have so much respect for them as professionals too.'

Paula Boston (2010) also writes in the 'Three faces of Supervision'; facing each other is about attending to group processes. These can often be fraught with complexities, despite little being written about them in the systemic literature. I learned of group processes from the work of Yalom (1983) and the tension of balancing the needs of the individual versus that of the group. By using the language of the forest metaphor, we can verbalise more readily how different trees in a forest have different forms and needs, but all form an intricate supportive network of the 'wood wide web'.

Branches

The branches represent our hopes and dreams for ourselves, the people we work with, our teams and our services. We thought about having short and long branches, the short branches asked questions about our hopes for the placement and time in the current supervision group and the longer branches connected to our dreams for our career and professional life. These questions helped us to reflect on our preferred directions and identity as a therapist. We connected it to the list of strengths and resources in the trunk and considered what new skills or experience we would like to add to these lists. We used future-oriented questions like 'imagine you have finished this placement and you feel this has been a worthwhile experience, what have you learned or experienced or noticed yourself doing more or less of? How would the rest of the group notice this?'

The fruits of the tree

This part asks questions about how we contribute to others in our work. I adapted this to think about the supervisees' previous experiences of supervision as gifts that they bring and what they had found helpful or not. This can be used to develop collaborative plans for supervision to meet their varying needs. 'Talking about my previous experiences of supervision, using safe non-challenging language such as fruits and flowers … was really helpful for me to think about my needs and to be honest about what doesn't work for me'.

The forest

After we have drawn and completed the trees, we are invited to share our trees with the group. This is based on the work of Barbara Myerhoff's (2007) outsider witnessing. It's not just about the retelling of the story, it's about the listening. Myerhoff describes it as 'transport and resonance' listening with two aims: firstly, to listen and think about what resonated with you and what images or words connected to you. Secondly, while listening to the professional tree stories, to consider where this took you to in your thoughts and think about what it made you imagine was possible.

Reflections from the sharing of our trees' exercises and voice entitlement

I invited the group to share their trees with one another. As usual, I reassured participants to only share what they feel comfortable with, and while listening, I noticed how differently they presented their trees. Some spoke with confidence and at length, while others finished hurriedly, almost apologising for taking up our time. I was therefore drawn to the theory of voice entitlement (Boyd, 2010) to address the significant meanings of having a voice. Voice entitlement in narrative practice refers to a history of speaking that is deeply embedded in our cultural, gendered, and educational experience. Thinking about voice entitlement, I appreciate and highly value questions like 'what were the messages in your family of origin about talking?'. These have significant power in shaping our relational understandings of speaking at work, in our supervision groups, interrupting one another and offering opinions. I expanded this conversation to explore these narratives asking the group questions such as 'do you think you do justice to your ideas when expressing yourself verbally? If this could be improved, what could contribute to that change? How do you find speaking in supervision, what could facilitate you taking more risks?' (Boyd, 2010)

Reflections from the forest ...

At this point we move from the identity of ourselves as trees to that of a collective team identity. We place the trees side by side to invite a collective retelling. This part reminds me of Peter Lang's 'we-identity' (2000) – that we are all part of each other's stories. We notice elements such as: the strong and firm roots that serve us as a foundation in our work, the hopes and dreams we have for our work, ourselves, the supervision team and our families, the people we are connected to who support us in our work and life. We then take a meta-view of ourselves and reflect, 'when we place ourselves side by side, can we think of ourselves as a forest'? 'What makes it possible to experience ourselves as a forest, and what is made possible for our work with our clients by our experience of being a forest'?

The relational knowing of each other we developed in the sharing of our trees and the connections we made to our voice entitlement narratives provide a clear link to the ideas behind positioning theory (Boston, 2010). Namely that the positions we take with one another in relationships and the different cultural, professional rules that bind those positions influence how we 'speak' to one another. We then wondered how and where a tree stands in a forest, what position is it taking to the other trees in the forest and why.

In nature, the trees position themselves very carefully in the forest; it doesn't happen randomly. Instead, the trees give each other enough space for the roots to grow, for the branches to spread out and not get entangled, and for the leaves to create an adequate canopy to protect the forest ecosystems.

One supervisee described themselves as a weeping willow, standing below the canopy, with leaves and branches drooping around as protection. They imagined that their tree was covered in moss that spread from one tree covering all the other trees to give them warmth and habitats for insects and places for other fungi to grown on. Another supervisee envisioned themself as a mango tree, and imagined the forest to be full of more mango trees feeding animals and giving energy and vibrancy to the ecosystem. Another talked about being a palm tree standing strong above the canopy, proud of their ability to sway and bend to protect the other trees in a storm. I saw my Douglas fir trees standing close enough to all the trees, my roots underground connecting to all the trees sending messages and nutrients to keep the forest communicating and healthy. By talking in this way within the metaphor of a forest, we were able to communicate complex and sensitive views about our relationships with one another. It also enabled us to describe and imagine our preferred ways of relating to one another in a way that developed our identities of strengths and competences to keep us aligned to our values.

Seeing the creation of our forest as a safe context for learning and growing is synonymous with Byng-Hall's (1995) ideas from Attachment theory about a secure base and placing most value on the relationships with one another for personal and professional development.

The group reflected that they felt so strongly connected to the tree metaphor that they were transported to an imagined forest/world. I likened this to a 'fifth province; a space of dialogical co-creations' as written about by Imelda McCarthy (2004). I appreciated the idea of seeing our supervisory space like a fifth province; place of inclusiveness, all lives embraced, no experts, only co-travellers; no certainty or righteousness, only various and unknown possibilities. 'An imagined place where different interests came together … a province of imagination … and possibilities' (McCarthy, 2004) McCarthy quotes Aristotle: 'a vivid imagination compels the whole body to obey it'. This supports the postmodern ideas of narrative therapy, that if we thicken our preferred stories, we can tell these stories and live these stories. Furthermore, the narrative ideas of scaffolding fit nicely with the concept of a forest of supervision and using others to support learning.

Storms

Another very important purpose of the forest is to prepare ourselves for hazards/storms in our work. Trees are more protected from storms when in a forest, and "every tree plays a different role to help protect the forest". This diverse response is critical as it serves to disrupt the storm, consequently minimising the damage. This speaks to reinforcing and valuing difference in our group and hopefully helps to create the safe context needed to weave in discussions on our social graces in our supervision.

We continued the PTOL exercise and considered 'like trees in a forest, there are also storms in our lives'. Questions asked included 'what are some of the storms you face in your systemic training, in your supervision groups, in your team and your work'? In narrative work with trauma, the trauma or the problem story is not privileged, but instead the response to the trauma. As such, questions around this ask: 'How do you respond to storms in your life and how can we help each other to hold onto these'?

We returned to our trees and our forest and reminded ourselves of our abilities and values as a demonstration of support for one another. We reflected that we could have delved deeper into these responses to the storms, by considering our family of origin scripts such as Mason's (2019) messages on how to cope with adversity, with pain, loss, and conflict or Fredman's (2007) ideas about exploring our relationships to help.

Final reflections ... new seeds planted

Overall our experience of using the PTOL as an approach, method, and technique (Burnham, 2010) for supervision that pulls from a range of systemic clinical theory, narrative therapy techniques, and reflective practice was very rewarding and fruitful (to stay with the metaphor!). At the core it privileges the relationships between ourselves as the mechanism for change in our personal and professional development. Bateson wrote and thought about these ideas throughout his career. In 'Steps to an ecology of the mind' (1972) he wrote about the importance of difference and seeing ourselves intricately related to nature (1979). The metaphor of the tree and forest has proved to be a gift that has kept on giving in our supervision groups. We have continued to use the language of nature especially in sensitive and difficult conversations and have named it 'eco-isomorphism'. Feedback from the group was that it helped us to connect to one another as we stared at each other through our screens and we have incorporated 'what kind of tree are you today' into our pre-session warm-ups before seeing our clients.

Using the PTOL to support staff teams

Background and development of the approach

Within our NHS mental health trust, the PTOL is one of several different staff support approaches that teams are able to access. With its emphasis on promoting resilience, a positive identity, reconnecting with shared values and purpose, the PTOL approach offers a powerful and effective way to build team cohesiveness and improve wellbeing. It can also support staff teams to manage the process of change and transition (Wonders and Lee, 2019). It's no coincidence that the PTOL has taken root within our Trust given the use of the 'Tree of Life' as a therapeutic intervention within inpatient and community settings.

The development of the PTOL approach described here arose from an initial pilot within a community mental health service where we were also developing a community-based Tree of Life group for service users. While our initial aim had been to 'warm the context' for the therapy group (i.e. establish the 'Tree of Life' approach within the service with the hope that conversations focused on 'personal' rather than 'patient' identity may take root), it also afforded us the opportunity to begin developing the PTOL as a staff support intervention. At the time, many staff within our service were struggling to cope with increasingly demanding workloads, understaffing, and high staff turnover. Teams were also anxious about a future service transformation. Moreover, there was no provision of regular reflective practice and a limited range of staff support interventions offered within the Trust. Therefore, the offer of staff support using the PTOL was readily taken up by the teams.

Overall, the PTOL pilot was well received and attended by the vast majority of staff within each team. We obtained positive outcomes from the evaluation of our PTOL pilot, using both qualitative and quantitative data (n = 58). Using a scale of 0–10 (with 10 being the highest), participants gave high ratings for their interest in the session and how useful they found it (average rating of 9 for both scales). We also enquired about what participants found most helpful about the workshops. Three key themes emerged as summarised below:

- *Team cohesion/team working*, e.g. feeling appreciated by the team, valuing other team members, a greater sense of 'team spirit', awareness of shared team values, sharing experiences as a team, feeling more connected to the team.
- *Self-development/learning*, e.g. greater self-awareness, opportunity for self-development and learning, being more accepting of change; validation – 'doing our best'.
- *Identifying storms and preferred responses*, e.g. specific ideas and actions (e.g. mindfulness), having an opportunity to find a way forward as a team, greater awareness of the 'storms' that affect the team.

In addition, we gathered feedback on what participants would change about the workshops or found least helpful. The main themes were as follows:

- The sessions not being long enough (i.e. less than 2 hours)
- Disruptions to the sessions (e.g. staff having to leave the session to attend to duty tasks)

- Lack of contribution from all group members (including senior members of team not being present).

This feedback, along with our subsequent experience of running these workshops, has helped to shape how we structure the workshops and the minimum commitment we expect from teams (discussed further below). We have found it helpful to make this explicit as part of our efforts to 'prepare the ground' in advance of the workshops, which is described in more detail below.

Preparing the ground

The importance of working collaboratively with the team to 'prepare the ground', in advance of the workshops, cannot be overstated. The purpose of this preparation is to maximise the participation and engagement, and establish a safe and contained way of working with the team. The process of preparing the ground starts at the point that a request to provide the PTOL workshop is made (often by team manager/leader or sometimes the team psychologist) and continues into the initial session. As the first point of contact, it's helpful to be curious about why the PTOL, as opposed to other approaches, is being considered (what is the history of the idea? How did the idea come about?), in addition to what the managers/teams expectations are (what changes are they hoping to achieve?). As facilitators, we aim to work collaboratively with the team and try to be as flexible as possible to accommodate the needs, while adhering to the key elements of the approach. There are various practical considerations to factor in, such as the size of the team, the format of the session (remote versus face to face), and who will be expected to attend. In our experience, teams benefit from receiving information about the workshop in advance, particularly as there may be concerns about the level of self-disclosure involved and the vulnerability this may bring. So it is helpful to emphasise that the focus is on professional identity and they should only share what they feel comfortable with, given their 'trees' will be displayed for all to see.

From the outset, facilitators should be transparent about the rationale and clear about minimum commitment required, which will be dependent on the service context. Based on the outcome of our pilot, as mentioned previously, we stipulate the following expectations: teams need to sign up for both parts to occur no more than six weeks apart (creating the forest and responding to the storm); sessions need to be at least 2 hours long; the sessions will be protected time and attendance is expected for those required.

Creating the 'team forest': A safe place to stand

Our PTOL approach was originally adapted from the work of Kis-Sines and Pluznick (2014) and developed through use with community-based staff teams. An adaptation of the approach for acute psychiatric wards has also been piloted as described in Box 11.5. The PTOL is a structured intervention delivered in a group format over at least two sessions. The sessions are always facilitated by at least two facilitators (with experience of Tree of Life approach and group work); this enables both the process and content of the group can be attended to. A broad outline of the two-session PTOL is shown in Box 11.2.

BOX 11.2: PTOL workshop overview

Session 1 – Drawing the trees and creating the 'team forest'

- *Introduction*
  - Introduction to the approach
  - Warming the context: what are some of your favourite trees? What meaning does this hold?
  - Establishing ground rules
  - Facilitators share their own PTOL and explain the different parts of the tree

- *Drawing the trees*
  - Each person draws their own individual PTOL

- *Retelling of stories*
  - Each individual given opportunity to share their tree with the group (sharing in smaller groups/pairs if needed)
  - Trees are displayed on a wall to create the 'team forest'
  - Participants serve as outsider witnesses for each other by noting something that stood out for them during each presentation and writing these on the trees.

- *Team forest: Collective retelling*

  Facilitators reflect on the following themes:
  - The strong and firm roots we all seem to have which have served as a foundation or preferred directions in our work and as team members

(Continued)

- The hopes and dreams we have for our service users, our work and our team
- The people who we are connected to who have taught us a lot of things
- The people who continue to support us in our work and life
- What is made possible in our work with services users and families by our experience of being a forest?

Session 2 – Responding to the 'storms'

- Welcome back and reconnect with the team forest.
- *Professional storms of life:* Facilitators ask the group to identify the storms, effects, and response to the storms

  - What are some of the storms that we face in our daily work?
  - What are some of the effects of these storms on your work, team, and life?
  - Are their ways you respond to these storms that help you to hold on to preferred directions in your work/life?
  - How does the team help you to respond in these preferred ways?
  - When you respond to storms in preferred ways, what difference does this make in the lives of service users and families? To your experience as a mental health professional?

- Identify action plan for implementing 'preferred responses' and agree review date with facilitator
- *Endings*: certificates to be written in pairs/small groups and presented in wider group
- Final reflections and evaluation questionnaires.

The initial session starts with 'warming the context' by everyone introducing themselves as their favourite tree. We find it helpful as facilitators to make reference to our own professional trees (which we prepare in advance) when explaining what the different parts of the tree represent.

Box 11.3: Handout for staff on parts of the PTOL

Questions to guide telling the preferred stories about our professional identity

Fruits and flowers: Contributions from and to others

- What has the team and others contributed to your development?
- What does the team most appreciate about your skills and knowledge?
- What would they say you have contributed to their work?

Branches of the tree: Hopes and dreams

- What are your hopes and dreams for the people you work with? For the work you do? For the team?
- What are some of the next steps in your career?

Leaves of the tree: Important people

- Who supports you in the work you do (past and present)?

The ground: The now

- How long have you been with this team?
- What is your role within the team?
- What values and commitments of the team are most meaningful to you? Why?
- How does this 'fit' with your preferred directions/values for your work?

Trunk of the tree: The skills you bring

- What skills and knowledge do you bring to your work with the team?
- What is the history of these skills and knowledge?
- Who in your life first noticed these skills and knowledge? Can you tell us a story about how it might have been visible to them?
- Who on the team is most aware that you have these skills? Is there an example of a time when these skills and knowledge would be most evident to that person?

Roots of the tree: Where you are coming from

- What brought you to this work?
- Who and what inspired or influenced you? It might be a person, an event, or something else.

Then we invite each participant to draw a 'professional tree' (refer to Box 11.3 for a handout of the parts of the tree which guide staff through the process) which is followed by the 'telling'. During the telling, participants share aspects of their preferred story they wish to highlight. In our experience, sharing the tree in the wider group helps to foster a greater sense of team cohesion and connection with shared values. However, as mentioned earlier, if the group is too large or there are other reasons for doing so, the trees can be shared in pairs or smaller groups. Regardless of the format, it is important for the sharing to be completed by all participants in the initial session so that the 'team forest' can be established ahead of the 'storms' session.

During the sharing, we invite those listening to act as outsider witnesses. This links a key principle of narrative therapy that 'a story told is a story lived, and a story lived is a story told' (Morgan, 2000). Once everyone has shared their stories, participants 'plant their tree in the forest', which is done symbolically by physically displaying the trees on a wall. This 'team forest' is the safe place to stand, or 'riverbank' position from which the difficulties, or 'storms' can be explored (Ncube-Millo and Denborough, 2007).

Following this, participants are given an opportunity to admire the 'team forest' and read over the trees, particularly if they have not had the chance to share in the wider group. Reflecting on their experience of outsider witnessing, participants are encouraged to write something that stood out for them on post-it notes, which are placed on the trees. An adaptation would be to invite participants to add 'flowers' to the trees, that is what they thought others offered to the team, and highlighting what they value most about their colleagues' contribution to the team (Wonders and Lee, 2019). At this point, facilitators do the collective retelling in which they reflect on the shared themes from the trees and highlight the strengths of the team forest, as described in Box 11.1. We mark the end of the session by giving participants their trees so they can reflect on the messages, and end with a comment from each participant about what they will take away from the session.

Professional storms of life

> *The problem is the problem, the person is not the problem.* (White and Epston, 1990)

The second part of the PTOL workshop focuses on how the 'team forest' copes with the 'storms', that is the difficulties and challenges we face in their work.

It's vital to explore these difficulties safely, because some participants may discuss traumatic experiences. To establish this sense of safety, facilitators must spend time at the start of the session reconnecting the group to 'team forest'. This re-establishes the safe place to stand and helps to foster the emotional containment needed for self-reflection. It's helpful for facilitators to recap on the collective retelling from the first session, that is the shared values, strengths, skills, and future hopes. Generally, staff should only attend the second session if they have completed the first (this dilemma and others are discussed in Box 11.4).

As a starting point, we list all the storms first on a flip chart and collaboratively agree with the group which ones to prioritise in the session (which may link to the reasons the initial referral was made). We then explore the impact of the storms (the 'effects') and what are the helpful ways to cope ('preferred responses'). Our general preference is to discuss storms as a whole group although it can be done in smaller groups to save time (each group is allocated a storm to explore). When undertaken as a whole group, it is important that enough time has been given to identifying the preferred responses for that particular storm before moving onto the next one. Exploring the storms can be a time-consuming process and teams can easily get drawn back into the problem-saturated story of the storms. When the group feels a bit stuck in the 'problem', it can help to ask questions about the unique outcomes such as 'what helps to have a good day at work? … when is the storm of X less present? … has there been a time when the storm has been absent/or passed completely? … when do you feel most connected to your values at work/to colleagues/ to clients etc.' This begins to outdraw ideas regarding preferred responses and connect to the preferred narratives represented by the PTOL forest. We may also wish to draw upon the connections and knowledge that participants have about each other, for example, 'who in the team would notice that you were having a good day?' … 'were being less affected by the storm?'…. 'What would they notice you were doing differently?' … 'who in the team supports your ability to cope with/ respond to the storm?'.

Once all the storms have been discussed, we ask the team to generate some specific actions they would like to take forward to help them hold onto the preferred responses. As there is often a lot of ideas, we encourage the team to focus making some small changes initially. To support this, facilitators should arrange to check in with teams at a later date (ideally within 1–2 months), to explore how these responses are taking root within their day-to-day work. Within our pilot initiative, we found that this follow-up meeting helped teams take responsibility for making changes and implementing preferred responses. For example, one team set up weekly mindfulness sessions as a result of the facilitator following up on how they were implementing preferred responses.

Endings, certificates, and celebrations

As is the case for the Tree of Life approach, our PTOL framework draws upon the narrative therapy practice of 'definitional ceremonies' to mark the ending and acknowledge the work of the group. Definitional ceremonies encourage the retelling of alternative and preferred stories to those within our network, as a way to further strengthen these stories (White, 2000). Within the PTOL, the ending ceremony involves participants being presented with a certificate which links to the preferred story about their professional identity. The certificate names the person's professional skills, strengths, and abilities; their future hopes; and the special people that have contributed to their professional life. There are different ways to complete the certificates although based on our experiences, the most effective way is for this to be done in pairs or groups of three. Once completed, participants present certificates to each other within the wider group. Facilitators then bring the session to a close, thanking everyone for their contribution and ensuring that no one has been negatively affected by the storms discussion.

Box 11.4: PTOL practice considerations, dilemmas, and reflections

- Adapting the model for large teams: our standard PTOL approach poses some challenges for larger teams (more than 20 participants). One solution is to split the team into two separate groups (with each group undertaking the two part workshop). There would then be some attempt to share to the whole team the themes from the 'forests' and preferred responses to the storms.
- Staff attendance: One common challenge is ensuring all team members attend and addressing significant absences, such as team leaders or consultants. Another dilemma is whether to include staff in the storms session if they didn't attend the first session. While our general rule is that staff are required to attend both, there may be times when exceptions have to be made. Facilitators need to consider how to ensure these staff who only attend the storms session feel

(Continued)

part of the 'team forest' (e.g. drawing a PTOL to bring to the storms session).
- Virtual versus in person sessions: While there are advantages to running the session online in terms of accessibility*, it makes several key aspects of the approach more challenging, such as creating/admiring the forest, participants being able to acknowledge each other's trees and facilitators being able to fully observe and connect with the group processes.
- Attending to therapeutic group processes: while adherence to the structure of the PTOL is important, underpinning the main task are the therapeutic processes inherent in group work which facilitators should closely attend to (Yalom, 1993). This includes attuning to the emotional temperature of the group, being aware of how each person is participating, noticing and responding to any resistance or challenging behaviour. For this reason it is essential that the workshops are run by two facilitators with the requisite clinical experience.

*At the time of writing (March 2022), NHS settings still required staff to socially distance.

Box 11.5: Case study: Inpatient mental health teams. Dr Claire McDonald

Inpatient psychiatric wards can be exceptionally challenging environments for staff and patients. Staff regularly experience difficult interactions with service users, increased risk of physical assault, low pay, and a lack of positive feedback. Research has highlighted the positive effects team-building interventions can have within healthcare settings, including improvements in team cohesion, staff interactions, and teamwork skills; however, pressures associated with mental healthcare can make inpatient wards difficult contexts to implement staff-based interventions. The present author and Dr Jessica Townsend (who was a psychologist in clinical training in the service at the time) designed, delivered, and evaluated a brief, stand-alone session for staff

(Continued)

to help foster connectedness and wellbeing within the team through co-development of a 'Team Tree'. We used a mixed-methods approach to evaluate feasibility, acceptability, and staff experiences of the session with 46 multidisciplinary staff (33 females; 13 males), across four acute wards. Some of our (unpublished) results included that the protocol developed was feasible to deliver to staff in under 90 minutes. Over 85% of staff found the session enjoyable, worthwhile and interesting. Quantitative results revealed statistically significant improvements in measures of self-reported mental wellbeing, team cohesiveness, and perceived social support following the session. Staff described the groups as a team-building experience and enjoyed the tree metaphor, sharing thoughts and discussing their teams' strengths, skills, and values.

"Very interesting and helpful."
"Team-building at its best."
"Beautiful."
"Reminds us of what we do well."

Each team consequently hung up their Team Tree in a staff area and some felt that they could use the tree going forward as a reminder of their teams' qualities.

Box 11.6: Case study: Using the PTOL in acute physical health hospital settings. Dr Amanda Mwale

Staff within physical health settings have experienced tremendous challenges, public scrutiny, pressure, and stress as a result of the COVID-19 pandemic. Supporting staff members to voice their distress and find ways of alleviating this in safe places has been an integral part of assisting them. Throughout the pandemic, staff have reported changes to their motivation and sense of purpose. In an attempt to address this, we used the PTOL to support staff who work in acute physical healthcare within both inpatient and outpatient teams.

The aim of engaging in the PTOL for staff within physical health settings is to encourage a team to participate in recognising who they

(Continued)

are as individuals and how much stronger they stand as a team which can be represented by the metaphor of the Forest of Life. Due to staffing challenges and limited time, the way in which team sessions are set up can vary widely, therefore it is important to seek feedback after sessions to understand the impact. This can then also be shared with managers and leaders who can offer more time and resources if required. Staff that included nurses and allied health professionals were offered the opportunity to produce individual trees that contributed to a forest, and for other teams with less time available, staff produced a collective team tree that represented a shared identity, experiences, hopes, and values. The PTOL has generally been well received and more specific feedback is offered below.

Experiences of the PTOL in physical health settings included the following formats:

Collective team tree. Twenty-nine participants working in small groups, with each working on one section of the tree (e.g. 'team's roots'; 'team's branches') before sharing the larger group.

"The session will affect us in a good way by being reminded to be kind/compassionate to ourselves and each other."

"The session will improve team closeness; improve our ability to empathise with colleagues; Make me appreciate the skills I can bring to the team."

Individual Tree Drawing, then using the Forest Metaphor to reflect as a team; between 6 and 12 participants

"What was useful was, the reflection on our careers and the team; the creative tree drawing; leaving positive comments about colleagues."

"I didn't really realise how much I needed this! I feel so much better about myself and my profession."

The use of the PTOL has allowed for staff to return to their 'Island of safety' in recognising the neglected and subjugated stories that affirm their identities. Being able to engage in this exercise has brought about a reconnection to their values, strengths, relationships, and hopes in a way that allowed them to think creatively about how they can move forwards in responding to the 'storms' presented by the ongoing impact of the pandemic.

Conclusion

The PTOL approach encourages us as staff to reflect on our relationship to work, the professional identities we share and co-create at work, and how we contribute to each other's working lives, the team, and the services. The stories gathered from a PTOL exercise can help teams to remember and reconnect to the values that brought them to the work, the individual skills and strengths of each team member, and the team as a whole. We argue that these are the stories that should continue to be told, strengthened, and privileged about people and teams in the NHS. The NHS and its staff are not only defined by narratives about waiting lists, under-resourced services, and too much paperwork, but by the people working in it every day and their positive stories about their work and each other. The PTOL uses the powerful metaphor of the tree and its forest to embody the statement 'we are greater than the sum of our parts' (Aristotle) or like trees in a forest we are stronger in a forest, and we stand together and support each other.

References

Bateson, G. (1972). Steps to an *Ecology of mind*. San Francisco, CA: Chandler Publishing Company.

Bateson, G. (1979). *Mind and nature: A necessary unity*. New York: E.P. Dutton.

Bertrando, P. & Gilli, G. (2010). Theories of change and the practice of systemic supervision, in Burck, C. & Daniel, G. (eds.) *Mirrors and reflections processes of systemic supervision*. London, Karnac, 3–22.

Boston, P. (2010). The three faces of supervision: Individual learning, group learning, and supervisor accountability', in Burck, C. & Daniel, G. (eds.) *Mirrors and reflections processes of systemic supervision*. London, Karnac, 27–46.

Boyd, E. (2010). "Voice entitlement" narratives in supervision: Cultural and gendered influences on speaking and dilemmas in practice, in Burck, C. & Daniel, G. (eds.) *Mirrors and reflections processes of systemic supervision*. London, Karnac, 203–224.

Burnham, J. (2005). Relational reflexivity: A tool for socially constructing therapeutic relationships, in Flaskas, C., Mason, B. & Perlesz, A. (eds.) *The space between: Experience, context and process in the therapeutic relationship*. London: Karnac, 1–18.

Burnham, J. (2010). Creating reflexive relationships between practices of systemic supervision and theories of learning and education, in Burck, C. & Daniel, G. (eds.) *Mirrors and reflections: Processes of systemic supervision*. New York, Routledge, 49–79.

Burnham, J. (2012). Developments in social GRRRAAACCEEESSS: Visible-invisible and voiced-unvoiced, in Krause, I. B. (ed.) *Culture and reflexivity in systemic psychotherapy: Mutual perspectives*. London, Karnac, 139–162.

Byng-Hall, J. (1995). Creating a secure family base: Some implications of attachment theory for family therapy, *Family Process*, 34, 45–58.

Denborough, D. (2014). *Retelling the stories of our lives*. New York: Norton, 121–143.

Dreyfus, L. H. & Dreyfus, E. S. (1986). *Mind over machine*. New York: The Free Press, 16–31.

Epston, D. (1994). Extending the Conversation, *Family Therapy Networker*, 18, 31–36.

Fredman, G. (2007). Preparing our selves for the therapeutic relationship: Revisiting "hypothesizing revisited", *Human Systems: The Journal of Systemic Consultation & Management*, 18, 44–59.

Harré, R. & Van Langenhove, L. (eds.). (1999). *Positioning theory: Moral contexts of intentional action*. Malden, MA: Blackwell.

Jordan, M. & Hinds, J. (2016). *Ecotherapy; theory, research and practice*. Dublin: Palgrave.

Kis-Sines and Pluznic (date unknown). Tree of life: Questions about professional identity for child and youth workers. Available at: https://dulwichcentre.com.au/wn npcontent/uploa ds/2014/01/tree-of-life-professional-identity.pdf.

Kolb, D. A. (1984). *Experiential learning*. Hoboken, NJ: Prentice Hall.

Krause, I. B. (2018). *Culture and reflexivity in systemic psychotherapy: Mutual perspectives*. London, Routledge.

Lang, P. (2000). *Personal communication. KCC workshop*. Available at: https://peterlangsystem iccommunity.com.

Liddle, H. A. & Saba, G. S. (1983). On context replication: The isomorphic relationship of training and therapy, *Journal of Strategic and Systemic Therapies*, 2, 3–11.

Mason, B. (1993). Towards positions of safe uncertainty, *Human Systems: The Journal of Systemic Consultation and Management*, 4, 189–200.

Mason, B. (2011). Supervising and the training context: Some thoughts and ideas about the ownership of knowledge in practice, *Context*, 116, 2–4.

Mason, B. (2013). Towards a culture of contribution supervision practice: Some thoughts about the position of the supervisor, in Burck, C., Barrett, S. & Kavner, E. (eds.) *Positions and polarities in contemporary systemic practice: The legacy of David Campbell*. London: Karnac, 107–126.

Mason, B. (2019). Re-visiting safe uncertainty: Six perspectives for clinical practice and the assessment of risk, *Journal of Family Therapy*, 41(3), 43–356.

McCarthy, I. (2004). The fifth province and spirituality: Co-creating a sacred space of love in therapy conversations, in Madigan, S. (ed.) *Therapy from the inside out*. Vancouver: Yaletown Family Therapy Press, 1–16.

Mckay, B. (2014). Making the most of multiple opportunities in group supervision: Using systemic and narrative practices to bring forth skilled clinical practice, in Lim, C. & Sim, E. (eds.) *Clinical supervision*. Singapore: Counselling and Care Centre, 98–115.

Morgan, A. (2000). *What is narrative therapy? An easy-to-read introduction*. Adelaide, South Australia: Dulwich Centre Publications.

Myherhoff, B. (2007). *Stories as equipment for living*. Ann Arbor, MI: The University of Michigan Press.

NHS. (2019). NHS long term plan. http://www.longtermplan.nhs.uk.

Ncube, N. (2006). The tree of life project, *International Journal of Narrative Therapy & Community Work*, 1, 3–16.

Ncube-Millo, N. & Denborough, D. (2007). *Tree of life – Mainstreaming psychosocial care and support: A manual for facilitators*. Randburg: REPSSI.

Reder, P. & Fredman, G. (1996). The relationship to help: Interacting beliefs about the treatment process, *Clinical Child Psychology and Psychiatry*, 1(3), 457–467.

Rober, P., Elliott, R., Buysse, A., Loots, G. & De Corte, K. (2008). Positioning in the therapist's inner conversation: A dialogical model based on a grounded theory analysis of therapist reflections, *Journal of Marital and Family Therapy*, 34(3), 406–421.

Schön, D. (1987). *Educating the reflective practitioner*. San Francisco, CA: Josey Bass.

Spencer, S. (2019). *Think like a tree*. Great Britain: Swarkestone Press.
White, M. (2000). *Reflections on narrative practice*. Adelaide, South Australia: Dulwich Centre Publications.
White, M. & Epston, D. (1989). *Narrative means to therapeutic ends*. New York: Norton.
Wilson, J. (1993). The supervisory relationship in family therapy training, *Human Systems: The Journal of Systemic Management and Consultation*, 4, 173–178.
Wohleben, P. (2017). *Hidden life of trees*. London: William Collins.
Wonders, S. & Lee, C. (2019). Exploring roots and fruit: Using the "tree of life" to help teams manage change, *Clinical Psychology Forum*, 315, 22–26.
Yalom, I. (1983). *Inpatient group psychotherapy*. New York: Basic Books.

12 The Heads and Hearts Model of Reflective Practice

Dr Arabella Kurtz and Dr Joanna Levene

> *Well I really do think that in order to live, in order to continue living, we have to have hope. What is hope? It is kind of the place of the future, it's the idea that you can move there, and that you will be able to move there.*
>
> – SIRI HUSTVEDT IN CONVERSATION WITH RAZIA IQBAL, THE HAY FESTIVAL, NOVEMBER 2021

In this chapter we present the Heads and Hearts Model of reflective practice groups, condensing and bringing the up to date material in Dr Arabella Kurtz's book *How to Run Reflective Practice Groups: A Guide for Healthcare Professionals* (Kurtz, 2020). Joanna Levene provides an extended example of a reflective practice session, showing the model in use with staff working in an acute medical setting in the wake of an unusual and very distressing event. We also consider how to adapt the approach for short runs of reflective practice, anything from one-offs to sets of two or three sessions, which we are increasingly being asked to provide.

It has been a great privilege and a pleasure facilitating reflective practice groups for healthcare colleagues over many years, learning about work full of human interest and variety, and sharing in moments of pain, confusion, clarity, pride, and joy. During the coronavirus pandemic in 2020 and 2021, we have witnessed intense distress and fear, as well as a strength of feeling about the value of clinical and care work and the importance of team support. We have found that reflective practice groups have helped us remain hopeful while facing up to difficulties, allowing a depth of engagement with the rich experience of our work, in all its colours, and keeping us grounded in a sense of purpose and professional identity. We have come to think of realistic hopefulness as one of the benefits of reflective practice.

Reflective practice: Its origins and current context

Reflective practice involves bringing emotion and intellect together in thinking about our work, and in developing skills and capacities. Reflective practice in groups draws on the resources and talents of a number of unique individuals, and thereby has the potential to build solidarity and support between colleagues with diverse experiences. Indeed, a diversity of backgrounds and viewpoints is definitely a positive in reflective practice, widening the range of resources – emotional, sociocultural, intellectual – available to the group. Reflective practice is also a useful way of reducing mistakes, highlighting and helping members think their way through areas of confusion and concern, as long as they feel safe enough to bring their work in the round, rather than an airbrushed version.

There has been enormous interest in reflective practice in health and social care in recent years, even more so since recognition of the vital importance of supporting staff in these sectors brought about by the coronavirus pandemic. But reflective practice is not new. Classical philosophy, and the Socratic approach to dialogue, teaches us to question the assumption on which inquiry is based, instead of marching ahead to answer a set of predefined questions. It holds that if we are too focused on the outcomes we want to achieve from the outset, we will be constrained in our thinking and limited in what we learn. We need to be ready to question the foundations of what we think we know.

The early twentieth-century phenomenological tradition in philosophy is another profound influence, and specifically the view that an open engagement with experience – the messy, complex, and surprising business of living as opposed to abstract ideas about it – is intrinsic to the learning process. It also grounds reflective practice in subjective experience, reminding us that we are individual beings who perceive and come to know the world through minds and bodies bound in space and time, and within particular biological, psychological, and social contexts.

Donald Schon, writing in the early 1980s, was the first person to coin the phrase 'reflective practice'. In his book *The Reflective Practitioner* he made the case for the reintegration of intuition and reflexivity into professional practice, which had been squeezed out by a narrow focus on technological expertise. He argued for the introduction of a form of creative and outside-the-box thinking about individual cases, to counter the dominance of standardised approaches (Schon, 1983). Schon described how reflection-on-action, meaning a kind of problem-solving based on close retrospective attention to specific work experiences and the use of diverse thinking and creative methods to understand them, leads to reflection-in-action, and an enhanced capacity to tailor practice to here-and-now work with the individual case. For clinicians, Schon brought together the art and the science in what we do.

The growing demand for reflective practice groups in healthcare is also partly the result of an increase in mental health awareness, making it possible for staff to be more vocal about the human and relational aspects of their work. But the situation is a complex one. On the one hand, there is a great deal of talk about the need for compassionate cultures of care, and about reflective practice as a means to achieve these. On the other, our modern healthcare organisations have never been less compassionate. They have been based since the 1980s on a target-driven hard business model, and heavily impacted more recently by the politics of austerity. In the UK, there are chronic staff shortages and colleagues are overworked and underpaid, and regularly report worrying levels of bullying and discrimination (West, 2021).

What this means is that those of us setting up and running reflective practice groups are working, to some extent, against the grain of modern healthcare systems. We operate in a context in which there is a high degree of organisational ambivalence towards reflective practice, and individual staff may not be consciously aware of this.

Development of the Heads and Hearts Model

Arabella developed the Heads and Hearts Model of group reflective practice (originally the Intersubjective Model) in response to requests from facilitators attending training courses. Imposter syndrome turned out to be rife in the reflective practice field. Colleagues thought they should simply know how to facilitate groups, despite never having been taught or shown. They were often afraid to ask for help or let anyone know how unsure they felt. Many had limited experience of attending a reflective practice group themselves or had not had a good experience if they had done so. The most common reason for this was a lack of clarity of purpose in the group, and the potential for it to become too personal and lose a work focus. A key aim, therefore, in presenting the Heads and Hearts Model, is to demystify reflective practice: to be explicit about its aims and approach so that colleagues have a solid basis for developing their work.

There are already a number of models of reflective learning available, all of which describe a three-stage progression from the description of experience, to analysis or critical reflection on it, to application or learning output (Stedmon

& Dallos, 2009). The Heads and Hearts Model is similarly based on a reflective learning cycle, with the aim of bringing relational thinking into increasingly marketised health and care systems. The model embodies recognition of the need to be our whole selves in healthcare and to have space to process emotional responses to our work. It is intended to bring together the intellectual and emotional aspects of practice, connecting our heads and our hearts as healthcare practitioners.

The model's theoretical bases are psychodynamic and systemic. The model is psychodynamic in its focus on emotional containment and interpersonal processes, including, where possible, exploration of previously warded off, unacknowledged and unconscious feelings. It is systemic in the value placed on attending to and developing organisational support. The model also draws on the psychoanalytic theory of organisations, and particularly Menzies Lyth's concept of the social defence system, with its dual emphasis on opening up thinking about practice at ground level and working at the same time to remove constraints on the direct care of patients in organisational processes and procedures (Armstrong & Rustin, 2017; Menzies Lyth, 1960).

Relevant research has also shaped its development and is fully reviewed in Arabella's book (Kurtz, 2020). Key influences include:

- Research on the impact of stress and trauma on the human mind and body, and in particular on the capacity to resolve knotty problems and empathise with others (van der Kolk, 2014)
- Evidence of the importance of organisational support in determining the effectiveness of reflective practice in improving clinical practice (White & Winstanley, 2010)
- Studies showing the importance of the quality of the supervisory relationship in determining colleagues' experience of learning at work, and whether they feel safe enough to talk openly about real issues of concern and confusion in their practice (Beinart & Clohessy, 2017; Ladany et al, 1996).

Overview of the eight stages of the Heads and Hearts Model

The Heads and Hearts Model consists of a series of eight stages, which represent the key ingredients of group reflective practice. They are shown in Figure 12.1 as

The Heads and Hearts Model of Reflective Practice

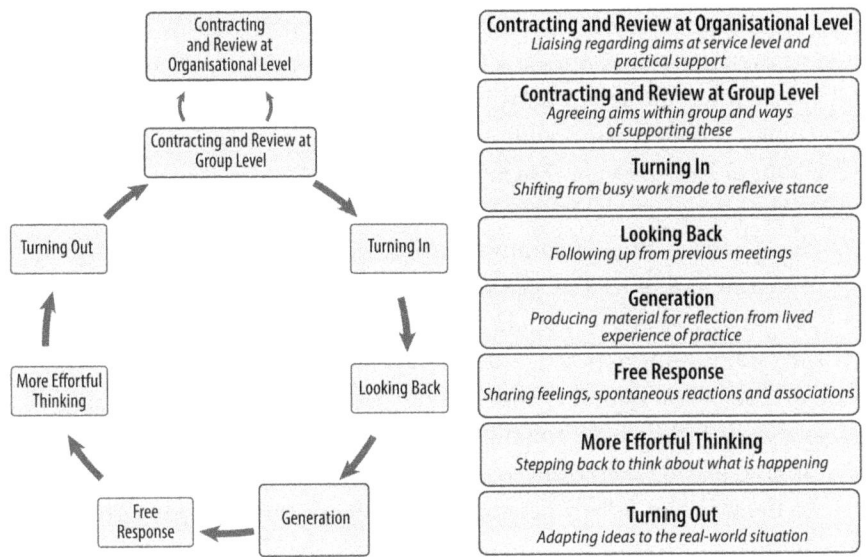

FIGURE 12.1: Diagram of the Heads and Hearts Model.

a single reflective practice group, which shows the structure and flow of a session. The stages do not necessarily need to be carried out in a set order every time the group meets; rather, the facilitator should feel free to introduce the various elements to a greater or lesser degree, depending on the needs of the group and their own style. The three core elements of the model are creation of a space for sharing lived experience of practice with colleagues, an opening-up space for the group to respond in a free and human way, and a gathering-together space for more concerted meaning-making. These correspond to the Generation, Free Response and More Effortful Thinking Stages described below.

We will now take you through the eight stages of the model, describing what the aim is from the facilitator's point of view and typical dilemmas and practice points.

Stage 1. Contracting and Review at the Organisational Level

This stage involves gathering information about the wider context for a request for reflective practice, and giving feedback at the service level about the work as it progresses. This includes liaising with senior staff to understand what the group is for and discussing the practicalities of setting it up, and keeping them in the loop about developments. This stage allows ambivalence towards reflective practice at the service level to be addressed and made part of the work, rather than trying to pretend it does not exist and having difficulties later as a result. This can happen when the group finds itself trying to operate without management support, or defining its aims without reference to the service context.

The aims at this stage are threefold:

- To open a channel of communication with managers to maximise their investment in reflective practice and support for it
- To educate senior colleagues about the value of reflective practice and its impact on clinical practice and staff wellbeing
- To discuss the resources and support needed for such a group, such as the need for a private room and the organisation of rotas so staff can attend, getting help from senior colleagues where possible and facing up to the fact that sometimes conditions are not sufficient for a group to go ahead.

Before starting a reflective practice group the facilitator is advised to discuss aims with service heads, getting a sense of what they want out of the group and establishing whether this is realistic. Sometimes these groups are idealised and seen as a way of magically getting rid of problems, and it is helpful to manage expectations from the start. It is also useful to give time to troubleshoot together, thinking about barriers to the smooth running of the group and sharing in resolving these.

This work on organisational contracting happens at the start, and going forwards at review points there should be feedback to service heads, involving them in the work and sharing responsibility for its support. Group members should decide together what to let managers know about, and communicate this in general and thematic terms, ensuring that it is not possible to identify any individual group member or person spoken about. The facilitator should make sure members feel they have ownership of this process, and that they are involved in thinking about when and how to give feedback to service heads on the work of the group.

Stage 2. Contracting and Review at the Group Level

During this stage, members of the group agree on what arrangements are needed within the group to support the work. This should be preceded by development of a shared understanding of the group's purpose, so plans are considered in relation to the task rather than in the abstract. It covers issues such as where and when the group meets and for how long, who is in the group, how to maximise stability of membership, and how to make the group feel safe enough for people to be open about real issues and dilemmas. Our research suggests that the concept of 'good enough safety' rather than absolute safety, adapted from Winnicott's reassuring notion of the 'good enough parent', is helpful here. Complete safety is neither realistic or possible, and learning at the edge of what is already known necessitates taking some risks (Biggins, 2019; Winnicott, 1973).

In our experience, discussion of contractual issues can often be unhelpfully brief or staff can get bogged down at this stage in trying to deal with every last thing which could possibly go wrong. Therefore, a key task of the facilitator is to help staff think sensibly about issues that are likely to come up without allowing the group to get overtaken by anxiety. We suggest a brief initial discussion (say 10–20 minutes in a first meeting), followed by a further conversation a few meetings in so arrangements can be reviewed in the light of experiences of working together, and regular reviews after that – say once every six meetings. A brief written contract should be shared after the initial review, and ideally this is produced by one of the group members and not the facilitator. Table 12.1 lists the main issues for consideration by the group at this stage.

Stage 3. Turning In

The Turning In Stage involves the transition from a busy, pressured work mode to a reflective one, which can be difficult when staff are working in stressful environments. Research into the biology of stress helps us understand why the shift can be difficult to make and also why it is important to do so, since the parts of the brain which mediate empathic responses, and which allow for linguistic communication and higher-level emotional processing, are deactivated under stress. Continuous stress is bad for anybody, but it is a particular problem for those involved in the work of caring for others. In addition, colleagues may understandably be anxious about opening up in front of each other. The task for the facilitator is to strike a balance between acknowledging that it might feel difficult to enter an open, reflective space and remaining firm in the value of doing so.

Sometimes staff in a reflective practice group are taken up with pressing external concerns, whether these are to do with what is going on in the service or their lives outside work, and do not manage to leave these behind. It can be

TABLE 12.1: Group contracting issues and summary of advice.

Contractual issue	Summary of advice	Points for consideration
Confidentiality for clients and discretion for professional colleagues	Material identifying clients should be taken out or changed; where possible identities of staff should be protected and discretion about professional matters encouraged	Is material being spoken about in front of people outside the clinical service, in which case confidentiality of patients should be ensured? Are issues regarding colleagues processed in a respectful and productive way?
Confidentiality for group members	The detail of what is discussed in the group should be kept in the group; communication outside the group, for example when feeding back to managers, should be thematic and general	Group members can find it hard to talk about safety within the group, so check on this at review points
Management of boundaries: when a safeguarding or performance issue needs to be raised outside the group	Talk this through with a supervisor or trusted colleague before acting; let the group know what is happening, discuss the issue separately with the group member concerned, lodge the issue with the relevant colleague and reinstate the group's boundaries as before	Is the issue sufficiently concerning to merit external consideration?
Stability of membership	Attendance should be voluntary with an expectation of regular and consistent attendance	The more stable the membership the better, but if staff cannot attend every time, specify minimum expectation of attendance and consider sharing thematic notes after sessions within specified group to develop a sense of belonging
Group membership	It is often best to separate managers and ground-level staff into different groups, although if they feel safe together reflective practice can then develop at the service level	Things can change over time and it is a sign of progress at the service level if managers and staff feel comfortable working together in a group when they did not previously

(Continued)

TABLE 12.1 (Continued): Group contracting issues and summary of advice.

Contractual issue	Summary of advice	Points for consideration
Length of each group session	1 hr minimum, 1.5 hr ideal (less than this can work if the group meets more often than monthly)	Is the time allocated long enough? If not consider meeting more frequently, or less often and for longer
Length of group overall	Reviews should be at least six monthly; arrange to meet initially for a year with plan for either an open-ended group afterwards or group for a finite period of 2–3 years	Is it best to set up an open-ended group or a time-limited one? Don't jump into offering an open-ended group too soon but base your decision on the resources available and the motivation of staff
Where will the group meet?	Regular use of a room that is set apart from a busy clinical environment is a basic requirement; a quiet, comfortable, and spacious room is ideal	Do consider rearranging the furniture so group members are as comfortable as possible
External/internal facilitation	External facilitation is usually best but if this is not possible the facilitator should (a) be someone removed from the day-to-day work of group members (e.g. by facilitators swapping to run groups across services), (b) and/or have access to supervision to help them keep in role	Has the facilitator, external or internal, got the support they need? An external facilitator will need good links with the service and the support of managers; an internal facilitator needs access to supervision to help them keep in role
Written record	It is best for the responsibility for a written record to be rotated among members, to describe discussions thematically rather than in detail, and to be kept for a year and then destroyed	What is the purpose of any written record? If it is to inform reviews and feedback to managers, it does not need to be kept beyond a year; remind members to destroy notes if they have been circulated during the year

tempting for a facilitator to go along with this state of preoccupation, particularly if they are internal to the organisation and share in the concerns. But if the group gets taken over by them for too long or too often, members can become frustrated and feel that they are missing out.

Techniques for enabling the transition to a reflective mode include:

- Moving straight into a focus on reflective practice, which tends to be easier when the facilitator is external and/or the group is well established

- Short mindfulness exercise, which is a popular approach but does not enable exploration of connections between external concerns and what is then brought to the group
- A systematic check-in, in which each member (including the facilitator) says something about how they are before starting the group
- A more general, informal check-in, in which the facilitator asks how people are, and members then contribute on the basis of want or need, but do not go round the group one by one.

The latter technique is the one we favour, since a systematic check-in can take too long and there is a risk of the group getting taken over by external issues without some selection of what is helpful to share.

Stage 4. Looking Back

This stage is when the group finds space for ripple effects, inquiring about thoughts and feelings which may have come up in response to the discussion last time, and allowing space for follow-up and follow-through. It often has a particular value for the person who shared material last time, giving them space to respond when they have had time to process the discussion and test ideas out in practice. It should be possible to bring afterthoughts from the last meeting, or from meetings before that, because afterthoughts come at their own time and pace.

This stage is easy to miss out, but it is a particularly important one. It aims to model and support the process of learning in a group over time, and to check the powerful and quite unrealistic impulse towards rapid and complete mastery of complex conundrums and emotionally impactful human situations. Facilitators have often spoken to me about the pressure they feel to come up with a solution in reflective practice, even when what is being shared is unfamiliar and complicated. Indeed, reflective practice groups can feel an enormous and unhelpful pressure to 'get on top' of a difficult or anxiety-provoking situation, rather than to move through it together, building a solid understanding of what is going on, even if this understanding is incomplete.

This pressure towards over-quick mastery has been particularly strong in the face of the out-of-control situation of a global pandemic. It is natural for us to react by trying to control the uncontrollable, and by seeking mastery – or the illusion of mastery – of the situation, whether realistic or not. This is what we might think of as a manic response to challenge. In the face of such a response, it is very helpful to have spaces and structures which support us in working at genuine solutions, such as the provision of regular reflective practice, which over time offers a growing and realistic sense of competence and control, instead of something which feels forced and empty.

The Looking Back Stage can be included as a brief, routine review of afterthoughts from the previous meeting. It is useful to have such a check, but it is also helpful for the facilitator to be flexible about allowing time to go over a difficult area as and when this comes up, if this does not push something else out of the way.

Stage 5. Generation

This stage involves the generation of material from lived experience of healthcare practice, usually by one member, for the consideration of the group as a whole. It is called the Generation Stage to draw attention to the choices we make in what we bring as material for reflective practice. It is deliberately not called the presentation stage to get away from the anxiety about performance associated with the idea of a presentation for work.

It works best if material is brought to reflective practice in a way that fits with its aims of developing thinking about clinical dilemmas by drawing on the intellectual, human and creative resources of the group, and through the exploration of feelings and experiences of relationships on the ground. The facilitator should encourage members to bring material that is as rich and detailed as possible, moving away from abstract description, technical language, and diagnostic labels, and with a focus on human interest and the experience of relationships in the clinical situation.

Some groups respond quickly to this invitation; others take longer to make the shift away from the usual professional discourse. We usually ask what the person generating material would like from the group before they begin to share and try to bring this back in at the More Effortful Thinking and Turning Out Stages. The generator can be encouraged to bring observations about interactions between themselves and the client, and the detail of what they did and felt (even if surprised by this), rather than focusing exclusively on the client. There should be space to name and explore associative links, and reactions that do not make sense at first but may shed a light on something useful as thinking develops.

Now to a key point of technique. Reflective practice groups work best when what is shared is lived ground-level experience, as opposed to abstract or thematic description. The closer this is to real life the better, and the more individual voices can be heard the better too. We try to avoid groupthink. Working with material close to the immediacy of subjective experience enables a meaningful and creative engagement, bringing the diversity of individual minds into one space. So we encourage individual ownership of material at the Generation Stage and we steer groups away from thematic or topic-based discussion, or too much discussion of a shared experience, in which the assumption can be that everyone thinks and feels the same. If groups want to think about a shared experience – say a patient known to all – we show an interest in the different experiences members will have had of the same person or event, and encourage one member to go into depth.

Members should take it in turns to generate material for reflective practice in such a way that over time all members participate, but that as far as possible members can use the resources of the group when needed. The best way of doing this is for the group to organise a loose rota, so someone takes responsibility for generating material each time, but members can swap with each other if it makes sense to do so.

Stage 6. Free Response

In this stage the facilitator invites group members to connect with their more immediate and intuitive reactions to the material shared, to begin to explore emotional responses, and to think together 'outside the box', sharing links and associations. Creative approaches can be helpful now and in the More Effortful Thinking Stage, and are described in Arabella's book. At this point it is critically important to guard against groupthink and the idea of a right way to respond, ensuring that individuals feel able to share their own reactions and to be as much themselves as possible. This is easier said than done, and the facilitator will need to be patient and work to free people up over time. They will also need to be sensitive to the diversity of backgrounds and viewpoints among individuals in the group, taking careful note of who might need support in speaking. We try to do this in a gentle way, modelling curiosity in a range of different thoughts and feelings, including offering our own when helpful, rather than putting any one individual on the spot.

In an apparent paradox, being invited to respond in an open and spontaneous way can feel unexpectedly difficult, particularly early in the life of a group, because it involves giving up professional habits. These include the pressure to instruct or move prematurely to a problem-solving mode, and an over-reliance on technical language or abstract description as shorthand, thus closing down thinking about a problem. But there is good reason for working at freeing up responses in healthcare colleagues.

It is also common for groups to find it hard to share emotional reactions to the work, perhaps feeling that it is unprofessional and reflects badly on them to do so. Facilitators will need to communicate confidence in the rationale for doing this, helping the group to understand as well as acknowledge feelings where possible, and bringing the focus back to the work situation during the course of the session. The facilitator should also attend closely to feelings of trust and safety in the group, and the need for members to receive a sensitive and respectful response to opening up.

It is often helpful for the person who has generated material for the group to sit out during the Free Response and More Effortful Thinking Stages, using a popular technique from the systemic model of supervision. This brings about a transition from the Generation to the Free Response Stage, ensuring that the group does something with what they have heard, rather than going back to their colleague for more information. It also allows the person who has generated material to benefit from listening to the way others respond.

Stage 7. More Effortful Thinking

The More Effortful Thinking Stage is about stepping back from sharing material and the group's more immediate responses in order to develop a coherent understanding, however partial, of what is going on. The emphasis should be on working from the ground up and using ideas where they make sense of experience, rather than on the top-down and full application of a particular approach – although it may be helpful for groups to try the latter from time to time. Formulation is certainly part of what takes place at this stage, but the focus is on meaning-making, and on theory-practice links where they enhance this, rather than the systematic use of a model. Ideas from any of the healthcare disciplines may be drawn upon, as well as from outside usual professional discourses.

Facilitators sometimes need to help get a balance between the Free Response and More Effortful Thinking Stages. Groups often move into an abstract mode too quickly, before they have had the chance to explore the situation presented to them. On the other hand, they can find it difficult to step back from emotional reactions to the work and shift into a thinking mode. It is also helpful for facilitators to support groups in achieving a balance between ordering material too much or too little. A group may be overly focused on gaining mastery, trying to gain a systematic understanding of what is going on at the expense of making some sense of the lived experience of practice. Alternatively, it is sometimes hard to move discussion beyond a mass of competing ideas. Facilitators should welcome a period of sustained, deliberate thinking by the group but not expect it to last for the majority of the meeting.

A group will sometimes expect the facilitator to offer a finished formulation and provide the answer to whatever question has been posed. This can be flattering, but generally speaking it is best to avoid taking up the expert position too firmly, thereby creating unrealistic expectations regarding expertise and limiting the extent to which members develop understanding for themselves. This is a key point, as we have heard many times from facilitators who spend the group working away at 'an answer'. The facilitator's task is to support the growth of members' capacity to reflect on their practice, not to do it for them. We do this by showing curiosity in how various members of the group are thinking and feeling, inviting them to respond to each other, and drawing out the distinct contributions of each person.

Stage 8. Turning Out

The Turning Out Stage involves making a bridge between what has gone on inside the group, and the real-world conditions of practice which influence application, offering both constraints and possibilities. This is the point at which the person who generated material rejoins the group if they have been sitting out, and is invited to give feedback as to how useful they have found discussions. There is also space at this point for the group to think about how an idea can be adapted for use in the external context.

This stage exists to bring each meeting to an end and help members orient themselves to activities outside. There can be a pressure to wrap things up too completely at this point and present the group with an answer. A light touch is helpful, modelling for the group an ongoing process of reflection and discovery as members apply ideas from the group to experiences in practice.

The task for the facilitator is to give enough attention to this application stage without the group becoming overly focused on what to do. Detailed action planning is something to take to supervision, or discuss with colleagues outside; but it is useful to begin to sketch out some initial lines of application, so the transition from inside to outside the group is not overly abrupt.

An example of a reflective practice group session using the model

The context was a monthly reflective practice group with a palliative nursing team working across the community and in an acute hospital. This group had been facilitated by a clinical psychologist, Joanna, over a number of years, and while the structure and format had varied, the monthly meetings with the team had been constant. *Contracting and Review at the Organisational and Group Levels* had taken place a number of times over this period and group level contracting had recently been reviewed due to the change in format necessitated by COVID-19. Despite these changes, the long-standing nature of the group had created a shared understanding, which made the ensuing conversation possible.

This particular group session at the start of the COVID-19 pandemic was exceptional in its medium – the then unfamiliar videoconferencing – and in the fact that only two team members were present due to work pressures: 'Jenny' and 'Sophia'. The session had begun with the *Turning In Stage*, a check-in on wellbeing. This moved seamlessly into the *Looking Back Stage*, since the focus of the previous group meeting had been on the impact on the nursing team of continuing to provide a service to dying patients and families during the pandemic.

The team had been offering advice and support to hospital staff unfamiliar with caring for large numbers of dying patients. The *Generation Stage* was initiated by Jenny, who mentioned that she had 'had to throw my shoes away' the previous day. Joanna questioned this curious comment and a story of a death unfolded. Jenny had visited a dying cancer patient on an acute ward, accompanied by a student nurse who was shadowing her. Jenny noticed that the patient was bleeding and realised that she was witnessing the start of a catastrophic bleed due to a tumour-related ruptured artery. This is a rare event which a palliative care practitioner may witness a few times in a career and results in rapid and unpreventable death. Management focuses on communicating calmly to the patient what is happening and ensuring they are as comfortable as possible, which usually involves sedation. Jenny described how she and a palliative colleague also visiting the ward took control, as this situation was entirely unfamiliar to the ward staff. This involved attempting to stem the blood flow with pressure, sorting out medication for sedation and summoning the patient's relatives. They also reassured the surgical registrar who was proposing a surgical intervention, fearing that he had not done enough to help the patient. Jenny then ran down to the entrance of the hospital to meet and prepare the family, visitors only being allowed in exceptional circumstances due to COVID-19. She returned with the family, by which time the area had been cleaned, the patient covered and in the last moments of life, just in time for her relatives to say goodbye. On leaving the ward, the student nurse burst into tears, clearly very distressed by what she had witnessed. Jenny comforted the student, who then asked: 'Why are you so calm?'. This shook Jenny, leading her to question herself: 'Am I hardened to suffering? Should I feel bad or ashamed of this?' With Jenny's permission, we started to explore her actions and expectations of her role.

With only one other participant, the *Free Response Stage* was brief. Sophia acknowledged how hard it is to witness such an event. Joanna was struck by the strong imagery of Jenny's narrative, particularly recalling her initial comment about her shoes. Joanna shared her own feelings of shock at Jenny having been thrown into such a traumatic situation and being expected to remain calm and expertly take control.

This quickly led to a discussion, the *More Effortful Thinking Stage*, about values and purpose. We discussed how a surgical or medical setting aims to treat and maybe cure or prolong life, whereas palliative care has different aims: to improve quality of life and alleviate suffering. Within this frame, Sophia reminded Jenny that the patient had died without distress and the family had seen her looking peaceful and with time for goodbyes. Jenny had done her job well and should feel proud of herself. However, we acknowledged that 'proud' might seem a strange emotion. How could pride be an appropriate feeling in the face of something so awful and distressing? How could we hold two such different interpretations of the situation – one a picture of a traumatic bloodbath and the other an example of excellent end-of-life care? This led to a discussion of how values, role and purpose differ depending on context. Using reflective practice allowed us to balance thinking and emotion, holding in mind and integrating these ambiguities – bringing the head and heart together.

As our discussion concluded, we reached the *Turning Out Stage*, with Jenny deciding to check-in with the student nurse in order to normalise feelings of distress, share the contextual understanding of what had taken place and offer support from the team and Staff Support Service if required. This was also a reminder of the support available to all staff should Jenny, Sophia, or other colleagues require it.

Adaptation of the Heads and Hearts Model for short-term reflective practice in response to significant events

During the pandemic we have done a lot of work supporting teams, and adapted our facilitation of reflective practice groups to provide one-, two-, and three-off sessions. This is partly because we do not have the resources to provide ongoing reflective practice to all who ask for it. But we have also found that a discrete set of reflective sessions is often what colleagues want. They ask for help in response to a significant event or series of events, and it is often more possible for staff in a busy service to accommodate sessions on two or three afternoons than to make a regular commitment. We now distinguish between ongoing and regular reflective practice, which builds capacity and team resilience over time, and short-term and responsive reflective practice.

Inquiries about reflective sessions in response to a significant event often include a request for support for trauma processing, and it is important to be guided here by the research on psychological debriefing. This suggests the value of clearly distinguishing a reflective practice intervention from one focused on the prevention of trauma or the repetition of mistakes. The former is aimed at enhancing support and solidarity within a team, facilitating natural healing through shared meaning-making; the latter will focus on basic care of staff in the aftermath of an event, and at the appropriate time, a thorough consideration of what has happened and the lessons to be learned (see chapter 18 on psychological debriefs in this book).

In summary, we ensure that a few days have passed after a traumatic event before we attempt a reflective session. We also attend to arousal levels, making sure people feel as safe and comfortable as possible, and getting a balance between exploration of a difficult experience and discussion aimed at making sense and gaining perspective. For this reason, it can be helpful to pace discussions across a couple of sessions. But if facilitating a one-off we go gently, aiming for some sharing of experiences and meaning-making, rather than a systematic account of difficult events.

Generally we have found that the principles of the Heads and Hearts Model are helpful in guiding more focused work, combining attention to emotional responses and differences within a team, with the creation of shared meaning-making and solidarity. Advice regarding the adaptation of the stages of the model is presented in Table 12.2. The key points are as follows:

- Contracting is important, even in one-off reflective sessions
- Adapt the Generation Stage to balance breadth and depth in the material shared, focusing more on breadth than in ongoing reflective practice
- Give more time at the end for Turning Out, and provide closure by reviewing the experience of the group.

TABLE 12.2: Advice for adapting the Heads and Hearts Model for short-term reflective practice in response to significant events or experiences.

Stages in order of introduction in a one-off session	Adaptations for responsive reflective practice
Contracting at Organisational Level	Brief but still important to establish what is wanted by whom, so worth having that extra conversation
Turning In	Keep this short and integrate with contracting: avoid checking-in with everyone and ask how people are feeling before contracting with group
Contracting at Group Level	Combine listening to concerns with practical suggestions: talk about what people need to make good use of group and make suggestions where necessary and review experience at end
Looking Back	Miss out in one-off groups, include in two- or three-offs
Generation	Combine breadth and depth: give some time to the group as a whole if they have all been through something, but move to consider more in-depth experience from one to three members
Free Response and More Effortful Thinking	Focus on listening and responding to individuals and broaden out later: if relevant lightly bring in links with others' experiences towards end
Turning Out	Give more attention to this for closure: discuss how to make use of thinking in group and ask about takeaway in last session
Contracting at Organisational Level	Incorporated into Turning Out Stage; consider feedback to organisation if relevant: facilitator's focus should be on thinking about whatever action is taken rather than doing it themselves

Contracting at the organisational level will often be minimal before embarking on a time-limited reflective practice intervention, but initial conversations about what is wanted and by whom are still important. Beware of being asked to provide reflective practice on behalf of someone else: if possible try to speak directly to the people you will be working with, and establish that they actually want what you are offering. We have found that it is useful to think about any action or feedback to others outside the group at the Turning Out stage, to give closure to the experience.

It is easy to miss out the group contracting stage in a one-off meeting, associating it with more leisurely set-ups, but in a group which meets only a couple of times it is not possible to build safety and trust gradually and so it is necessary to talk explicitly about how to ensure 'good enough safety'. We do this by combining consideration of what the group wants with our own suggestions, keeping contractual discussions brief and returning to them at the end for review. We ask, 'What do we need to put into place to make it feel possible for people to talk as openly as possible, and make good use of the group today?' We address practical matters at this point, closing doors and turning off bleeps, and also setting ground rules for keeping identifying information within the group and treating each other with sympathy and respect. We finish each group in a short intervention with a review, asking about experiences of the meeting.

If a group is meeting once or twice to process something they have all been through, it often does not make sense for just one person to share an experience from practice. However, if everyone tries to share their experience, the group can become overwhelmed and individual voices get lost. We aim for a balance between breadth and depth, hearing initially from everyone and then asking if a couple of people would like to share their experiences in more depth. We try to help members listen to others' experiences, rather than everyone jumping in with their own. Even in one- or two-offs this can work well, helping the group to learn about the varying experiences of individuals.

During the Free Response and More Effortful Thinking Stages, we try to help people make links between the experiences of others and the material shared, but not at the expense of considering it in as much depth as possible. In one-off sessions, the emphasis tends to be on breadth rather than depth of experience because the group will not be used to working together and needs to develop solidarity and connection. We go with this, encouraging participants to be curious about the diversity of experiences in the group where possible.

Conclusion and future directions

The Heads and Hearts Model was developed before the pandemic but has been consolidated and adapted in response to the intense pressures faced by healthcare staff during this time. The problems which result from subjecting colleagues to ongoing stress and trauma have never been more evident. Extreme levels of anxiety and low mood are widespread, as are tensions in teams and between colleagues at service level. We can see clearly how difficult it is for staff to make use of supportive and reflective spaces when in greatest need. But we have found that when a reflective culture already exists in a service it has been possible for colleagues to make significant use of these spaces, drawing on already established and trusted relationships. This makes perfect sense – why would you go to unfamiliar people when things get difficult? – and is a strong argument for a preventative approach, involving widespread cultural change and embedding staff support and reflective practice in health and social care settings.

The extent to which manic defences kick in when things are especially difficult has also become apparent; by this we mean going beyond a coping mode into something more heightened and extreme, making vulnerabilities and problems hard to look at. We have worked with many groups, particularly of senior colleagues, in which there has been a marked reluctance to look at anything negative or concerning, at a time when it is especially important to do so. This underlines the importance of the facilitator being able to hold onto a realistic sense of hope and belief in the constructive value of the work, while also helping groups to look at feelings of sadness, hopelessness, and desperation. An understanding of how to deal sensitively but robustly with defensive processes, especially as these manifest in groups, is invaluable.

The model's attention to the question of when and how to provide organisational feedback has also been helpful: staff are often struggling with extreme difficulties in their external work environment, and keeping reflective practice entirely closed risks collusion with work practices which are at best unhelpful and at worst harmful. We are working with staff in reflective practice groups to consider when and how an issue should be taken up outside, with whom and by who. It will be important in future to develop and evaluate protocols on how and when to provide this type of organisational feedback. Generally speaking, the facilitator should not be the person to take specific actions regarding feedback, as this compromises their role, and it is better if this process is owned by the group in some way. Another key issue is the need to protect the reflective practice group, or at least a significant part of any meeting, as a place for looking at thoughts and feelings, free from external constraints and the pressure to act. The structure of the model is key here, demarcating the three core stages of Generation, Free Response and More Effortful Thinking, and the application stage of Turning Out. The safe, explorative space at the centre of any reflective practice session should mean that members are not worried that what they say will be taken outside the group, or have consequences on actions taken without this being considered by all.

At the core of the Heads and Hearts Model is a focus on containment: on allowing difficulties from practice to come into the open, however unexpected, confusing or upsetting, and on doing something with what emerges, enabling the group to process lived experience of practice and to gain perspective on it. This focus has been useful when working with staff facing so much distress and uncertainty. It has given us a realistic sense of hope, which we have tried to pass on to others.

References

Beinart, H. & Clohessy, S. (2017) *Effective Supervisory Relationships: Best Evidence and Practice.* Chichester, West Sussex: John Wiley & Sons.

Biggins, A. (2019) Does group reflective practice change practitioners' understanding of clients? An interpretative phenomenological analysis of the impact of monthly reflective practice groups within clinical psychology training. Unpublished dissertation: University of Leicester.

Kurtz, A. (2020) *How to Run Reflective Practice Groups: A Guide for Healthcare Professionals.* London: Routledge.

Ladany, N., Hill, C.E., Corbett, M.M. & Nutt, E.A. (1996) Nature, extent and importance of what psychotherapy trainees do not disclose to their supervisors. *Journal of Counselling Psychology*, 43(1): 10–24.

Menzies Lyth, I. (1960) A case study in the functioning of social systems as a defence against anxiety: a report on a study of the nursing service of a general hospital. *Human Relations*, 13(2): 95–121.

Schon, D. (1983) *The Reflective Practitioner: How Professionals Think in Action.* Farnham, Surrey: Ashgate Books.

Stedmon, J. & Dallos, R. (Eds) (2009) *Reflective Practice in Psychotherapy and Counselling.* Maidenhead, Berkshire: Open University Press.

West, M.A. (2021) *Compassionate Leadership: Sustaining Wisdom, Humanity and Presence in Health and Social Care.* The Swirling Leaf Press.

White, E. & Winstanley, J. (2010) A randomised controlled trial of clinical supervision: selected findings from a novel Australian attempt to establish the evidence base for causal relationships with quality of care and patient outcomes, as an informed contribution to mental health practice development. *Journal of Research in Nursing*, 15(2): 151–167.

Winnicott, D. (1973) *The Child, the Family, and the Outside World.* London: Penguin Books.

13 Psychological support for healthcare workers in India

Using a reflective lens

Professor Poornima Bhola, Dr Rathna Isaac, and Dr Chetna Duggal

The Indian healthcare system is vast and complex. The National Health Policy (2017) aims to address the healthcare needs of the country's large and varied population through the 'Health for All' mission. As healthcare workers (HCWs) work to fulfil this mission, they themselves experience significant stressors that impact their health and wellbeing outcomes. In this chapter, we present an overview of the healthcare system in India and discuss research trends spotlighting the mental health needs of the community of HCWs. We highlight the growing attention to the development and strengthening of psychosocial support frameworks for HCWs, and how these efforts have been bolstered in the context of the COVID-19 pandemic. We then explore exemplars of current initiatives and innovative efforts towards providing psychosocial support for HCWs, with particular reference to the power of reflective practice. We reflect on the processes and experiences in the provision of psychosocial support and distil themes to guide practice pathways and shape future possibilities in protecting the wellbeing of this vital segment of professionals.

The Indian healthcare context

The public healthcare system operates at three levels: primary healthcare is provided in rural areas through sub-centres, primary health centres, and community health centres, while secondary care is delivered through district and sub-district hospitals. Tertiary care services are extended at regional/central level institutions or super-specialty hospitals located in urban centres. An interface between the community and the primary healthcare system has been created through a community health workers team consisting of auxiliary nurse midwifes (ANMs), accredited social health activists (ASHAs), and Anganwadi workers (AWWs). As part of the National Rural Health Mission, ASHA workers are selected from within the community and function as health promoters to build awareness about healthcare services, facilitate service delivery pathways and mobilise community action, particularly in economically deprived and underserved areas. AWWs are responsible for the dissemination and documentation of health information, particularly related to maternal, newborn, and child health such as nutrition, family planning, and immunisations. ANMs are village-level multi-purpose female health workers who work at the grassroots of the primary healthcare system, who focus on maternal and child health, sanitation, nutrition, and first-aid or treatment of minor injuries. ANMs review and guide the work of ASHA workers and also have expanded responsibilities in remote areas of the country or during health emergencies and natural disasters.

Private healthcare services form another layer of care and account for a large proportion of the healthcare infrastructure in the country. The concentration of private healthcare services in urban areas is associated with an urban/rural and public/private divide in the reach and quality of services. The uneven geographical distribution of healthcare human resources is compounded by the overall inadequate numbers of trained HCWs. There are only 19 health workers (doctors, nurses, and midwives) per 10,000 people in India, against a World Health Organization recommended norm of 25 health workers (Chhina et al., 2017).

Psychosocial support needs of HCWs in India

Overburdened with high patient load and working with limited resources, HCWs in India experience unique and ongoing stressors, and these may be further exacerbated by the locus of work. For instance, in conflict-affected areas of the state of Assam, community health workers feared for their physical safety and experienced personal loss and displacement, concerns that they felt were not recognised by seniors and officials (Rajbangshi et al., 2021). Women ASHA workers may be particularly vulnerable, as they carry out unpaid labour at home in addition to the healthcare work, without a fixed salary and adequate benefits (Ved et al., 2019).

While there has been some recognition of the psychosocial support needs of HCWs, the COVID-19 pandemic brought this issue into sharper focus. A spate of recent research on the needs and challenges faced by Indian HCWs revealed heightened stressors in the work environment. Frontline health workers witnessed loss and suffering and experienced societal stigma for being exposed to the virus, with many unable to meet their families for months at a time (Chakma et al., 2021; Pulagam & Satyanarayana, 2021). Younger, junior professionals and women with caregiving roles at home were particularly vulnerable to developing mental health concerns (Chakma et al., 2021; Purwar et al., 2021). Several researchers outlined recommendations for developing stronger support mechanisms to process trauma and address stress, both at individual and systemic levels.

There are wide variations in conceptual frameworks and delivery modes for offering accessible psychosocial support to HCWs in India, ranging from webinars to tele-counselling or drop-in mental health services (Gupta et al., 2021). Manuals have also been developed to respond to frontline workers' psychosocial concerns in the context of post-tsunami work (WHO Country office India, 2006) and during the COVID-19 pandemic (e.g. Government of India & Department of Psychiatry, NIMHANS, 2020; Indian Council of Medical Research, 2021; Janardhana et al., 2020). The creation of reflective spaces and the use of reflective practice in the self-care of HCWs are evolving in India, with the pandemic providing added impetus.

Current practice and innovations in psychosocial support for HCWs

Reflection is a tool that helps us further our learning and foster our personal and professional growth. Engaging in reflective practice involves building capacities to reflect more deeply on our thoughts and feelings to develop new insights and understandings about our work and ourselves. Reflective work can be an individual activity for personal goals and enhancing self-care, but it can also be a powerful tool for the support and growth of groups and collectives. This section brings together a series of practice examples that have integrated reflective practice within psychosocial support for HCWs. Since there was little documentation of these initiatives, we interviewed relevant stakeholders to learn about their experiences and processes.

Listening circles: Creating spaces for solace and solidarity

The act of 'listening' creates a space for reflection, as it indicates an openness and willingness to meet people where they are and explore where they would like to go. We explore three initiatives that experimented with creating reflective listening spaces for HCWs: Caretharsis Listening Hours by First Drop Theatre, Listening Circles by Indian Network of the Diaspora for Essential Aid and Relief (INDEAR) and by Sangath.

Caretharsis Listening Hours[1] for doctors and nurses began during the pandemic and are held online. The Listening Hour was conceived by Jonathan Fox, who is also the co-founder of Playback Theatre. These circles often begin with a theme (e.g. pulls between work and family) or a prompt to activate awareness like visualisation, movement, or grounding exercise. Participants are then invited to reflect on what comes up for them, and tune into what resonates as they listen to others' reflections. The work is informed by reflective methods drawn from the experiential and expressive arts, including mindfulness and image work. Key to the Listening Hour is the principle of *emergence*, which brings out connection, meaning, and resilience in the stories shared. In the closing phase of the *reprieve*, the facilitator binds together the patterns of what was shared, but really it is the participants who own this reflective process.

Listening Circles by INDEAR[2] is a collective of volunteer mental health professionals across the globe who partnered with healthcare colleagues in India to support their work in the COVID-19 crisis. They provided free psychological first-aid and related mental health support, and each listening circle usually had a topic or focus (e.g. balancing work with family life). Participants included HCWs, mental health practitioners, and also community volunteers, who shared their experiences of grief at the proximity and scale of death, and anger at inadequate or inaccurate media depictions of their realities. Some participants expressed resentment that they were mandated to continue working as part of essential healthcare services and did not have any work-from-home options. Themes centring on inadequate systemic acknowledgement and response to their psychosocial needs also emerged within these sessions. More detail on this can be seen in Box 13.1.

---

[1] We spoke to Ms Radhika Jain, of First Drop Theatre, who is an Expressive Arts therapy practitioner, Accredited Playback Theatre Trainer, and a certified Listening Hour Guide, to learn about the *Caretharsis* Listening Hours.
[2] Initiated by Radhika Bapat and Uma Chandrika Millner, both clinical psychologists who joined hands across India and the USA. We had conversations with Radhika Bapat, Uma Chandrika Millner, and also with three facilitators of the Listening Circles, Jayoti Soor, Mona Klausing, and Laura Himmelstein, to learn about how a reflective lens was used to inform how their initiative was framed and positioned and also to support their facilitators.

> **Box 13.1: Reflecting on doing**
>
> *I feel self-care is a very colonised space and we need to change the narrative to it being community care as well. We call it self-relational-community care so we can include all aspects. You can take a warm bath …. but relational care is about connecting with others those who are your chosen community …. and community care is about taking care of others in your community.* – Uma Millner, INDEAR Listening Circles

Facilitators were given access to a reflective space where they could meet before and after each listening circle. This allowed them to share their impressions about the process and make changes (e.g. addressing de-escalation of conflict in healthcare setting, grief work) that were more responsive to participant needs. These meetings were a holding space for the facilitators' own responses to the intense expressions of anger and grief from some participants. These opportunities to meet and reflect together also helped them appreciate how some HCWs may struggle to be vulnerable in such an unfamiliar and temporary space. During their interactions, the facilitators shared ideas about what processes were working, what needed to be strengthened and what needed to be changed. Through these exchanges, they recognised the need to hold back from rushing into problem-solving, allowing for reflections and varied perspectives to emerge.

Listening Circles by *Sangath*[3] (a non-governmental, not-for-profit organisation working in Goa and other Indian states) were initiated in response to the COVID-19 pandemic. This involved 75-minute, small-group, online, fortnightly sessions for frontline healthcare and essential workers in both English and Hindi. Their tagline 'Listening is the doing at our circles!' was also evident in the thoughtful development of methodology, with practice listening circles first held within the team, followed by internal listening circles for Sangath staff at all levels (which included lay health workers/field workers too). These learnings were used to prepare a manual to guide facilitators, providing them with both standardisation and support. Box 13.2 considers facilitation of these spaces. Participants in the Sangath groups tended to speak more about their personal lives or work–life balance concerns rather than their work lives in iso-

---

[3] We interviewed Aarushi Agarwal, project coordinator, Speak Your Mind Project at Sangath India and Pooja Nair, intervention coordinator at Sangath.

lation. Perhaps this was stimulated by the merging of the personal and professional experienced during the COVID-19 lockdowns. In both the INDEAR and Sangath initiatives, varied pathways of care were provided in addition to the listening circles, including toll-free helpline/websites to access one-to-one counselling/support sessions and other wellbeing resources.

Box 13.2: Facilitating Listening Circles

The idea behind all the listening initiatives was to encourage sharing among HCWs about their personal and work lives, to provide emotional support and validation, and to experience solidarity in response to COVID-19 challenges.

All three reflective practices emphasised the creation of a safe and confidential space to listen, be vulnerable, and share emotions and stories. As these initiatives were online, people from different geographical locations could join, choose to stay anonymous, keep cameras off, text in the chat box, speak or just listen, and this flexibility of choice in how deeply to engage with the process seems important.

Facilitators clearly positioned themselves as witnesses to the reflective process rather than as experts. Apart from using a few prompts to help participants open up or stepping in if any participant experienced the process as emotionally overwhelming, facilitators allowed stories to emerge naturally. The participants were encouraged to reflect on and link stories, experiences, and emotions, and open up possibilities within the group.

While the primary focus remained on creating a reflective space, specific skills like breathwork or mindfulness were also taught. Healing is supported when we find a witness to our stories and *Listening Circles* demonstrate both the power of listening and the compassionate presence of group members.

Enacting change: Using applied theatre methodologies

Storytelling and theatre have been used by First Drop Theatre as an innovative way to support HCWs in coping with the stress of their professional lives and is described in Box 13.3. This *Playback theatre* approach is an exploratory reflective process within a contained space, grounded within a humanistic philosophy.

> **Box 13.3:** *Taking Centre Stage*: **Using playback theatre with nurses**
>
> Radhika Jain, of First Drop Theatre, shared her experiences with nurses in the high-demand areas of palliative care and elder care. She spoke of how getting nurses to shed their inhibitions and enter into 'play-mode' was a gradual process. Gentle reflective prompts such as 'How are you feeling?', 'Where is this feeling sitting inside you?', 'What does this moment mean to you?' supported nurses in becoming the 'tellers' of their stories. Jain noted how "those who are listening may recognise that 'this is my story too!' or that 'I have a different story …' and in this way they are already connected as they listen and see the reflection."
>
> During these sessions, expressive arts methods were also used in continuation to the playback theatre performance to work on the concerns that emerged from person stories shared by nurses. The use of like 'imagine your safe space' helped deepen experience and teach self-care methods.
>
> Nursing work involves emotional labour and the session themes were often related to emotional experiencing and communication, including difficult emotions like anger and painful experiences around death and dying. Jain shared an observation, "Many nurses come from a Christian community where caring is important. So, there is guilt and shame when they are angry with or feel disconnected from their patients. Especially in India … when I even think about it, I am going against my God."
>
> The feedback from the nurses indicated benefits from expressing difficult emotions and their own needs, which translated into more empathy for their patients. Some nurses experienced increased confidence in addressing issues within the organisational hierarchy which they had previously been silent about.

The idea of personal sharing is taken even further with communication and reflection stimulated through the medium of embodied stories. In this collective journey, strength is drawn from sharing in pairs, groups of three or the wider group, and from the sense of community that emerges. The facilitator (called the *conductor*) listens for the stories from the participants rather than directing them. Trained actors, who are listening, begin to improvise and perform both the stories and the embedded feelings for participants to observe and experience. They may use creative approaches such as poetry, metaphors, images, or even scarves to express and reflect it back, often bringing out what is hidden, unsaid, or longed for. For instance, coloured scarves may be used metaphorically as an abstract depiction of emotions or feelings, or as representations of elements integral to the teller's story. The conductor links the emerging stories through the process of *narrative reticulation* and slowly evokes deeper stories (Fox, 2020).

Doctors for Doctors initiative

The Doctors for Doctors or D4D[4] initiative was launched in 2019 by the Indian Medical Association (IMA) to foster the wellbeing of medical students and doctors. The initiative was launched to promote mental health and wellbeing of doctors, prevent burnout, and reduce suicide rates especially among medical trainees. The goal was to create systemic and policy level changes to improve working conditions and prevent violence towards doctors, and to ensure sustainable psychosocial support for those who might need it. The context of the pandemic brought mental health needs of doctors to the forefront, and the D4D initiative became even more critical. Focus group discussions were held to understand the needs of doctors and identify where and how to target mental health or wellbeing efforts. These suggested a strong felt need for mental health support, with participants describing a range of personal and professional stresses, and symptoms of depression and anxiety. Box 13.4 offers a powerful example of this.

Through the pandemic, workshops and seminars conducted as part of the initiative were accessed pan-India by doctors across different phases of professional development. The fact that the initiative was under the umbrella of a national association with a strong network of professionals helped in mobilising participation. There have been efforts to initiate reflective groups for psychosocial support to address the diverse needs of healthcare practitioners (e.g. groups for obstetrician/gynaecologists). These collective experiences carry tremendous potential to strengthen the role of reflective elements in medical training and practice.

---

[4] We spoke to Dr Nilima Kadambi, a paediatric surgeon and the chairperson of the IMA National Committee for Emotional Health and Well-being of Medical Students and Doctors. We also interviewed Dr Sandip Deshpande, Dr Suhas Chandran, and Dr Ashlesha Bagadia, psychiatrists from Bangalore, who have been working towards better mental health for HCWs, both independently and as part of the D4D programme.

> **Box 13.4: The power of the personal**
>
> In our conversations with practitioners who had initiated psychosocial support and reflective processes for the medical fraternity, the personal underpinnings of their commitment were evident. We share one such story to illustrate how individual journeys can often pave the path for collective movements.
>
> During her residency, paediatric surgeon Dr Nilima Kadambi found herself overwhelmed with grief when she lost a young patient with leukaemia. Her reaction met with a lot of disapproval from her seniors and she shared her reflections:
>
>> Unfortunately a lot of us senior doctors sometimes make young medicos feel guilty about emotions. … We are first and foremost human beings … and then we have professional training and experience and knowledge that builds layers on top to help us cope. … It is the person of the doctor that connects with the patients and if you didn't have that human connect, I don't think we'd really be good doctors.
>
> As she experienced personal crisis in her life years later, her belief in the power of experiential learning and reflective practice was strengthened. Dr Kadambi is now the chairperson, IMA National Committee for Emotional Health and Well-being of Medical Students and Doctors.

Working within the community

Atmiyata[5] is a mental health intervention that works with community volunteers (including ASHA workers, leaders of Sakhi Mandals,[6] and AWWs) from parts of rural India to deliver 4–6 counselling sessions to people with distress and common mental health conditions. The model is an innovative, low cost, high impact, community-based model to reduce the mental health and social care gap. The intervention employs a stepped care approach, using community-based volunteers, known as 'Champions', who are identified, trained, mentored, and

---

[5] We spoke to Dr Kaustubh Joag, from the Centre for Mental Health Law & Policy, Pune, India.
[6] Sakhi Mandal Yojna is an initiative by the Government of Gujarat, a state in India, to empower women in rural areas.

supervised by community facilitators (CFs). The training is based on participatory and reflective approaches, and the CFs meet Champions twice a month to support their work using a range of participatory and reflective approaches to build peer support and motivation and prevent burnout. During the refresher trainings and reflective discussions, encounters with gender, violence, substance abuse, and caste-based discrimination in the community were reported as determinants of psychosocial distress among the Champions themselves.

These varied initiatives spearheaded by individual practitioners, mental health and professional organisations, and government agencies have coalesced to catalyse a movement of sorts. While these developments are gathering momentum, the participation and sustained engagement from the healthcare community has not kept pace with the vision and scope envisaged in these diverse initiatives. The recognition of the value of reflective practice in Indian healthcare for professional growth and personal wellbeing is waiting to be realised.

Key practice points

In this section, we elucidate key practice points based on the learnings distilled from the diverse practice exemplars and from our own professional experiences. We highlight both the challenges and the growing opportunities for reflective practice and psychosocial support in healthcare.

Navigating space and safety concerns

Finding a protected space and time for either personal or group reflective work may be a serious challenge in a lower-middle-income country like India. HCWs may also be overwhelmed by healthcare practice challenges and any opportunity of support and reflection may first be seen as an avenue to problem-solve for stressors associated with it. Beyond the barriers of lack of privacy and work burden, there may be some inhibitions related to the idea of finding value in sharing personal experiences or revealing distress. Contextual beliefs about HCWs, particularly doctors being an 'avatar' of God, are deeply entrenched in the Indian psyche and can be equally oppressive for HCWs themselves. They might feel pressured to live up to the image and expressing concerns and vulnerabilities might be incompatible with this. They may also feel very uncomfortable with making 'time for themselves', an act that might be seen as 'selfish' or 'indulgent'. The emphasis on duty has been particularly strong during the pandemic, when HCWs were celebrated as 'heroes' around the world. The limited permission to express personal vulnerabilities within the professional community can further 'invisibilise' their internal struggles. It is possible that when the role and the person are separated too much, the role gets glorified, and the person dehumanised. It is this personal and professional divide that may need to be first questioned in reflective spaces. Entering though different doors, for instance through the use of movement, yoga, or experiential activities with varied degrees of reflection, may create the space for acceptable practice models. These diverse options may feed into each other or reach different people.

There is also perhaps a 'culture of privacy' around sharing familial/emotional concerns and concerns about confidentiality: a collective silence rather than an individual one. A respectful acknowledgement of these concerns and addressing issues around safety and confidentiality is essential. A group process that models reflective listening and gently encourages sharing and reflection, rather than questioning or answering, might help participants find their own comfort with the process. The use of a strengths and resilience-based approach that builds on narratives of hope, rather than operating through a deficit lens, might allow participants to connect with their personal and interpersonal resources in meaningful ways. Combining formats for both shared and private reflection can also be useful, with issues explored within groups and others through journals and creative self-expression.

At a more fundamental level, the notion of building a culture of reflection and attention to emotions within the healthcare profession, right from training years, is critical. The role of senior practitioners, health administrators, and supervisors cannot be overstated, and the more open they are to discussing their challenges and concerns, the more this allows other HCWs to do so. When leaders own and support psychosocial support initiatives, this can help circumvent any time, space, and resource-related constraints. A culture that promotes cooperation and mutual support among colleagues in the same profession can also help reduce the associated stigma and help nurture a safe, supportive, reflective space. This might cascade to overall improved psychosocial wellbeing for HCWs, the communities they care for, and also open pathways to care for those who might need further support.

Questioning the outsider gaze

Who can speak for what HCWs need and want? While mental health practitioners are often positioned as providers of psychosocial support, it is important to recognise and acknowledge the outsider gaze. Involving HCWs in the programme development and conducting periodic needs assessments and audits can support a deeper and nuanced understanding of the challenges, strengths, and experiences of HCWs. Being an outsider can create barriers to sharing but this may sometimes also lend an advantage; HCWs could be more comfortable sharing their vulnerabilities with those outside their professional circle.

We recommend a 'listening-observing-not-knowing stance' to help build trust and engagement and develop responsive programmes. The need for such reflective inquiry is accentuated in a diverse country like India, with sharply distinct rural–urban healthcare systems, 22 official languages, complex caste and class structures. When psychosocial initiatives involve international facilitators or seek to borrow from psychosocial paradigms used in other countries, we need to ensure that local knowledge and strengths are recognised and incorporated. Box 13.5 reflects on ways to decolonise practice.

> **Box 13.5: Decolonising practice**
>
> Uma Chandrika Millner shared her experiences in setting up listening circles with facilitators who were from the Indian diaspora, South Asian, and from other nationalities, "As we progressed, the things I started to see was, a lot of internalised colonisation or colonised perspective entering in. Like 'I want to save the situation', or here is this white psychiatrist wanting to teach meditation to doctors at a time when they are barely making it."
>
> Such reflections impelled the team to guard against a re-enactment of this perspective with attempts to change or replace the mental health support systems in India. Instead, this was seen as a partnership for collaborative efforts during the challenging pandemic situation.

Addressing diversity and inclusion

In a country where individuals speak in different languages and dialects, programmes need to be delivered in local languages to ensure equitable access. Initiatives that focus on English-speaking urban professionals with digital access may be exclusionary and have circumscribed impacts. HCWs in rural and resource-constrained regions may not be as well connected via digital mediums and some women community workers might not have easy access to the family mobile devices. We recommend the use of innovative ways of disseminating information and mobilising participation; perhaps through community radios or street plays, the embedding of messaging about the value of psychosocial support within other programmes within the community and effective liaison with influential community leaders.

The impact of social locations (e.g. gender, class, caste, religion) is experienced more often than acknowledged or expressed in individual and group spaces in healthcare settings. Psychosocial support services need to sensitively acknowledge differing experiences and needs across intersectionalities and how this influences subjective wellbeing, without deepening divisive fault lines – not always an easy balance to achieve. Recent research has indicated that the caste of the AWW and other frontline workers can have a significant impact on the acceptance from the community they are assigned to serve. It can affect the trust given by the community members as well as the trust she creates by either perpetuating or challenging caste divisions through her own service delivery actions. These caste tensions can manifest in perceptions of bias, a hostile environment, and even risk of physical violence against the AWW, consequently interfering with both work and wellbeing (John et al., 2020).

There is no denying the existence of power differentials and hierarchies within healthcare systems and this may percolate into group processes. While planning psychosocial support services, it is important to consider if participants will feel less constrained in homogenous groups or when the facilitators are also drawn from their own cadre or group. It is also possible that inviting facilitators from outside the system may be experienced as freeing. Conversely, the promotion of dialogue between members in heterogeneous groups can potentially encourage mutual learning, respect, and a culture of inclusivity. There may be much that an ASHA worker from a village could share with and teach a surgeon in a big city. Addressing universal experiences can create a bridge that allows members of diverse backgrounds to connect with each other. The recognition of all being a part of the same larger healthcare family could have deep and powerful impacts on each of their identities and ways of viewing their professions.

Opening Pandora's box: The personal and the political

HCWs may begin their support journeys by focusing more on systemic issues which are easier to access and discuss rather than delving into more personal emotions and experiences. However, a skilled facilitator may enter through this door to draw out the personal impact of these systemic experiences and enable greater emotional awareness, in addition to advocating for systemic change and empowerment.

There are times when tangible changes in the organisation culture and healthcare system are viewed as vital for psychosocial wellbeing. For instance, community HCWs who are part of the public healthcare system in India prioritised their needs for health insurance, fixed work hours, facilities (e.g. clean drinking water, restrooms in rural or remote areas), and issues of bribery and corruption in obtaining their own payments (BehanBox, 2021). HCWs in urban areas or in the private sector may have a different set of challenges. We recommend that a space be created for these difficult conversations and efforts made to amplify the voices of the marginalised to create the change needed.

As we open safe reflective spaces, we may encounter the unexpected: questions, revelations, and needs expressed by HCWs that we feel ill equipped to contain and work with. We recommend sensitisation and training in trauma-informed approaches for first-level responses to disclosures of any personal trauma, abuse, harassment, or violence. We can expect post-traumatic sequalae stemming from cumulative experiences in the healthcare sector during the extended COVID-19 pandemic and need to be prepared to conduct rapid risk assessment and facilitate mental health referrals through well-established support and referral pathways.

Built to last: Developing sustainable initiatives

One of the bigger challenges in providing meaningful and consistent reflective spaces relates to the scalability and sustainability of initiatives, particularly those that began in response to pandemic-related stressors. The limited mental health human resources in India (e.g. 0.7 psychologists per 100,000 population; World Mental Health Atlas, 2017) necessarily impose constraints on the degree of involvement in leading psychosocial support initiatives for HCWs. We recommend the use of cascading models to involve and train members within the healthcare communities who would also serve as role models. Working through healthcare organisations rather than reaching out to individual HCWs and partnering with professional organisations may help embed initiatives within systems.

Most of the current initiatives in India are running without any monetary support and there are challenges to long-term sustainability of such voluntary initiatives. Collaborating with partners for grant support might help create sustainable and scalable programmatic roadmaps to expand the scope and reach of such initiatives. Developing contextually responsive frameworks that factor in the unique stressors that HCWs experience might also ensure programmes are well received and meet the needs of all segments of the professional community.

Conclusion

We propose a multi-tiered reflective practice framework that is contextually responsive to respond to the psychosocial needs of the HCWs in a resource-constrained country like India. At the core of the reflective practice framework lies self-exploration through an intersectional lens, that is embedded in the discourses of the medical professional community and further in the socio-economic-political context and zeitgeist. A process of reflective inquiry that incorporates experiential and creative tools makes it possible to deliberate on the diverse realities and needs of each group of HCWs. Through collaborative faciliatory styles, that are situated in frameworks of empowerment and inclusion, values of social justice and equity may be brought to life. Delivery frameworks complemented with guidance documents that chart out suitable time frames and logistics using cascading models might be helpful in realising the goal of this framework of integrating reflection as a tool for promoting psychosocial wellbeing and resilience and prevent burnout and other risks. This framework could be scaffolded with interventive modalities of care delivery – for those who might need further support – through collaborations between the various professionals working towards mental health services and care. Processes of feedback, documentation, and evaluation can be integrated through reflective spirals to strengthen and evolve dynamic frameworks of care for the healthcare community in India.

Key points

In this chapter, we introduce the public and private healthcare system in India and describe the varied needs, resources, and contexts of HCWs.

We outline exemplars of psychosocial support initiatives using participatory and reflective approaches, such as listening circles, applied theatre, group work, and community-based mentoring models.

We recommend the use of strengths and resilience-based approaches, creative and experiential methods, and early integration into training frameworks to address barriers to the expression of personal vulnerabilities.

The development of sustainable delivery frameworks built on values of social justice and equity with cascading training models can target both individual and systemic change.

References

Behanbox (2021) *Female frontline community healthcare workforce in India during COVID-19* [online]. Available at: https://behanbox.com/wp-content/uploads/2021/03/APU-Report-Final.pdf.

Chakma, T. *et al.* (2021) Psychosocial impact of COVID-19 pandemic on healthcare workers in India & their perceptions on the way forward – A qualitative study, *The Indian Journal of Medical Research*, 153(5), 637–648. doi: 10.4103/IJMR.IJMR_2204_21.

Chew, N. W. S. *et al.* (2020) Asian-Pacific perspective on the psychological well-being of healthcare workers during the evolution of the COVID-19 pandemic, *BJPsych Open*, 6(6). doi: 10.1192/BJO.2020.98.

Chhina, Rajoo S. *et al.* (2017) Health Manpower Planning, *Current Trends in Diagnosis and Treatment*, 1(1), 53–57. doi: 10.5005/JP-JOURNALS-10055-0013.

Fox, J. (2020) The Playback NR Workbook, *Guidelines for Mastering Narrative Reticulation*. New York, Tusitala Publishing.

Gupta, S. *et al.* (2021) Feasibility and effectiveness of telecounseling on the psychological problems of frontline healthcare workers amidst COVID-19: A randomized controlled trial from central India, *Indian Journal of Psychological Medicine*, 43(4), 343–350. doi: 10.1177/02537176211024537.

Government of India & Department of Psychiatry, NIMHANS (2020) *Caring for health care warriors – Mental health support during COVID-19* [online]. Available at https://covid19.india.gov.in/document/caring-for-health-care-warriors-mental-health-support-during-covid-19/

Indian Council of Medical Research (2021) *Guidance document for the psychosocial support for health care workers during COVID-19 pandemic*. Indian Council of Medical Research.

Janardhana, N., Joseph, S. J., Kanmani, T. R., Kumar, A., Chand, P. K., Desai, G. and Cherian, A. V. (2020) *Psychosocial care for frontline health care workers: An information manual*. Nimhans Publication 81.

John, A. *et al.* (2020) Factors influencing the performance of community health workers: A qualitative study of Anganwadi workers from Bihar, India, *PLOS ONE*, 15(11), e0242460. doi: 10.1371/JOURNAL.PONE.0242460.

Nanda, P. *et al.* (2020) From the frontlines to centre stage: Resilience of frontline health workers in the context of COVID-19, *Sexual and Reproductive Health Matters*, 28(1). doi: 10.1080/26410397.2020.1837413.

Pulagam, P. and Satyanarayana, P. T. (2021) Stress, anxiety, work-related burnout among primary health care worker: A community based cross sectional study in Kolar, *Journal of Family Medicine and Primary Care*, 10(5), 1845–1851. doi: 10.4103/JFMPC.JFMPC_2059_20.

Purwar, S. *et al.* (2021) Online survey to assess psychological problems among frontline healthcare workers during the first wave of SARS-CoV-2 (COVID-19) pandemic and their psychosocial determinants: An Indian perspective, *Disaster Medicine and Public Health Preparedness*, 1–6. doi: 10.1017/DMP.2021.290.

Rajbangshi, P. R., Nambiar, D. and Srivastava, A. (2021) Community health workers: Challenges and vulnerabilities of accredited social health activists working in conflict-affected settings in the state of Assam, India, *BMC Health Services Research*, 21(1), 829. doi: 10.1186/S12913-021-06780-Y.

Ved, R. *et al.* (2019) How are gender inequalities facing India's one million ASHAs being addressed? Policy origins and adaptations for the world's largest all-female community health worker programme, *Human Resources for Health*, 17(3), 1–15. doi: 10.1186/S12960-018-0338-0.

WHO Country office, India (2006) *Resources for psychosocial support in disaster management: Psychosocial support for tsunami affected population in India* [online]. Available at: https://apps.who.int/iris/handle/10665/206307.

14 Open Dialogue, Dialogical Leadership, and Staff Support

Dr Lisa Monaghan and Cathy Thorley

Hello! How are you?
Would it be ok if we started with a few questions?

- How did you get to be reading this chapter today?
- How would you like to learn and gain from reading this chapter today?
- What are you feeling in your body having been asked these questions today?

Well, now you have thought about yourself in this moment, let us start with a quote that inspired the development of Open Dialogue in its birthplace:

For the word (and, consequently, for a human being) there is nothing more terrible than a lack of response.

(Bakhtin, 1975)

Open Dialogue is an approach that originates from Western Lapland and is a network-based method of helping those experiencing mental health crisis. It is based both on responding and reflecting, on hearing every voice, and responding to every person's communication (verbal or non-verbal) in the present moment for it to be a truly dialogical interaction (Rober, 2005). A person's network is defined in this approach to be anyone the person at the centre of concern (PCC) deems it to be, so may not be just immediate family or next of kin. In this chapter, we will describe how the Open Dialogue approach is part of the ongoing global paradigm shift in mental health services, and how we have both continued to evolve its application within our dialogical working practices and within our organisations, to support staff in mental and physical healthcare settings.

We propose that working within and using this approach is just as supportive for staff as it is for those they are supporting. However, due to the more emotive aspects of the approach, and how professionals are expected to bring a more personal resonance to the work, it requires greater levels of support, self-reflexivity, and supervision for staff to maintain their wellbeing and engagement in the approach. We have gone on to use this as trainers and supervisors, in building new services and developing established teams, in many areas from inpatient wards in mental health and acute hospitals to community arenas and globally with other practitioners. We will discuss these aspects using practical examples later. We will first outline the Open Dialogue approach and its history, then explore theory and research related to this approach, before turning to practical applications.

As we considered the request to write this chapter, we were aware of the dichotomy of providing an instructive construct others could use in their work with staff, without losing the ethos of the approach itself. Dialogism is not a method or a set of techniques, it is an outlook based on acknowledging and respecting – and reaching towards – the otherness of the Other (Seikkula & Arnkil, 2014). So, while other models may ask you to focus on formulating, mapping and employing formal tools and techniques that professionals 'use' in the work, we would like you to focus on yourself and your embodied reactions to your time spent with us in this space. We hope that the following history and descriptions of our ways of orientating and applying this approach in our lives and work enable you to have a richer understanding of it and how you might wish to enact it in yours. In short, the dialogue *is* the action.

Open Dialogue is currently spreading globally as a movement trying to change the way in which mental health issues are viewed and treated. The Open Dialogue approach has elements of Social Network, Systemic, and Family Therapy theories at its core and from the very first contact. Dialogical practice uses responsive listening combined with professional's reflections to enhance the experience of the network and create a space where untold stories can be shared. Reflecting, in this approach, refers to the way the professionals talk about their own ideas and resonances in front of the family (Andersen, 1991). In practice, it involves meeting with the PCC and their network on a regular basis from the point of crisis with the same practitioners involved (where possible) for the life of the problem.

The crisis becomes an opportunity to generate new stories, in which the experiences emerging in the form of symptoms are clothed in words. (Seikkula & Arnkil, 2006)

Background theory and research

We will give a brief overview of the evidence for the approach and encourage you to use our references to further your curiosity in this area. The results from Western Lapland had been overlooked for many years arguably because they were in such opposition to the rest of the Western world's experience and findings (Seikkula et al., 2003, 2006). The success and positive results on reduced numbers of inpatient admissions, shorter lengths of inpatient stays, lower levels of medication needed, as well as high levels of patients returning to work or education were seen as outliers or anomalies. A 19-year follow-up study (Bergstrom et al., 2020) found similar results.

Open Dialogue would seem to be an approach in stark contrast to health systems (Jackson, 2012; Razzaque, 2014; Razzaque & Woods, 2015), based on a medical model, with siloed services that treat patients in isolation from their social network (Campbell, 1985). Having a social network has been shown to be associated with more favourable clinical outcomes and a higher quality of life in those with mental health presentations (Giacco et al., 2012), thus, working to enhance social networks has clear advantages. An extensive review of the evidence base for Family Therapy and Systemic practice found that systemic therapies are effective, acceptable to clients, and cost effective (Stratton, 2016). The Open Dialogue: Development and Evaluation of a Social Network Intervention for Severe Mental Illness is a large-scale randomised control study being undertaken in the UK evaluating the Peer-Supported Open Dialogue (POD) approach.

It works on two levels.

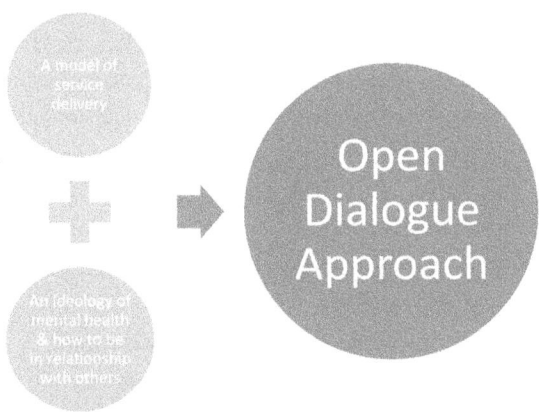

FIGURE 14.1: Ideology and delivery of the Open Dialogue Approach.

TABLE 14.1: The 7 principles and 12 key elements of the Open Dialogue approach.

The 7 principles	The 12 key elements
1–5: Organisation of the service 6 and 7: Practitioner embodiment of approach	How to be present in the space
• Immediate help • Social network perspective • Flexibility and mobility • Responsibility • Psychological continuity • Tolerance of uncertainty • Polyphony and dialogism	• Two (or more) therapists in the team meeting • Participation of family and network • Using open-ended questions • Responding to clients' utterances • Emphasising the present moment • Eliciting multiple viewpoints • Use of a relational focus in the dialogue • Responding to problem, discourse, or behaviour in a matter-of-fact style and attentive to meanings • Emphasising the clients' own words and stories, not symptoms • Conversation among professionals (reflections) in the treatment meetings • Being transparent • Tolerating uncertainty

Source: From Olson et al. (2014).

The importance of organisations in supporting staff welfare

A social network model must, in our opinion, at its core, reflect the society it seeks to connect with and cannot be separated from that social context. Open Dialogue is a need-adapted approach that must adapt to the needs of the culture it is serving. With multiple pressures a daily reality for health and social care staff, how can Open Dialogue work at a strategic and local level to support them? When working in this way, both organisations and facilitators need to consider how to adequately support staff undertaking this type of work and maintain their wellbeing in the long term. We postulate that the dialogical methods within this approach can support all those involved in this work, whether facilitation, participation, or organisation.

Laloux (2016) developed a model of stages of organisational change which is a way for organisations to move away from practices that are hierarchical, and reductive, moving towards more compassionate organisational cultures.

> **Box 14.1: Beginning a meeting**
>
> A crisis is seen as an opportunity in OD but this way of working can be used in any team meetings. Bringing a team together soon after a difficult experience or time, when people are more emotionally connected to the situation, can allow new knowledge and helpful stories to emerge that enables change to occur.
>
> Mindfulness has been incorporated as part of the UK training to address the pressurised contexts teams are working within, as it has been shown to support the tolerance of difficult emotions and reduce rushing into solution-focused decision-making.
>
> When opening a session, facilitators should undertake a mindfulness exercise (brief) to ground staff into the space and enable all to be present with their embodied experience. This enables staff to 'put down' what they are sitting with and engage and focus on the space they are currently working within. OD necessitates that each person is asked about their journey to the meeting and what they would want to use the space for.
>
>> What is the history of you being here today? (If this is the first time of coming together this way)
>> What would you like to use the space for today?
>
> Allowing space to open up to all voices moves away from blame, eases tension, and can help make visible new ways of working and managing that worry, conflict and service pressures and meeting objectives have hidden.
>
> Respectful conversations: if a person is absent, speak as if they were not, hear the conversation from their perspective – this stems from the nothing about me without me principles of care.

Increasingly, leadership and management organisational models highlight not just the need for compassion, but also the business and human factors sense in adopting these evolutionary, non-hierarchal approaches. The Buurtzorg approach recognised that care is not mechanical, and the best care comes when staff are trusted and have the freedom to provide the high-quality care they aspire to. These ideas are not new, and studies have repeatedly found that staff wellbeing and high-quality patient care are intrinsically linked (Johnson et al., 2017; Hall et al., 2020; Mistry, Levack & Johnson, 2015; Salyers et al., 2016; West, 2012).

We propose that Open Dialogue as a need-adapted network approach can bridge the gap in being able to provide care to those working in and using services, while incorporating other areas of professional and social knowledge and understanding, in a culturally sensitive and effective manner that seeks to flatten the hierarchy.

Dialogical organisational practice

During the acute phase of the pandemic, I (Lisa) was asked by a panel during a Mad in America (MIA) forum[1] how I was using my OD skills in my work in the respite centres we had created and in supporting frontline staff. At that time, my response focused mostly on my ability to sit with and be comfortable with being uncomfortable; to sit with the sixth OD principle of uncertainty. This for me presented one of the greatest challenges for staff and the general population, but it helped me in my role of supporting staff, the organisation, and the larger shared services. Being able to stay in that space enabled me to slow down and help others to do the same, to stop, to hear, to think in a time where everything was on fast forward and changing repeatedly. Working long term with people who had chronic mental health conditions and their families also allowed me the perspective of being able to appreciate 'small' but meaningful successes. With this always in mind I was able to:

- Support responses to incidents and COVID-19-related experiences in all areas of the hospitals
- Enable safety and peer connections
- Generate spaces for all to be heard
- Avoid premature decisions
- Modelling tolerance of painful emotion

---

[1] MIA is a non-profit organisation that is rethinking psychiatric care in the US and abroad. It provides news on psychiatric research, as well as the lived experience of those who have been diagnosed with a psychiatric disorder and calls for profound change to what they suggest is a failed drug-based paradigm.

- Allowing space for contradictory perspectives to exist side by side
- Explore situations of moral distress and ease the impact of the uncontrollable
- Not burnout myself.

Dialogical skills are particularly valuable when working with difficult team dynamics. In dialogical practice when a system is stuck, we can intervene. This often entails someone coming into the system to interview members involved in the 'stuckness' in front of each other. This allows an active listening position as well as an active reflective stance to be taken by all parties. This can start with the therapist, manager, or dialogical team member being interviewed by another not linked to the system about their views and experiences of being stuck. This can help to shift the system from a blaming position which can personalise the 'stuck issues' to one encouraging consideration of the system context. Being curious in a meeting about areas, such as what was going on for individuals so they can establish what held them back, what was triggering for them, and what their intentions are for the space and time, is helpful in addressing how to move together beyond the problems holding them in place. Being in tune with ourselves and open and transparent in our reactions in the moment can help others to take a risk and be more vulnerable in the space.

Ruptures and collective connectedness

Dialogical reflective practice is useful in many organisational contexts and can be incorporated into any stepped care approach to support staff. This space can be helpful when ruptures and collective traumas are experienced. We have used this approach to help services reflect on issues of racism from patients, to process the COVID-19 pandemic and in regard to the vaccination as a mandatory condition of employment legislated by the UK government, among others. As this type of space can feel very new or even alien to many people working in health and social care, we have used the following explanation in the communication and arrangement of these type of groups. This example refers to the group support offer for managers relating to the mandatory vaccination process in 2022.

> **Box 14.2: Written invitations**
>
> "In Dialogic Reflective Practice we create a space where each participant feels heard and responded to, the starting point of a dialogical meeting is that the perspective of every participant is important and accepted without conditions. Everyone attending will have their camera on and each person will have time to speak to their experience. The facilitators will reflect on the conversation as it grows and will use some grounding techniques to help everyone feel safe and contained. It is a confidential space, and anyone can seek help individually afterwards if needed. With an emphasis on listening and responding, Open Dialogue fosters the co-existence of multiple, separate, and equally valid 'voices', or points of view, within the meeting. In the context of a tense and severe crisis, it is important to be able process the impact on us personally and professionally. Sitting with the context and tolerating the uncertainty we are still experiencing is difficult but connecting with others and coming to some shared understandings can be helpful in managing these experiences. There is space for each voice, in a collaborative exchange weaving new, more shared understandings to which everyone contributes an important thread. This results in a common experience without rank that aims to reduce distress and allow each person to move on in a way that is right for them."

Current practice and innovation in staff supervision and wellbeing

Supervision or Intervision (as it is referred to in the UK POD teams) allows for exploration of experiences and counter-experiences in relation to the families. At another level it can also further develop these relationships and understanding within a team. In addition, it can be a useful tool for managers to test the temperature of a team routinely and can act as a way of resolving differences, helping to resolve organisational frustrations and difficulties at a team level. However, this should be cautiously and carefully facilitated. Working with staff at this deeper level of mutual knowing and with the expectation of additional personalisation beyond normal professional boundaries can have detrimental effects on staff who are unprepared and left uncontained afterwards. Follow-up and inclusion in stepped care approaches to staff support is needed to manage engagement and wellness throughout. The intensity of interaction with patients and their families may add to the vicarious burden of professionals. It is also possible that more personalisation in Intervision increases the likelihood that working practice issues, when emerging, are personalised rather than seeing it as a systemic issue (Monaghan, 2018). This also can have further ramifications for peer support workers and those experts by experience.

> **Box 14.3: Supervision and online considerations**
>
> Intervision space was created to have a deliberately less hierarchical nature than 'supervision'. The practitioners that are bringing an issue can become a smaller group within the group, given space to reflect on their experience while their colleagues actively listen. The dialogical focus is not on what happened, but rather attunement to how the work is making them feel, what is impacting on them, and its relationship to their own history.
>
> During the COVID-19 pandemic, it became necessary to work using virtual forums.
>
> When this is carried out online, the speakers keep their cameras on while the listening team members switch off their cameras, which are only switched back on when the speakers stop and invite the listeners to reflect. These reflections focus on the listeners' resonances, images, and body sensations while they speak about what they have heard; they ensure that they speak about the people listening rather than directly to them so that they can stay in a listening position. This process can happen once or twice before the team come back together and reflect as a whole on the session with the people who brought the issue always having the last word.
>
> "When my colleagues reflected on what I had experienced at work, I felt truly heard and understood, maybe for the first time. I realised I wasn't the only person who felt like I did." Nurse in acute healthcare setting (participant in OD pandemic support group).
>
> Using reflection in difficult conversations, facilitated conversations, and performance discussions can enable all parties to slow down, move away from policies and towards human connection. It allows everyone to be in an actively engaged position and can remove the shadow of
>
> *(Continued)*

> hierarchy and power dynamics that impinge staffs' ability to speak freely and in a productive and respectful manner.
>
> What appears to be significant in the process of intervision is having the space to explore the feelings and thoughts that arise for the practitioner about their own family of origin. This seems to open possibilities and ideas to position themselves differently to their colleagues and work context.
>
> "I didn't think so much would have opened up for me, this is such a different way of looking at things from our normal meetings." (Medical Doctor. Group Participant)

The network style OD, reflective space, and format may be a way of all team members having better knowledge of each other, enhancing compassion and trust in each other, thus enabling better clinical ways of working. West (2012) suggests that to build a culture of engagement, managers must show the same level of engagement and give genuine commitment to the intervention and the team. This can be made visible by Dialogical approaches such as being present, transparent, and participating openly and fully in team Intervisions.

We have used dialogical reflective practice sessions in various contexts. These are based on reflecting team principles (Andersen, 1991). Overall, the space is opened to talk less about the content (case details/team-specific dynamics) of a situation but rather of the impact of it and of personal and professional connections to this. Often, other staff in the group are invited to reflect on what a speaker has brought to the meeting and of any resonances and connections they make. The speaker then is invited to have the last word and speak of the experience of hearing the reflections.

This practice has been used with a wide variety of acute hospital teams and services to process and manage team objectives, caseload pressures, work-related stress and trauma, issues relating to and caused by the recent pandemic, team away days/future planning, and training with redeployed staff to manage both their and the system's anxiety. "I feel energised and that I have more options now. I don't feel so hopeless and exhausted" (Allied health professional, pandemic support group 2020). Reflective practice has also been successfully used with psychology trainees on placement in various services to process their experience, clinical work, and personal career journeys. Finally, it is used in group supervision sessions with groups and teams who are working directly with individuals, families, and networks to help them to process what is arising for them in their work and support their own processes and family of origin resonances.

Dialogues across boundaries

Just as Professor Kimmel (2016) described privilege as being invisible to those that have it, so we have found that power is often invisible to those that wield it. We feel that it is our individual and collective responsibility to create safe spaces for all people and voices to speak up, particularly when we are the ones in the powerful positions, wherever that may be. Our use of benign curiosity can enable difficult conversations to be held without enacting blame. People shut down and can become fixed in their positions or opt out of the dialogue altogether if they feel blamed. People do not change from a position of blame. Curiosity allows the possibility of change through the dialogue. For example, noticing and being curious about, why more men are speaking in a meeting than women, allows visibility of powerful discourses, creating opportunity for more voices to be heard. Exploring power dynamics without blame can allow new meaning to emerge, bringing forth new ways of understanding the issues at hand.

Service design

In 2016, I (Cathy) was tasked to set up and manage an England-wide NHS service offering an Open Dialogue style service to individuals with mental health difficulties and the people important to them. In order for all staff to feel supported and connected to the service, it was important that not only the people who were part of the new service, but everyone connected to it had a space to talk about it and have any concerns heard and responded to. This involved deep listening and being present for individuals right from the start.

I also quickly learnt that it was the power of a relationship that was the key in getting the infrastructure in place such as HR systems and new referral and note-keeping systems. Meetings were face to face ideally and listening to and respecting each person involved helped to get the necessary systems in place more smoothly. There was a connection made that was deeper than sharing professional expertise. In order to connect more deeply, we brought more of ourselves into the conversation, personal discussions about our own lives and predicaments. What might traditionally be seen as wasting time became key to building trust in the relationships, helping all to feel supported and ultimately to get the job done.

Trainee forums

In one of our teams, we offer a large number of regular placements to doctoral psychology trainees from a wide variety of London courses and across all years of training. Due to the nature of the service and the environment in which it is situated, the team has always had to think of ways to reduce isolation and increase connection across the service. One way we have done this, for the trainees working with us, has been to offer a monthly forum where they all attend. This is facilitated by a qualified member of staff and supports them to reflect on their work, the impact on themselves, and their experience of the training itself. In the dialogical forums, trainees are exposed to the Intervision techniques available from this approach. The impact we have found is multifaceted. Having this space is welcomed and valued by the trainees as a space to connect with each other, understand other peer experiences, achievements, and worries. It is an opportunity for them to practice reflecting skills, embodiment, and attunement as well as dialogical questioning in a psychological safe space. It also enables the qualified team in assessment progresses, undertaking observations of trainees and vice versa and teaching therapeutic skills they will use throughout the placement in co-facilitating groups. This grows personal and professional confidence as well being a place that personal worries can be noted and taken up outside of the group with individuals. The variety in trainees allows visibility of otherwise less dominant voices; the polyphony of the approach enables trainees to become aware of their own resonances, triggers, and way of being in the room with clients that enhances professional growth.

Owning our own worries

Seikkula and Arnkil (2014) write about approaching difficult situations that are of a worry to us in a dialogical way and of doing this early on before difficulties have become more significant. They write that we can often hesitate to act early because of a fear of how a meeting to discuss problems will be received. They suggest that often when we have a worry that it can be hard to sit with uncertainty and that we can easily slip into thinking we know what needs to change and speak from that position. At that point we have lost our ability to truly listen to the other from their own unique position and lost our trust in the process that new perspectives and ideas will arise.

They suggest that when we have a worry about another that we think how we can thank the other for what they have done or what has been done together about the issue. Then be clear to express our own worry and sincerely ask for their help in lessening the worry with an expectation that something will emerge from the dialogue where both will be helped.

A recent example of this was when a manager noticed that one of her staff members had stopped attending team meetings and was sitting separately to other staff who she usually spent time with. Her work was also not of her usual standard. The manager was invited to consider her way of approaching this. Previously she would have spoken to the person and told her that her not coming to meetings was not acceptable and that her work was not up to scratch, and she needed to work harder.

Instead, she approached her employee with genuine curiosity and said that she was sitting with a worry and asked for her help with it. An open conversation happened where the employee was able to share that she felt overwhelmed and had increased caring responsibilities. Through the dialogue, ideas and possibilities emerged. The employee said that the experience of being noticed and having a conversation where there was a genuine interest in what she could bring to the thinking made all the difference to her. Upon review, we found that the issues for both members of staff were resolved.

Box 14.4: Ending

Open dialogue meetings strive to end with a final question about how to continue the sessions and work together. All voices, in the same way as the opening of a session, are asked for their input into this and perspective. Everyone is asked if they want to meet again and if so in what way and when.

In a meeting, final thoughts from all the team are gathered about where the experience has taken them. Asking staff to state where they are now, even with one word, enables the facilitator to check risk, enhance safety of the group, and mitigate any barriers to further sessions.

Conclusion

We believe that the same processes and skills from Open Dialogue are easily transferred from the network meeting to wider organisational staff support and enhance leadership capabilities. The mental health network approach can be conceptualised for teams and organisational work, but one must consider the skills to be alongside each other in the process at every stage.

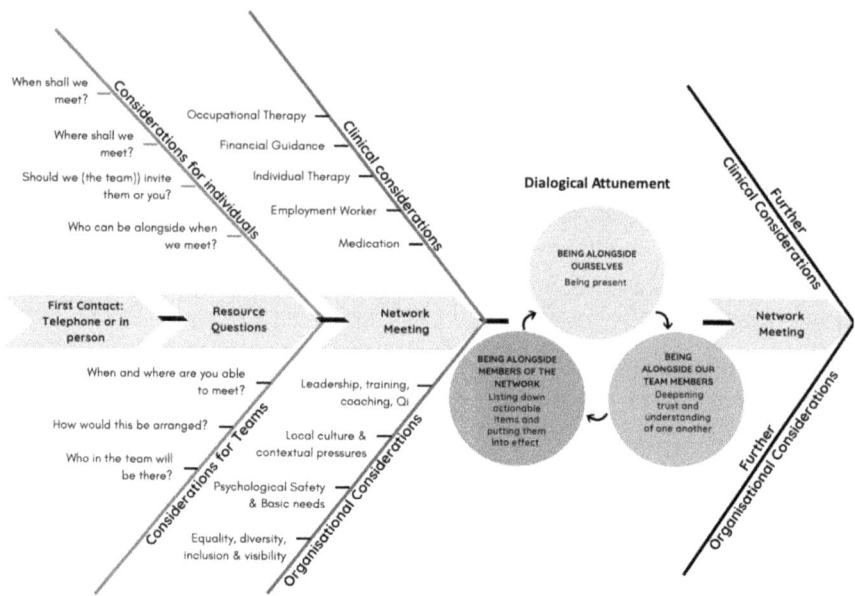

FIGURE 14.2: Network diagram with dialogical attunement integration.

Does Open Dialogue and dialogical leadership have a place in organisational and team discourse, in healthcare and social care symposiums? We would argue that it not only fits well with the many health and social care agendas and initiatives but can also sit within the multilayered Organisational Development tools already in use. Bringing dialogical skills into these arenas, while not easy, could support the foundations of health and social care work. When staff are able to remain true to their values, it has a positive impact on their professional identity, countenance, and personal wellbeing. This is supported when they are able to see their organisations address system issues that are undermining the very work, they are set up to do, bringing both into alignment and sustaining each other.

Objective-driven and pressured timelines can create a cycle of both physical and emotional exhaustion. Staff stuck in this relentless cycle often feel the need to drive forward in threat mode to solutions that ultimately act to fatigue them on all levels. If as Seikkula (2011) suggests, we need to become aware of what is occurring in us before we give words to it, we need to find ways for staff to pause to do this. Thoughts of fixed and static forms must be given up for fluid and dynamic relational interactions. Self-attunement and reflection supports us to distinguish between merely hearing what a person is saying and truly listening to what they are actually trying to say. Leading to expressions of connection and deeper understanding, not opinions of what *we think*, is the best course of action.

As you have read and reflected on this approach today, what have you underlined as important to you to remember? What has stood out for you to take away into your life beyond these pages? How is it connected to your own and others wellbeing? What support do you need to enact this new knowledge?

Open Dialogue challenges us all to listen to our inner voices, to bring the personal and the professional together. In developing this self-reflexivity which can aid cultural change and value-driven interventions in teams and organisations, it can support staff in the long term. When the world and work is overwhelming, having any space at all to reflect and connect together as a team is precious and supportive of staff wellbeing. Being dialogical is a way of being in the space between each other, in the room, in the meeting, and in life. So, what do we recommend if you want to be a dialogical leader and use these tools and ideas to support staff? Slow down, less is more, breathe, listen with all of yourself, be present with all of your senses, reflect from your own internal and external experiences, and remember the embodiment of love and humanity in our connections.

How could I talk in a way that increases others' desire to listen. How could I listen in a way that increases others' desire to talk?

(LYOTARD, 2014)
(https://lup.be/products/100320)

Credits: Alencia Kerdezia Trim, Assistant Psychologist

References

Andresen, R., Oades, L. and Caputi, P. (2003). The experience of recovery from schizophrenia: Towards an empirically validated stage model. *Australian & New Zealand Journal of Psychiatry*, 37(5), 586–594.

Andersen, T. (1991). *The reflecting team: Dialogues and dialogues about the dialogues*. New York: W. W. Norton.

Bakhtin, M. (1993). *Toward a philosophy of the act*, trans. Vadim Liapunov. Austin: University of Texas Press.

Bergström, T., Taskila, J. J., Alakare, B., Köngäs-Saviaro, P., Miettunen, J. and Seikkula, J. (2020). Five-year cumulative exposure to antipsychotic medication after first-episode psychosis and its association with 19-year outcomes. *Schizophrenia Bulletin Open*, 1(1), sgaa050.

Campbell, P. (1985). 'From little acorns – The mental health service user movement'. In: Bell, A. and Lindlay, P. (Eds.). *Beyond the water towers: The unfinished revolution in mental health services*, 2005, 73–82.

Giacco, D., McCabe, R., Kallert, T., Hansson, L., Fiorillo, A. and Priebe, S. (2012). Friends and symptom dimensions in patients with psychosis: A pooled analysis. *PLoS One*, 7(11), e50119.

Hall, L. H., Johnson, J., Heyhoe, J., Watt, I., Anderson, K. and O'Connor, D. B. (2020). Exploring the impact of primary care physician burnout and well-being on patient care: A focus group study. *Journal of Patient Safety*, 16(4), e278–e283.

Jackson, V. (2012). Developing open dialogue. Available at: http://developingopendialogue.com/ [Accessed 30 March 2022].

Johnson, J., Louch, G., Dunning, A., Johnson, O., Grange, A., Reynolds, C., Hall, L. and O'Hara, J. (2017). Burnout mediates the association between depression and patient safety perceptions: A cross-sectional study in hospital nurses. *Journal of Advanced Nursing*, 73(7), 1667–1680.

Laloux, F. (2016). *Reinventing organizations*. Lannoo Campus: Nelson Parker.

Lyotard, J. F. (2014). Complete collection Jean-François, Lyotard. In H. Parret (ed.), *Writings on contemporary art and artists* (Vol. 1–6). Leuven: Leuven University Press.

Mistry, H., Levack, W. M. and Johnson, S. (2015). Enabling people, not completing tasks: Patient perspectives on relationships and staff morale in mental health wards in England. *BMC Psychiatry*, 15(1), 1–10.

Monaghan, L. (2018). What are the themes of developing peer-supported open dialogue in the national health service in England? Unpublished dissertation.

Olson, M., Seikkula, J. and Ziedonis, D. (2014). *The key elements of dialogic practice in open dialogue: Fidelity criteria*. Worcester: University of Massachusetts Medical School.

Razzaque. (2014). *Introduction to peer-supported open dialogue*. London: North East London Foundation Trust.

Razzaque, R. and Wood, L. (2015). Open dialogue and its relevance to the NHS: Opinions of NHS staff and service users. *Community Mental Health Journal*, 51(8), 931–938.

Rober, P. (2005). The therapist's self in dialogical family therapy: Some ideas about not-knowing and the therapist's inner conversation. *Family Process*, 44(4), 477–495.

Rober, P., Elliott, R., Buysse, A., Loots, G. and De Corte, K. (2008). Positioning in the therapist's inner conversation: A dialogical model based on a grounded theory analysis of therapist reflections. *Journal of Marital and Family Therapy*, 34(3), 406–421.

Salyers, M. P., Bonfils, K. A., Luther, L., Firmin, R. L., White, D. A., Adams, E. L. and Rollins, A. L. (2017). The relationship between professional burnout and quality and safety in healthcare: A meta-analysis. *Journal of General Internal Medicine*, 32(4), 475–482.

Seikkula, J., Aaltonen, J., Alakare, B., Haarakangas, K., Keranen, J. and Lehtinen, K. (2006). Five-year experience of first-episode nonaffective psychosis in –open-dialogue approach: Treatment principles, follow up outcomes and two case studies. *Psychotherapy Research*, 16(2), 214–228.

Seikkula, J., Alakare, B., Aaltonen, J., Holma, J., Rasinkangas, A. and Lehtinen, V. (2003). Open dialogue approach: Treatment principles and preliminary results of a two-year follow-up on first episode schizophrenia. *Ethical Human Sciences and Services*, 5(3), 163–182.

Seikkula, J. and Arnkil, T. (2006). *Dialogical meetings in social networks*. New York: Karnac.

Seikkula, J. and Arnkil, T. (2014). Open dialogues and anticipations: Respecting the otherness in the present moment national institute for health and welfare, Vantaa, Tampere.

Seikkula, J. and Trimble, D. (2005). Healing elements of therapeutic conversation: Dialogue as an embodiment of love. *Family Process*, 44(4), 461–475.

Stratton, P. (2016). The evidence base of family therapy and systemic practice. Association for Family Therapy and Systemic Practice UK.

We are the NHS: People plan for 2020/21. London: Stationery Office, July 2020. Available at https://www.england.nhs.uk/ournhspeople [Accessed 8 December 2021].

West, M. A. (2012). *Effective teamwork: Practical lessons from organizational research*. London, John Wiley & Sons.

15 Strategic Working and Supporting Leadership within a Healthcare Context

Dr Julie Highfield and Dr Adrian Neal

Fundamentally, psychologists' training and understanding are within the broader realm of people. Do we need to limit our understanding to mental health, or can we utilise our expertise more widely to understand motivation, performance, team dynamics, and how to get the best out of people?

In settings such as primary care and adult mental health, psychologists are not the only psychologically trained team member, and it can feel difficult to find our own voice and contribution. Conversely, in medical settings, psychologists often find themselves the only psychologically trained team member among a team of medical, nursing, and allied health professionals. These teams look to the psychologist for advice and guidance on the care of their patients; however, they also look to the psychologist for how to shape the wellbeing of staff. Additionally, there has been an increased invitation to consider the psychological wellbeing of the staff providing healthcare, and, in the UK, an increase in roles specific to staff wellbeing.

Practitioner psychologists have traditionally found themselves employed with a remit to provide psychological intervention to individuals and groups. In emerging healthcare staff wellbeing roles, it would be tempting to continue to follow this model. Often the position considered for psychologists is that of providing intervention: through the provision of psychological interventions to reduce work-related stress or resolve the psychological impacts of work such as work-related trauma. There are calls for us to 'teach resilience' and yet resilience is not a fixed characteristic or a skill but a dynamic interaction between the person and their environment.

The UK Health and Safety Executive considers the approaches of education and psychological intervention to be useful, but 'secondary' or 'tertiary' – treating the resulting ill health rather than dealing with the causal factors. There is increased recognition of practitioner psychologists' wider ability to offer consultation and advice. When it comes to the realm of staff wellbeing in healthcare, if we simply offer psychological intervention, we may be selling ourselves short.

In this chapter, we will explore the concept of influence as a practitioner psychologist, considering a number of healthcare settings, and comparing and contrasting formalised roles of staff wellbeing and authorised influence versus other more traditional roles for psychologists and informal influence. This chapter focuses on the evidence and opportunities for psychologists to have influence, work strategically, and how they may both be leaders, but also support leaders within a healthcare context. We encourage psychologists to move away from the idea of supporting staff wellbeing, to the concept of supporting a positive experience of work and enabling the core conditions to thrive at work.

Background theory and research

Providing care and treatment to people is inherently psychologically demanding. Healthcare staff, in particular nurses, have among the highest rates of work-related stress every year (Health & Safety Executive, 2015). In the NHS staff survey, 40.3% of NHS staff reported that they suffered from work-related stress (NHS Staff Survey, 2020). In a systematic review, multiple studies provide evidence that both wellbeing and burnout are associated with patient safety (Hall et al., 2016).

Interest in workforce wellbeing particularly increased following the 2013 Francis Inquiry. The inquiry linked patient errors and deaths to toxic culture and dysfunctional leadership, and it was concluded that to mitigate the risk the NHS needed to move towards a culture of compassion. This sentiment was echoed by the 2013 Berwick report. In 2014, the Care Quality Commission in England took this into account by shifting towards considering staff wellbeing and staff engagement in their assessment. This led to an increased rollout of employee wellbeing initiatives, but mostly focusing on individual approaches to self-care and self-management.

Thankfully, many important papers and guidance have sought to rectify this individualistic approach. For instance, the 2015 *NICE Workplace Health: management practices* recommendations focus on leadership competencies and practice for the wellbeing of the workforce. The 2017 British Psychological Society paper, *Psychology at Work*, emphasised the need for us to focus on the psychosocial working environment. The Health Education England commissioned document, *Workforce Stress and the Supportive Organisation*, takes a Systemic approach to workforce wellbeing. In the 2017 Stevenson–Farmer Review, there was a move away from individualistic wellbeing and a call to provide the core conditions to thrive at work. More recently, reports from fellow psychologists on the mental health of nurses and midwives (Kinman et al., 2020) and of doctors (Kinman & Teoh, 2018; West & Coia, 2018) have emphasised the need for improving the core conditions of work to improve staff wellbeing and patient outcomes. Indeed, the rapid guidance for supporting healthcare staff in the COVID-19 pandemic advocated leadership and systems approaches above psychological therapies (Highfield et al., 2020).

There are now a significant number of national publications since the Francis Report, which indicate the success of healthcare, and the success of caring for staff is beyond the individual, but lies within teams and culture. A golden thread that runs throughout these is the importance of good leadership.

If one were to read through the leadership literature, one would be struck by how large and diverse it is. There is limited evidence about which leadership approach is the most effective, and there is cultural variation in what are thought to be the positive traits of leaders. Throughout the range of approaches, there is one agreement: that it involves relationships.

Current practice

Given the evidence for leadership and culture in the influence upon staff experience, and interest, how do we as psychologists practically offer support to healthcare leadership?

1. **The position to allow influence to happen.**

The first, most challenging way to put this into practice, is to be in any position to influence.

Role definition and description have a significant impact on what the psychologist has permission and is authorised to offer.

For example, many roles will be designated like 'Practitioner Psychologist In …', with the setting defining the first sphere of influence. So a psychologist within cystic fibrosis (CF) firstly finds themselves only in a position of influence in the CF team. This role may have been funded initially for people with CF and their families. They may find themselves 'invited in' to offer teaching, reflective practice or clinical supervision, which may start to afford them the wider position of influencing the system. Over time, as relationships and with increased trust and credibility, the psychologist, as a 'safe pair of hands', may be invited to offer more thought to the strategic direction of the CF service, and they may find themselves able to offer ad hoc or routine support and ideas to the leadership roles. However, the bounds of the CF service may be the bounds of their influence, unless recognised for their work and invited to work beyond the bounds of the service they are employed for. One can take the example of *Practitioner Psychologist in Cystic Fibrosis*, and exchange for any other subsystem of healthcare, often characterised by conditions (e.g. nephrology, eating disorders) or location or healthcare need (e.g. critical care; primary care).

Other roles are more overt in their invitation for working within the staff system. There are increasing roles which are Trust or Healthboard wide. Such a title naturally lends itself to a wider sphere of influence. However often the starting point is to provide the secondary and tertiary inputs such as education, psychological intervention, and reflective practice. Staff who find themselves early within these roles, just as the example above, need to build relationships, trust, and credibility before being able to offer a lens on the wider organisation through supporting leaders. The strategy is to take the time to prove your worth, and slowly take time to influence.

2. What does supporting a leader look like?

Note the word 'invitation' utilised in the section above. As we understand from the world of therapeutic work, our clients need to be in a position of readiness and invite us in to work with them through engaging with psychological therapy. So too is the work with leaders and systems. We may offer our services; however, we need to be invited to deliver them or await the leader to take us up on our offers. Just as in therapy, this can take considerable time, readiness (to change), and potentially being willing to be vulnerable.

So in being supported or helped, what form does this take? Well, most often this takes the form of a one-to-one conversation. Unlike models of psychological therapy or coaching, it is unlikely to be steered by one core model of approach, and more likely to take the format of working through each dilemma as it arises. That said, we can still follow a core model of assess, formulate, and intervene, although the assessment is likely in the format of a conversation, the formulation is in the format of ideas and hypotheses, and the intervention may be in the format of ideas for action, advice, or consultation. For instance, the leader asks 'what do you think about how I manage a particular employee?'.

The psychologist would then evoke more information and potentially offer their thoughts based on a psychological formulation.

At other times, supporting leadership may take the format of working alongside the leader, such as being alongside them in meetings, and offering thoughts and support. Or potentially facilitating a team meeting alongside the leader or a teaching alongside the leader.

Another way of supporting leaders we often refer to as 'being a stagehand', where, symbolically speaking, the leader is the actor on the stage, and psychologist acts as a stagehand, offering possible next lines of the script. This specialist advisor role is possibly the most powerful position to hold and comes with many potential pitfalls, so is only offered in the most trusting of leader–psychologist dyads.

3. How to make the most of it – what is the work of influence?

A first important part of influence is to be known. To have a reputation and track record is helpful, alongside the position described above. The bedrock of this is the ability a practitioner psychologist has developed to form nurturing and enabling relationships. One must walk the fine line of when to say yes: if you are known for being helpful but are not authorised to help, it is tempting to state work boundaries and not respond to requests. Although it is imperative to have professional boundaries, being able to show willing and availability builds reputation, but also builds a soft 'power' which can lead to more formal authorised positions being established. For example, a psychologist working with the Cardiology team may offer some sound advice to the Clinical Director, who then recommends a conversation with the psychologist to her colleague, the Clinical Director of Gastroenterology. It would be tempting to state 'that's not my role'; however, a one-off helpful conversation could lead to increased positive reputation. The boundaries of the role can still be stated 'that's not usually my role, but I'm happy to be flexible within these limits'.

We need to consider *how* we have supportive conversations with various leaders and their teams. As far back as Aristotle, we have reflected upon how to make an argument that will be heard. Aristotle outlines three core parts of the argument The source (ethos) which is the properties of the person, the pathos or the feelings provoked by the arguer, and the logic (logos) or the properties of arguments. To argue well, all three need to be equally considered. Often as psychologists we may be drawn more to emphasise the logic to our argument, when operating outside of the therapy room. We need to be reminded of our relational aspects of therapy and also consider how we are perceived as an arguer and what feelings we provoke. Nickerson (2021) considers the component core qualities of the influencer as follows: their level of prestige, attractiveness, similarity, relationship to the audience ('I am like you'), their core knowledge in the domain, and their ability to encourage perspective taking. In order to make the most of our influence, we need to consider in each interaction how we are received in each of these areas.

Often as psychologists we can take a position of 'inside and outside', where we can take a participatory role within a meeting or group, and also an observatory role. This is where we utilise our skills of 'reading the room'. This can refer to the room itself, or more widely and symbolically to the team, system, or organisation. Part of our skills as a psychologist is to determine the readiness and motivation towards change or movement in each part of the system, and the embedded politics within this. We can utilise this knowledge in supporting leaders, guiding them on when to act, what part of the system needs more attention or focus. We can also apply the same knowledge to how we approach whole systems; for those psychologists positioned at an organisational level such as overarching staff wellbeing services, we can consider when sub-parts of that system are ready only to refer staff for one-to-one psychological therapies, and when there is an increased awareness of the need for team-based interventions. Often in healthcare, the invite to join the whole team is often in the immediate aftermath of a crisis point, hence the call for staff wellbeing psychologists to offer 'debriefing'. There is much speculation as to the quality of psychological debriefing summarised elsewhere (e.g. van Emmerik, 2002); however, supportive conversations with willing team members after significant events can often be revealing of other issues and can often create an entry point to working with the team. However, many teams can seal over after such events and are not yet ready to engage in next stages. In the systems equivalent of Vygotsky's zone of proximal development, we can identify when it is possible to push things where they are willing to go, and when it is wiser to take a tactical retreat.

4. The reality of working with leaders and systems

In the reality of working alongside busy leaders in complex systems, limitations arise. The following are some key examples.

- **Framing the relationship**

Most practitioner psychologists embedded in clinical work are skilled in therapeutic work. That is not the limit of our skills; however, time and time again a barrier to us having supportive conversations is that others will frame this as psychological therapy. Although informed by all of those skills and the associated experience, part of negotiating the leader–psychologist dyad is to define the boundaries of the relationship and to define them away from psychological therapy. (That said, we may at times offer psychological therapy to leaders if that is what we are invited and contracted to do.) Helpful frames, depending on the content, may be (a) an advisory role, (b) consultancy, (c) coaching, or simply framing it as (d) offering support as a psychologist.

- **Cognitive bias**

Leaders often have a position of responsibility for large numbers of people or systems. They find themselves having to make difficult decisions, sometimes with very limited time and potentially conflicting information. They will inevitably make mistakes, and it is possible that in response to these mistakes they will deploy cognitive dissonance and confirmation bias to ad hoc justify their actions. There are, however, instances of the cognitive bias of leaders being self-serving and potentially narcissistic in quality. An important part of working with leaders is to notice these and work with them, as simply bringing these to attention may be perceived as a threat and lead to disengagement or discrediting the psychologist. The work by Tavris and Aronson (2015) explores such biases in greater detail.

- **System design**

One of the most dominant and useful relationship-based approaches to examining leadership is leader–member exchange (LMX) theory (for an overview, see Bauer & Erdogan, 2015). LMX theory postulates that those leader relationships that focus primarily on what is written in the contract of employment are characterised by low trust, interaction, and rewards. When we think of our typical ward environment, where we have one nurse managing a team of 25–50 staff, the relationship can be somewhat transactional and characterised by a focus on the employment contract in this way. In high LMX relationships, the exchanges extend beyond the job description and high LMX followers are more likely to be given interesting work activities, receive more supervisory support, and obtain more opportunities for advancement. LMX quality positively correlates with a wide range of work-related attitudes and behaviours (Dulebohn et al., 2012) and work performance (Martin et al., 2016). In the context of our hospital environments, these high LMX relationships are more likely to happen in smaller teams, where there is more flexibility in role. These high LMX relationships naturally lend themselves to more collaborative or compassionate leadership styles. However, the reality is that healthcare systems are often designed to create the conditions for low LMX relationships.

- **Learned helplessness and burnout**

The interest in workplace wellbeing has also led to interest in burnout, which is not a diagnosis but an occupational phenomenon as a response to the social and work environment, as now recognised in ICD-11. It is a chronic state of being emotionally exhausted, cynical, and discouraged. The burnout of individual workers says more about workplace conditions than it does about that person. Of course, leaders are not immune to burnout, and working with leaders, psychologists need to recognise these symptoms in both the leaders and their teams to work out which way to work most effectively. If the leader shows evidence of emotional exhaustion, they are likely overextended, so delegation and better work boundaries may be the intervention. However, if their team is showing signs of emotional exhaustion, it is likely the team require a better management of the workload, which, with limited healthcare resources, is harder to manage. The leader may be showing signs of depersonalisation and cynicism, therefore is likely to be feeling disengaged, either from their team or from the wider system. Helping the leader to reconnect with their team or re-engage with their core purpose may be helpful. A cynical team too requires the work of engagement and feeling valued, often by their leaders. The leader who feels a lack of personal accomplishment may have felt continuously discouraged or thwarted by systems issues; this thwarting can in turn leave the team feeling discouraged, and learned helplessness is the risk. The intervention is likely at the level of system blocks, which may have some simple human factors solutions, or may be more politically embedded.

- **Wicked problems**

A wicked problem is a problem that is difficult to resolve due to contradictory and changing requirements. They may sometimes be difficult to recognise and there is no single solution. It cannot be removed from its environment, solved, and returned without affecting the environment; there is no clear relationship between cause and effect; and there is no endpoint. Wicked problems are different to tame problems, which are considered to have clear solutions. Healthcare workplace wellbeing is a wicked problem. Indeed, providing healthcare is also a wicked problem. If we tackle wicked problems in a decisive and single focused way, we are trying to manage it as a tame problem, often when we try to resolve wicked problems other compound problems emerge (Grint, 2010). For example, if a staff member is under stress at work, the solution may be to offer time off; however, if all staff took time off, there would be a workforce crisis, and if we kept staff in work we would be left with problems of presenteeism. If we offered teaching on better stress management, some staff are likely to gain awareness that their job is causing them stress and choose to leave for a less stressful role. We know from the debriefing and reflective literature that not all staff wish to come together to discuss the impact of work, that for some this in fact puts them at higher psychological risk. We can offer all of these solutions, yet some people will still struggle with the nature of the work due to excessive workload, poor relationships with team members or managers. Therefore, when advising and guiding leaders on the health and wellbeing of their workforce, we have no single solution to offer, and no endpoint in the problems being resolved. However, many approaches are invited to follow a 'surgical model': assess, intervene (remove), resolution. We perhaps instead need to take a chronic illness model of awareness, management, and damage limitation. Grint points out that "the uncertainty involved in Wicked Problems imply that leadership ... is not a science but an art – the art of engaging a community in facing up to complex collective problems" (Grint, 2008, p. 13).

Examples for practice

The example of Intensive Care

One author of this chapter has been the lead for Adult and Paediatric Intensive Care in her hospital since February 2015. She was also the Associate Director for the service from December 2017 to March 2020. Within her role she has had a designation as the lead clinician for Organisational Health, therefore formally authorising her position as systems advisor and implementer on staff wellbeing and experience. Since July 2020 she has been seconded two days per week to direct a national project on behalf of the UK Intensive Care Society – a charity which represents the different professionals working within intensive care.

Intensive care is a high-stakes, high-reward environment which has been characterised by poor staff wellbeing (e.g. Highfield & Parry Jones, 2019; Vincent et al., 2019; Highfield, 2021) and great need for an integrated approach for staff sustainability (Highfield, 2018). Before the pandemic, intensive care demands were increasing, requiring more capacity and workforce, but also troubling levels of turnover with 10% of units indicating turnover in excess of 20% (CC3N, 2018). The pandemic has unfortunately exaggerated these problems, particularly for nurses, as staff have been forced to breach ratios and stretch standards to meet the high level of demand.

Highfield frames her work around four key principles as highlighted in her 2018 paper:

1. Wellbeing at work is relationally based – one of the most important relationships is with the line manager
2. For all stress, demands should not exceed resources, therefore staff need to be provided with the core conditions to thrive at work
3. Critical care is emotionally challenging and some staff have learned maladaptive ways of managing this emotion
4. Change must happen at a systems level – one-to-one help only helps one person to realise the system is bad for them!

As Highfield (2018) outlines, we therefore need to manage emotional demands, increase emotional resources, and choose and support leaders who can drive these processes. In her work in intensive care over the years, she has moved to the authorised invited-in position to increase the emphasis on the support of leaders, and becoming a leader herself, to support these system changes. A shift came when she was invited to do this at a national level. Again however, as a charitable organisation this was a new system to navigate. She had to start from the tertiary approach of producing resources and gateways to psychological support, while slowly becoming known and moving her position to supporting leaders more actively, and taking a systems approach. Figure 15.1 illustrates the programme approach that the national project took, with year one focusing at

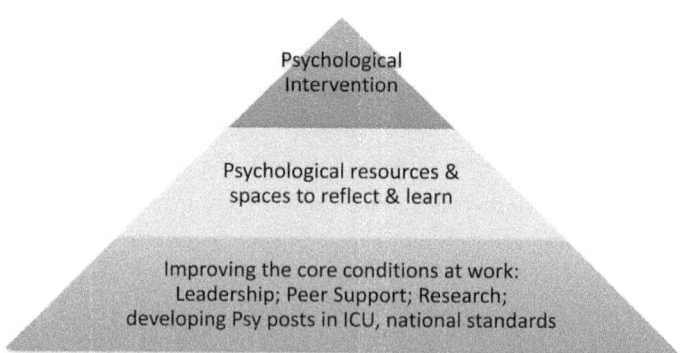

FIGURE 15.1: The Intensive Care Society Wellbeing Project.

the top of the triangle and in year two moving to the base of the triangle – moving the work from wellbeing to core conditions to thrive. In essence, what this looked like in practice was lots of webinars and written resources in the first few months, then a move to create a peer support training programme, embedded psychology posts in units, leaders' reflective sessions, and then at the next stage creating the Best Practice Framework (Highfield, ICS, 2020) and the Assurance and Improvement tool (Highfield, ICS, 2021) and advising at the Operational Delivery Network level. She again had to negotiate problems of systems design, individual and group bias, taking her time reading the room and deciding when to act and when to step back. At point of publishing, the project had been highly commended in the *British Medical Journal* awards and had a reach of over 90,000 points of contact.

The example of a Welsh Health Board

Moving any established organisational narrative is challenging, as many practitioner psychologists will know. Illustrated by the struggle we have had in challenging the dominant medical narrative to equitably include evidenced psychological and social factors. We also know that organisational narratives don't always respond to logic and an evidenced argument. Establishing an evidenced-based psychologically informed organisational wellbeing narrative is no different.

This example maps out how since 2015 a group of like-minded employees (led in kind by the head of Wellbeing, a practitioner psychologist) within a large NHS organisation (ca. 15,000) have collaborated to embed a new narrative, with mixed success.

It is import to point out that this process, which is ongoing, wasn't driven entirely by a single strategy; rather, it has evolved through some strategic planning, significant opportunism, political alliance building, dedication, collaboration, and also good fortune. This section will map out the key components of this process.

i. *A new narrative and getting into a position to influence*

The Head of Wellbeing post in this example was held by a practitioner psychologist and located within Workforce and Organisational Development (WOD). This post was responsible for managing an existing small staff psychological therapy service, and a clinical case load, but importantly was not attached to Occupational Health (OH). Being located within WOD and not OH has offered a distinct advantage in that it inadvertently authorised work beyond the focus away from individuals towards the wider system. As such, very early on, a new narrative was formed and its establishment seen as a long-term ambition. This narrative was as follows:

> *Workplace wellbeing is a complex multi-factorial biopsychosocial phenomenon, and we need to move away from an individual reactive focus towards a proactive systems focus.*

This new narrative was framed as being evidenced based and used in an early wellbeing strategy paper, but most importantly it was adopted by a key group of like-minded colleagues, including practitioner psychologists, OD practitioners, and senior WOD managers. With the support of these individuals, and from this position in the organisation, the new narrative felt authorised, and influence possible.

ii. *Building the new narrative through influence, relationships, and reputation*

The new narrative was subsequently spread across the organisation by colleagues which led to a snowballing effect. This process, though not initially part of a strategy, was slowly recognised as an essential. Central to this was the emerging reputation and profile of the Employee Wellbeing Service and its lead. This reputation was deliberately protected and developed as an intervention in itself; specific focus was given to the service's profile with senior managers and organisational leaders. At all times the desired narrative would remain simple and tethered to evidence-based practice. It was however also linked at an early stage to organisational objectives until then not explicitly addressed such as performance, patient safety, staff turnover, and quality while links to sickness absence were deliberately minimised (to link employee wellbeing interventions to sickness and absence are troubling metrics; there are times when it is better for all if an employee to leave the organisation or to take some time off, but in sickness absence measures, this would be deemed a failure). To support the development of organisational trust and reputation, specific emphasis was placed on the service and its lead being responsive to the needs of the organisation and a trusted 'safe pair of hands'.

iii. *Strategic(ish) use of systemic resources*

A range of initiatives (devices) to support the emerging narrative were rolled out over a number of years: these included both the established (e.g. Schwartz Rounds) but also the novel and locally developed initiatives (e.g. Taking Care

Giving Care Rounds). Other initiatives that have subsequently become standard 'wellbeing support' offerings include a focus on quality improvement work, leadership development, clinical innovation, team development, psychological debriefing, peer support, mentoring, and coaching. In many ways much of this work developed spontaneously when opportunities presented themselves. Although in many ways these initiatives developed without formal authorisation, they blossomed in an environment which encouraged innovation, positive risk taking, and where employees were given the agency to do so. Each of these initiatives has at its core the DNA of our original narrative, and we have no longer needed to be as explicit in promoting it. However, the resurgence of the 'resilience and individual toughness narrative' during the pandemic has required us to turn up the volume of our intended narrative from time to time.

iv. *Pivotal update to the strategy – Employee Wellbeing Framework*

In late 2019, authorised by the Director of WOD, a small group of colleagues developed a tool that would combine in one place the authorised organisational approach to both wellbeing and engagement. This new tool was entirely congruent with our original 'new' narrative, and for the first time offered managers and staff alike a practical tool to map out the core psychosocial conditions evidenced to support thriving at work. The authorising of this tool allowed us to move the narrative further away from health and individuals towards prevention and psychologically healthier working environments. This development also firmly recognises as an organisational ambition the intention to make the experience of work positive. In many ways this represents an evolution of the original narrative around wellbeing, given a much clearer focus on the work that is needed to make it achievable. One of the impacts of the pandemic has been that this work has been delayed. The focus on emergency response to acute needs has required a more transactional and reactive position, though with the organisation now looking to the horizon and recovery the Employee Experience Framework (EEF) is again being looked to as a useful resource. What's more the framework has been adapted for national (Welsh) NHS and Social Care use which should help the evolving narrative both consolidate and spread.

v. *Using data to support the narrative*

An important factor in the development and fostering of a new narrative has been its strong association with evidence, both evidence-based practice and practice-based evidence. The narrative in this case study would have been significantly limited if this position had not been adopted. Organisations feel reassured by data. Even though we know there is no inherent link between quality and data collection, it is nevertheless an important organisation need to be aware of. Offering reliable data supports the reputation of the service and its associated interventions and fosters reputational development. The more trust develops, the more agency is offered allowing for expansion and the taking of organisation's risks. It also supports, one might argue, the organisation's value in its internal wellbeing leadership.

In addition to the strategic use of data collection, the banner of evidence led/based practice can help authorise the use to wider more powerful data collection methodologies. Quality data collection will both offer up invaluable data about wellbeing, but also indirectly communicate the narrative. That the factors being asked about are important to the organisation and indeed tethered to its values. During the pandemic we have developed an organisation-wide survey asking about coping, fatigue, inviting opinions and around what resources might help, and then asking about the conditions people need to thrive using the EEF factors (i.e. control, belonging, trust, fairness, purpose). Data (and organisational trust in the data) from these surveys now numbering approx. 15,000 individual responses has helped shape a major organisational re-engagement initiative called 'People First' which will see executive and senior leaders regularly meeting with staff on the ground to understand their experiences, solve the problems they can't solve, and to rebuild trust and hope.

This case study illustrates how a new narrative around workplace wellbeing was seeded in an organisation and how over time it has been imperfectly fostered allowing it to evolve and take root. It is important to stress that this process continues, is vulnerable, and requires regular strategic and emotional investment from those in positions of influence, and moral authority in what is untimely a very hierarchical, complex bureaucratic and at times toxic system, the NHS.

Conclusion

Practitioner psychologists are more than just therapists – there is added value of psychologists as organisational consultants in healthcare systems. One of the key ways in which they can offer consultation is through their direct work with leaders, and this is a way of influencing wider organisational strategy and culture. That said, this work is complex; it takes time to build relationships and reputation, we need to be authorised and invited to do the work, and we meet with many obstacles along the way. We need to consider how we are perceived, how we read the room and are able to influence. We need to consider carefully how we frame the relationship to work with bias and vulnerability. Given the strong evidence base that leaders influence staff experience of work and their work-related wellbeing, if we can influence the leaders, we can hope to help a wider range of staff beyond our therapy room.

Key points

1. Our work as practitioner psychologists is people – not just mental health. Our staff wellbeing work should look beyond mental health.
2. A golden thread running through staff experience and wellbeing literature is the influence of good leadership.
3. Practitioner psychologists can support leaders in the way they think about themselves and think about the people they lead.
4. To do this, practitioner psychologists need to be aware of politic, position, soft power, and their ability to influence. The leaders do not always overtly identify in the same way that clients would.

References

Aristotle., Roberts, W. R., Bywater, I., & Solmsen, F. (1954). *Rhetoric*. New York: Modern Library.
Bauer, T. N., & Erdogan, B. (Eds.). (2016). *The Oxford handbook of leader-member exchange*. Oxford. Oxford University Press.
Berwick, D. (2013). *Berwick review into patient safety – Publications – GOV.UK*. Available at: https://www.gov.uk/government/publications/berwick-review-into-patient-safety [Accessed 29 November 2021].
Dulebohn, J. H., Bommer, W. H., Liden, R. C., Brouer, R. L., & Ferris, G. R. (2012). A meta-analysis of antecedents and consequences of leader-member exchange: Integrating the past with an eye toward the future. *Journal of Management, 38*(6), 1715–1759.
Francis, R. (2013). Report of the Mid Staffordshire NHS foundation trust public inquiry *Publications – GOV.UK*. Available at: https://www.gov.uk/government/publications/report-of-the-mid-staffordshire-nhs-foundation-trust-public-inquiry [accessed 29 November 2021]
Grint, K. (2008). Wicked problems and clumsy solutions: The role of leadership. *The New Public Leadership Challenge, 1*(2), 169–186.
Grint, K. (2010). The cuckoo clock syndrome: Addicted to command, allergic to leadership. *European Management Journal, 28*(4), 306–313.
Hall, L. H., Johnson, J., Watt, I., Tsipa, A., & O'Connor, D. B. (2016). Healthcare staff wellbeing, burnout, and patient safety: A systematic review. *PLoS ONE, 11*(7), e0159015.
Health & Safety Executive. (2015). *Work related stress, anxiety and depression statistics in Great Britain*. Available at: www.hse.gov.uk
Highfield, J. (2019). The sustainability of the critical care workforce. Critical care nursing. British association of critical care nurses, 24(1), 6–7.

Highfield, J. (2020) Intensive care as a positive place to work: Workforce wellbeing best practice framework. The Intensive Care Society. Available at https://www.ics.ac.uk/Society/Wellbeing_hub/Workforce_Wellbeing_Framework. [Accessed 29 November 2021].

Highfield, J. (2021). How are our healthcare staff now? *Critical Eye, 19*, 26–27.

Highfield, J., Johnston, E., Jones, T., Kinman, G., Maunder, R., Monaghan, L., Murphy, D., Rao, A., Scales, K., Tehrani, N., & West, M. (2020). The psychological needs of healthcare staff as a result of the Coronavirus pandemic. *British Psychological Society*. Available at: https://www.bps.org.uk/sites/www.bps.org.uk/files/News/News%20-%20Files/Psychological%20needs%20of%20healthcare%20staff.pdf [Accessed 29 November 2021].

Highfield, J., & Parry-Jones, J. (2019). Professional quality of life in intensive care medicine- The 2018 faculty of intensive care medicine workforce survey. *Journal of the Intensive Care Society, 21*(4), 299–304.

International Classification of Diseases, Eleventh Revision (ICD-11), World Health Organization (WHO) 2019/2021 https://icd.who.int/browse11.

Kinman, G., & Teoh, K. (2018). *What could make a difference to the mental health of UK doctors?* Society of Occupational Medicine. Available at: www.som.org.uk

Kinman, G., Teoh, K., & Harriss, A. (2020). *The mental health and wellbeing of nurses and midwives in the United Kingdom*. Society of Occupational Medicine. Available at: www.som.org.uk

MacDonald, I., Burke, C., & Stewart, K. (2006). *Systems leadership: Creating positive organizations* (1st ed.). London: Routledge.

Martin, R., Guillaume, Y., Thomas, G., Lee, A., & Epitropaki, O. (2016). Leader–member exchange (LMX) and performance: A meta-analytic review. *Personnel Psychology, 69*(1), 67–121.

National Institute for Health and Clinical Excellence. (2015). *Workplace health: Management practices. NICE Guideline NG13*. Available at: www.nice.org.uk

Nickerson, R. S. (2021). *Argumentation: The art of persuasion*. Cambridge: Cambridge University Press.

NHS Staff Survey. (2020). Available at: www.nhsstaffsurveys.com

Stevenson, D., & Farmer, P. (2017). Thriving at work: The Stevenson/Farmer review of mental health and employers. Available at: www.gov.uk

Tavris, C., & Aronson, E. (2015). *Mistakes were made but not by me: Why we justify foolish beliefs, bad decisions, and hurtful acts* (2nd ed.). Boston: Mariner Books.

The National Workforce Skills Development Unit. (2019). *Workforce stress and the supportive organisation*. Health Education England. Available at https://www.hee.nhs.uk/sites/default/files/documents/Workforce%20Stress%20and%20the%20Supportive%20Organisation_0.pdf [Accessed 29 November 2021].

van Emmerik, A. A., Kamphuis, J. H., Hulsbosch, A. M., Emmelkamp, P. M. (2002). Single session debriefing after psychological trauma: A meta-analysis. *Lancet, 360*(9335), 766–771.

Vincent, L., Brindley, P. Highfield, J., & Innes, R. (2019). A national survey of burnout in UK intensive care staff. *Journal of the Intensive Care Society, 20*(4), 363–369.

Weinberg, A., & Doyle, A. (2017). Psychology at work: Improving wellbeing and productivity in the workplace. *British Psychological Society*.

West, M., & Coia, D. (2018). *Caring for doctors, caring for patients:* How to transform UK healthcare environments to support doctors and medical students to care for patients. Available at: www.bps.org.uk

16 Brief Interventions with Senior Healthcare Staff during the Pandemic

Dr Penelope Cream and Professor Mike Wang

The Association of Clinical Psychologists (ACP-UK) is a member-led professional body set up to represent the work and interests of clinical psychologists in the UK. Its members represent all the different specialties of clinical psychology practice, including adult mental health, physical health, children and families, the psychology of ageing, and forensic and legal work. When the COVID-19 pandemic hit Britain in early March 2020, the ACP-UK and its members rapidly agreed to provide specialist psychological support to NHS clinical staff and those working in social care contexts. One of the groups they particularly reached out to was the most senior staff, including hospital consultants, clinical leads, and senior managers and those in executive positions, as well as to the clinical psychologists working with the hospital staff caring for some of the sickest patients. It was known to many of the ACP-UK members that senior staff are often the least likely to ask for help. In this chapter we outline the background to this decision and the narratives and literature on help-seeking in senior staff and psychological staff.

Contexts to the programme's development

From the outset of the pandemic in 2020, some ACP-UK Board directors who had worked in acute medical settings were specifically concerned about critical care medical and nursing staff. Mike, for example, had a long-standing research and clinical collaboration with some intensive care unit (ICU) consultants and was known for his work on accidental awareness during general anaesthesia: he had a prominent role on the Royal College of Anaesthesia's (RCoA) National Audit Project 5 (Pandit et al., 2014). In April 2020, Mike reached out to the RCoA Faculty of Intensive Care Medicine, proposing that ACP-UK might offer senior-level psychological support given the severe and expected impact of the pandemic on critical care. During the early part of the pandemic, it will be remembered there was a great deal of emphasis on COVID-19 respiratory complications and the need for mechanical ventilation and body rolling, mainly on ICUs. ICUs were filling up, and there was a huge drive to increase critical care capacity, with consequent demands on critical care staff. Nevertheless, some members of the ACP-UK Board thought we ought to focus on the needs of less prominent and influential healthcare workers such as porters, cleaners, and HCAs.

ACP-UK had been involved in planning for the NHS England national response from an early stage, and we were aware that the planned staff support 'resilience' hubs would be focused especially on nursing and general care staff (including porters and cleaners). We reasoned that it was actually the most senior medical staff who would not be provided for, given the inherent barriers to support-seeking. We felt that only an offer from the most experienced and qualified senior clinical psychologists who were familiar with acute healthcare environments would make any impression at all on senior medical staff. These assumptions have since been vindicated with evaluation data and qualitative feedback from those who accessed ACP-UK's support service.

At the same time, PC had proposed to ACP-UK the need to support clinical psychologists, the core members of the organisation. At that time, clinical psychologists were one of the only UK clinical professions whose welfare was not supported by a central professional organisation. This need was further emphasised when the pandemic started and clinical psychologists working in medical settings and elsewhere were rapidly redeployed to staff support roles, often in environments that were new to them, such as intensive care, respiratory medicine, and elderly medicine wards. It is all too easy to overlook caring for the supporters, especially when those supporters are in a minority role in a large organisation, as was usually the case at the start of the pandemic for many clinical psychologists in physical health. Many hospital trusts did not have specific staff support teams, and a large proportion of ICUs did not have clinical psychology input. It was a steep learning curve for all, and it has turned out to be one of the fastest leaps into the public and media consciousness for the role of psychology within medicine that we have ever experienced.

The staff support schemes were put to a vote and ACP-UK's membership elected to start schemes to provide one-to-one support for its members and senior frontline staff and managers on the basis that they were unlikely to seek help from more established sources. In addition, the members voted to offer free webinars on a variety of psychological aspects of managing during a pandemic and understanding its impact on critical care.

As a result, ACP-UK very rapidly set up three staff support scheme streams all aimed at supporting the supporters. One stream was for its full members (both qualified and trainee clinical psychologists), another focused on providing support for frontline senior ICU staff, and the third offered sessions to senior NHS and social care managers. As the pandemic progressed, critical care and the meaning of 'frontline' quickly expanded beyond the traditional ICU environment and acute hospital settings. Frontline came to mean the interface between staff and patients directly affected by COVID-19. ACP-UK responded by offering support to all frontline senior clinical and social care staff and managers.

Physician heal thyself – Why focus on senior staff?

The belief that clinicians should in some way be infallible to the same problems and illnesses that they help their patients manage (Klitzman, 2008) can prove a barrier to seeking support. This concept runs through many clinical and helping professions, including medicine and mental health clinical psychology. Reading through the many COVID-19 guides on team working and staff support, as well as those on clinical decision-making, it is striking how often the need for leaders to be visible, active, compassionate, available, and accessible is mentioned (e.g. DCP guidelines, 2021). Leaders are described as needing 'to tolerate and manage uncertainty for yourself and your staff' (BPS Covid-19 Staff Wellbeing Group, 2020) and how 'more senior managers should keep an eye on more junior ones' (Greenberg et al., 2020). This is all excellent advice but almost nowhere is there a description included of the particular needs of those same senior leaders, who experience illness, sadness, despair, and personal bereavement like anyone else, and potentially to a higher degree especially if from a Black, Asian, and minority ethnic background disproportionately affected by the pandemic (Women and Equalities Committee, 2020). The impact on leaders who are themselves in need of care is likely to be significant. This includes clinical psychologists who, particularly in these days of the pandemic crisis, are likely to have been stepping into newly visible staff and patient support roles, on a background of an already highly stressed and under-resourced workplace (BPS Membership Survey, 2019).

Clare Gerada's book *Beneath the White Coat* (2021) discusses in detail the reluctance that doctors experience when needing help, especially when this assistance is based within their own workplace or with colleagues they know. This is particularly prevalent in psychiatrists, 90% of whom reported that they would not consult another mental health professional (White et al., 2006). Interestingly, the ACP-UK scheme has had a number of senior staff from mental health services using the service.

Shame at not appearing to be the knowledgeable professional, at letting down colleagues, and a fear of jeopardising their careers have all been cited in studies as reasons for low rates of help-seeking in medical doctors (Gerada, 2021; Jones, 2005), as well as stigma at not coping or having psychological difficulties (Miller & Jones, 2005). The ACP-UK scheme, unlike some other medical support schemes, does not report practitioners for seeking help (although will act rapidly in the case of risk as in any other mental health setting). It makes it explicit from the outset to the doctors, nurses, managers, and other professionals that it cannot become involved with registration body tribunals or hearings.

A group statement published early on in the pandemic reports that 'psychological professionals will need to take care of themselves and each other physically, emotionally and psychologically as they respond to a high level of need. Supervision, time off and other self-care will be more important than ever, to allow psychological professionals to continue to serve effectively' (Guidance for Psychological Professionals during the Covid-19 pandemic, 2020).

A King's Fund report recommends that 'the role of leaders is to truly listen to those they lead, to genuinely strive to understand the challenges they face, to feel with them' (Bailey & West, 2020). In order for those in senior roles to be able to carry out this task, we need to be ready to support them, in the background should they prefer that support to be discreet. We specifically offered out of region and different specialty working, and one large health trust asked that this be a condition of our sessions with their staff in order to help them feel comfortable seeking support.

There is a culture of needing to appear strong, almost invincible at times, particularly in the face of junior staff or even other senior colleagues, and so help-seeking tends to happen more easily in a location where the person is not known and where there is a sense of additional confidentiality. Amy Edmonson's (1999) study on team learning and psychological safety focuses in part of leadership characteristics and behaviour. She quotes Roger Brown (1990) who described a series of behaviours among leaders such as asking for help, seeking feedback and admitting fault that posed a 'threat to face'. Fiona Lee (1997) drew together research that indicated a reluctance to see help even when that help is provided and clearly needed and that help-seeking was perceived as linked to appearing incompetence, dependence, and powerlessness.

The scheme format

All the schemes centred around the same model of brief multi-modal interventions delivered flexibly over a maximum of six sessions by experienced clinical psychologist members of ACP-UK. In the UK, all clinical psychology training is at postgraduate level. The clinical psychology doctorate training, which is a government-funded NHS competitive training route, takes three years of a mixture of clinical, research, and academic work. Depending on the routes taken with additional postgraduate experience and further degrees, it takes between 7 and 12 years to become a fully qualified clinical psychologist. Post-qualification grades range from 7 (newly qualified) to 9 (Departmental Head). We invited ACP-UK members with considerable experience of Band 8 and above to apply to be part of the team, with a minimum of two years working at Band 8. We also looked for some experience of working in physical health and also working with traumatic experiences. We welcomed a broad range of senior work grades as we were also supporting not only the hospital medical staff but also our own members, some of whom were trainees and who could be supported by more recently qualified colleagues. It was important to have a significant number of clinical psychologists in the team who were accustomed to working at a very senior leadership or management level to provide sessions to the executive or consultant grade staff members who contacted us.

The clinical psychologists provided the sessions voluntarily, many as an extension of their full-time clinical roles. As the scheme gathered pace, it came to the attention of two large NHS trusts who offered funding to provide additional spaces for the senior managers whose needs they recognised as substantial. ACP-UK was also successful in receiving a charitable award to assist with the administration of the scheme and the related webinar series and has since received an additional charitable grant to provide dedicated continuing professional development (CPD) sessions for the staff support team. These funding contributions allowed the lead of the staff support schemes to move from a voluntary role to a partly funded role, and for ACP-UK to offer the possibility of paid sessions to some of the volunteers. The schemes still continue at the time of writing, and the option to work on a pro bono basis suits many of the staff support team who often incorporate the sessions into their ongoing clinical roles, many of which are based on acute medical trusts. The staff support team psychologists came from a variety of specialties and included a large number already working in physical health settings. Some of the non-physical health psychologists in the scheme expressed some nervousness about whether they were taking the right approach, how to understand the different environments, and how to work flexibly. The clinical psychologists working in physical health were very accustomed to the sudden pivots and brief encounters that are typical of acute medical environments where time is short and many therapeutic interventions happen in a brief ward or corridor conversation.

The schemes were advertised in a variety of places, including the ACP-UK website and newsletters, the RCoA Faculty of Intensive Care and within NHS England's staff hub, as well as by means of direct staff letters from Chief Executive Officers and other senior executives. Word of mouth was also a very effective method of promoting the scheme and various social media groups recommended the scheme as well.

Staff looking for support self-referred using a form linked to the ACP-UK website. They then received a rapid acknowledgement of their request from the scheme lead (PC) and an information sheet about the scheme. This information included details of the level of expertise and training of clinical psychologists, risk management, cancellation processes and evaluation and feedback methods, and contact details for the scheme lead if they had any questions or concerns. PC was determined to offer a personal and rapid response, being very aware from her own work in acute medical teams that asking for help is not an easy or even normalised process within medicine, and that once someone reaches that point it is important to acknowledge this step with a speedy and welcoming response. Those asking for help were sent a personalised acknowledgement email from the scheme lead within 24 hours, or 48 hours at the most if the referral arrived over a weekend. We have never needed to use a waiting list.

The scheme users were matched with a clinical psychologist who then made contact and arranged a convenient time for the first session. Scheme users were invited at the point of self-referral to express a preference for various criteria, including an out of area psychologist, or one with particular characteristics of gender, ethnicity, religious faith, or spirituality. Introductions between clinical psychologist and scheme user were made in nearly every case within five days and usually within 48 hours of first referral. The responsiveness of the staff support team members in confirming their availability has been one of the most important parts of being able to run the scheme in this rapid response format.

The flexibility of how sessions were delivered was important in being able to offer sessions to the frontline staff around their work commitments and ever-changing shift rotas. Flexibility was also a feature of how the sessions were scheduled, and appointments offered at weekends, evenings, or in the daytime and at intervals to suit the scheme users proved very popular. Some were seen weekly and others had sessions with several weeks or even months between each appointment. This stands in contrast to the more traditional model of weekly or fortnightly psychology sessions. The majority of scheme users asked to 'bank' their final sessions for some weeks or months in case the pandemic pressures increased, and this was fully supported by their clinical psychologists, many of whom talked of how refreshing they found it to be able to work in a way that responded to client need rather than imposed systems.

The staff support team

Setting up a staff support team rapidly from scratch across the UK in the middle of a pandemic lockdown would normally prove a challenge but the enthusiasm and the desire to give generous amounts of time and energy by the ACP-UK clinical psychologists made the process a rewarding one. The fact that most of the association's members tend to share common goals and an understanding of how they can use their skills flexibly made this scheme less difficult to administer than if it had involved a need for basic training.

One benefit of drawing upon the membership of ACP-UK to provide the support sessions meant that the entire staff support team was already experienced in working with various psychological models, in assessing and managing risk, liaising closely with a professional lead, and in thinking sensitively with the scheme users about further sources of help should this be appropriate. The clinical psychologists were also experts at understanding the NHS contexts in which the scheme users were working, and in thinking with them about the impact of systemic or interpersonal difficulties. Importantly, clinical psychologists are trained in when to offer trauma-focused work and when this is inadvisable (COVID Trauma Response Working Group, 2020) so the team was able to gauge the pace of each session without the risk of exacerbating distress.

At the start of the pandemic, social media was busy with people wanting to set up ad hoc support services. Some of these, such as Frontline-19, have been very successful in using trained counsellors, and their target users may have been rather different staff groups to the ones we were helping. However, we were aware that social media posts by other groups did not want to undertake important checks such as qualification verification and DBS (police check) certification. It was important to us that we explained that we were providing a highly qualified, highly skilled and experienced team with the most stringent level of national mandatory accreditation available.

The clinical psychology team is made up of approximately 60 psychologists from a broad mixture of applied roles, all of whom have considerable experience in adult assessment, treatment, and multi-modal approaches. The majority come from physical health settings, with others working across all other clinical psychology specialties. The clinical health psychologists were immediately familiar with the challenges described by the scheme users and are used to working in very flexible ways as often required in hospital environments. Some of the team members from other specialties requested and received additional refresher materials and training updates, but these were minimal once people had gained confidence and realised that their core clinical skills were eminently transferable.

Supporting the supporters

Many of the clinical psychologists were volunteering their time and often working with the scheme at evenings and weekends. We wanted to give something back to the psychologists in the team in exchange for the time they were donating, and also to find activities that would promote a sense of belonging to a team. This is particularly important when no one has met in the non-virtual world but where everyone is working towards a common and demanding goal. Membership of the team was flexible so that the psychologists could take cases when they had availability and when their other work allowed.

There was no minimum or maximum number of cases and this flexibility worked very well in allowing people to participate in CPD and supervision even when between cases. The scheme lead arranged regular peer supervision groups on Zoom for up to 10 psychologists at a time, and also engaged specialist speakers to provide CPD webinars, for example cognitive behavioural therapy approaches for sleep disturbance as the majority of scheme users reported sleep problems on their initial CORE-10 measures. Team members are invited on a regular basis to suggest topics that they would find useful for CPD sessions. They all have access to a shared resources folder held online, and they are welcome to add material to this. One-to-one case discussion supervision is also available with the team lead.

A one-to-one supervision 'buddy' system is being piloted currently for those who want ongoing individual peer supervision in addition to the larger group discussions. In addition, a regular team newsletter is sent out with updates about the scheme, the latest referral numbers and recommendations for reading, training, videos and relevant radio and television programmes, as well as details of any public presentations done by the ACP-UK Chair or the scheme lead, who have both been invited on various occasions to speak about the schemes at conferences and to other organisations.

The intervention

We have often reflected as a group on the difference between brief intervention and more traditional therapy. Apart from the number of sessions, the main components that differentiate brief support sessions tend to be:

- The multi-model style, with an assortment of useful techniques drawn from across psychological approaches, without needing to work through a full therapy process
- The flexibility of session timing, with space between appointments to allow people to implement ideas from the sessions in their real-time workplaces, or – conversely – to be seen frequently in the early stages and then 'bank' the final sessions
- The 'banking' of sessions offering people reassurance that they could still seek help if infection rates rose sharply at a later date, so increasing work pressures once again with the likelihood of re-traumatisation
- An element of peer-to-peer conversation, particularly with the most senior levels of staff
- An underlying awareness of the systemic and organisational issues exacerbating many of the difficulties.

The clinical psychologists were free to draw on the psychological models that they felt were best suited to their allocated scheme user's presentation, and – in keeping with the usual way of working in clinical psychology – benefited from being experienced users of a range of different approaches. They reported in their feedback forms using a wide range of models including:

- CBT, including Third Wave Approaches
- Cognitive Analytic Therapy
- ACT
- Compassion-Focused Therapy
- Grounding techniques

- Psychoeducation
- Trauma-informed models
- Narrative and Systemic approaches
- Normalising
- Solution-Focused approach
- Reflective space
- Relational model to consider death and dying
- Relaxation work including use of online apps
- Coaching models
- Mentalisation
- 5Ps formulation model.

Many of the team members reported that the scheme users were very responsive to information, education, and the providing of strategies in particular, as well as normalising and the provision of time for reflective listening. Many scheme users explained that this was the first time they had had the experience of feeling listened to and supported without the fear of being judged. This multi-model approach was very practical within the time limitations of the brief six-session intervention, and it was useful to see how much could be achieved by motivated people seeking help at a time of extreme constraints on their time and energy. Some of the scheme users also used the sessions to reflect on earlier or complex difficulties and how these might be impacting on their coping methods during the additional pressures of the pandemic. As part of their sessions, some people explored whether they would like to go on to have longer-term psychological input beyond the ACP-UK scheme and how this could be arranged. In this way, the staff support scheme had the added function of signposting people to additional and sometimes highly specialised psychological support, as well as providing a positive experience of speaking with a clinical psychologist.

Evaluation

We used a cross-methodological approach to obtain the richest possible data. The scheme users were asked to complete a point of entry questionnaire that gathered contact details, workplace role and location, why they had selected this particular scheme, and an indication of the main difficulties they would like to address, along with a baseline CORE-10 questionnaire. This measure includes risk assessment factors and if these were selected a pre-allocation interview was carried out by the lead of the support schemes in order to make sure the clinical psychologist supporting the higher risk clinician was alerted to any additional risk factors and offered extra one-to-one supervision sessions with the scheme lead if required.

At the end of their series of sessions both scheme users and psychologists were invited to provide feedback about their experience of the scheme, about what worked well, what they would like to see done differently, and any other comments they would like to provide. The clinicians were also asked what type of support they would like from ACP-UK and from the scheme lead. A follow-up CORE-10 was administered at the end of the sessions, together with a self-rated improvement scale for the main difficulties the scheme users described. Additional data were gathered on the time taken to allocate each scheme user to his or her clinical psychologist, the number of sessions, types of model used, and perceived outcomes.

An additional and unexpected outcome that emerged in the feedback from the scheme users was their enhanced understanding of the role that clinical psychologists hold and the breadth and scope of their work and experience, from individual support to organisational and systemic consultation. A cascade effect started to emerge where scheme users reported taking their new strategies back into their teams, or where they approached their managers and boards to recommend and request clinical psychology input within their trusts or organisations or throughout their departments.

As the pandemic progressed and the stressors built, a growing number of scheme users reported wanting to consider whether to stay in their NHS or social care roles, and the painful tensions they were experiencing of feeling unable to remain in a career that they held dear. At the end of their time in the scheme, a number of people reported that the staff support sessions had helped them stay in their jobs, and that the clinical psychologists' first-hand understanding of their work contexts had helped greatly with the conversations and decision-making processes. One person explained that he had decided to leave his role. This was not described as a failure but as a considered, supported decision. To be able to take such a decision in a neutral, non-judgemental environment can be as important as assisting someone to stay in a job, and potentially leaves open the possibility of returning to a different clinical or managerial role in due course.

Enhanced confidentiality

The pandemic has brought many restrictions to our normal ways of working but also new opportunities, including flexible working and easy nationwide collaboration. The ability of the ACP-UK scheme to provide senior staff with psychological support outside their region or specialty allowed additional reassurance about confidentiality for people who may be reluctant to seek support from existing occupational health or staff assistance programmes. Many sites did not have such services at the start of the pandemic or in some cases tend to refer on their more senior cases due to a lack of psychologists with a similar level of leadership experience. At the time of writing, the scheme is still ongoing but interim analysis of the feedback data indicates that the most frequently stated reason for choosing this scheme was 'confidentiality – I wanted support from outside my work setting' (38%; n = 39), followed by 'I wanted support specifically from a senior clinical psychologist given their expertise' (34.5%; n = 35). This fits with additional feedback from scheme users which mentioned the fact that clinical psychologists use evidence-based approaches:

> *My psychologist was brilliant, clearly very experienced at dealing with senior clinicians. She took everything back to an evidence base.*

Reflections on the scheme and lessons learnt

ACP-UK is a young organisation. The pandemic occurred just below halfway through its existence when it was less than one and a half years old. The 22 months since the start of the pandemic have brought increasing membership numbers and the staff support scheme has been discussed as a member benefit, a way of giving back and being involved.

> *I'm so proud of being part of ACP-UK – it's been an amazing experience and professionally rewarding.*

The scheme has provided the opportunity for working differently and innovatively, as well as responding to individuals' needs. People accessing the scheme are welcome to request a clinical psychologist of a particular gender, ethnicity, religious faith, or spirituality. A small number of people have so far requested by gender and two by ethnicity. Beyond specific requests where the scheme user and the clinical psychologist were from a minority ethnic background both parties expressed in their feedback that this had been advantageous in considering the difficulties taking place in the workplace. More consideration of how to encourage preferences more freely may be useful, especially in an ostensibly equitable context such as the NHS where such a preference may not feel comfortable or appropriate.

Referrals come in at very varying rates, depending on the stage of the pandemic, promotion of the schemes by organisations and teams, and – most markedly – public holidays and holiday periods. It could be that frontline staff employ the coping strategy of pushing through while in work, and when they take a break they have time to experience the psychological effects of the work they have been doing. Referral management needs to be flexible as the majority of referrals arrive in the early hours of the morning, which is not a surprise given the levels of sleep disturbance and stress being reported in the intake questionnaires. Where word of mouth is a factor in people learning about the scheme, groups of referrals from the same location tend to arrive at once. The referral form has an option for requesting team input but even with multiple staff members requesting help from the same organisation only one consultant requested this.

Flexibility and doing things differently

The unusual circumstances of the pandemic have thrust clinical psychologists into the limelight, along with some of the reality of the working lives of healthcare staff. It has also in some instances brought the opportunity to work as we would like to, rather than as we have to, and this scheme set out to enable people to connect differently with their clients, their colleagues. Many clinical psychologists have long been used to working in set patterns, whether by dint of their chosen psychological model or by the constraints of funding, environment, and patient need. This scheme has offered the psychologists something a bit different, a chance to innovate and to focus from alternative perspectives. It has also provided an additional sense of teamwork, which has been particularly welcomed by those who are lone clinical psychologists in teams made up of other disciplines or who work predominately in solo independent practice. A bonus has been the reports of feeling proud of the work they are doing within the scheme, and how they have been able to feel they are 'giving back' when that sense might have been missing for some.

A great deal can be accomplished in a small number of sessions. However, it is not possible to please everyone all of the time, so as scheme organisers we need to remain open minded and flexible in our approach. The feedback for this scheme so far indicates that some of the staff members would like more than six sessions, while the data show that a proportion have been happy with only two or three. Some of the clinical psychologists wanted a longer number of sessions, some want less CPD, some want more, some want more guidelines and some like communicating very little. Overall the scheme team feels harmonious and the majority draw on their own practice which suits them well.

An unexpected benefit that has emerged from the scheme is the frequent expression of how rewarding and enjoyable the team psychologists have found the work. They talked of finding new satisfaction in their work even after many years in practice and that they have been enabled to work innovatively and flexibly with a different client group to that which they would normally be caring for.

COVID-19 as proxy

People ostensibly approached ACP-UK for help via the COVID-19 support scheme for reasons related to the pressures of the pandemic such as COVID-19-related low mood, anxiety, intrusive thoughts, and burnout. However, it quickly emerged during their sessions that many of the issues they described were long standing and exacerbated by the pandemic. These included difficulties such as organisational pressures, intra-team issues, management relationships and attitudes, bullying, and discrimination. This suggests that COVID-19 has been a proxy for enabling people to seek psychological help where previously this did not happen. The coronavirus crisis has provided an acceptable or normalising reason for people in clinical roles to seek help and to address wider and more systemic issues that are often not discussed but which cause ongoing distress. The opportunity to explore these with the clinical psychologists in the team has in some cases led to those in senior managerial or leadership roles being able to open up conversations with their own managers in turn. It also provides the opportunity for clinical psychologists working in staff support to draw attention to and provide assistance for the wider and underlying systemic issues within health and social care.

Future developments and impacts

The opportunities for future working are broad and exciting. There are at least some organisations that now have a new or indeed a first glimpse and experience of the work that clinical psychologists can contribute to staff as individuals and as teams, and to an organisation as a whole. COVID-19 may bring about a deep evaluation of the systemic and organisational issues that underpin each individual's contribution and provide the framework for compassionate leadership (Docherty, 2020), by the very people that we have been supporting in these schemes.

At the time of writing (February 2022), the scheme has received more than 200 referrals and continues to be open to new cases. This scheme would not have been possible without the generosity of time and spirit and thanks go to all the clinical psychologists in the ACP-UK COVID-19 Staff Support Team, the many people who have responded to or promoted the offer of support, the Board of ACP-UK for providing moral and practical support, and the funders and generous charity contributions that helped us continue longer term what everyone began in the heat of a crisis.

> **Key points**
>
> This chapter highlights how work with senior staff has given us the opportunity to demonstrate the expertise of clinical/practitioner psychologists and demonstrate the breadth of our skills.
>
> Further benefits have been:
>
> - Senior staff take back what they learn to pass on to their teams
> - Managers may request more psychological support after experiencing our input
> - Enhanced co-working opportunities after winning trust.
>
> Brief multi-modal intervention versus therapy
>
> - Allows psychologists to combine the appropriate parts of various models
> - Agreed short-term working focuses the sessions on immediate help
> - Scope for discussing and signposting on to longer-term therapy
> - An acceptable 'taster' of psychological work for those who may be reluctant or fearful.
>
> Targeting a hard-to-reach group like seniors
>
> - Offers similar or more senior-level support
> - Emphasises confidentiality
> - Understands the working and organisational context and pressures
> - Offers flexible sessions around shifts and emergency working
>
> COVID-19 as 'permission' to seek support
>
> - The pandemic normalised trauma, burnout, and anxiety
> - Open discussion of work pressures helped to destigmatise help-seeking
> - Expect staff members to bring long-standing difficulties to the fore by COVID-19 pressures.

References

Bailey, S., & West, M. (2020). *Learning from staff experiences of Covid-19: Let the light come streaming in.* The King's Fund. www.kingsfund.org.uk.

Brown, R. (1990). Politeness theory: Exemplar and exemplary. In I. Rock (Ed.), *The legacy of Solomon Asch: Essays in cognition and social psychology*, 23–37. Hillsdale, NJ: Erlbaum.

CORE-10 measure, CORE Systems Trust. www.coreims.co.uk.

Division of Clinical Psychology. (2021). *Building a caring work culture – what good looks like*. British Psychological Society. Available at https://www.bps.org.uk/sites/www.bps.org.uk/files/Member%20Networks/Divisions/DCP/Building%20a%20Caring%20Work%20Culture.pdf.

Docherty, M. (2020). *What has Covid-19 taught us about supporting workforce mental health and wellbeing?* The King's Fund. www.kingfund.org.uk.

Greenberg, N., Docherty, M., Gnanapragasam, S., & Wessely, S. (2020). Managing mental health challenges faced by healthcare workers during covid-19 pandemic. *BMJ, 368*, 1211.

Guidance for planners of the psychosocial response to stress experienced by hospital staff associated with COVID: Early Interventions. (2020). COVID Trauma Response Working Group. Available at www.traumagroup.org.

Guidance for psychological professionals during the Covid-19 pandemic. (2020). National Psychological Professions Workforce Group. Available at https://www.ppn.nhs.uk/resources/ppn-publications/31-guidance-for-psychological-professionals-during-covid-19/file.

Jones, P. (2005). Themes from the stories. In P. Jones (Ed.), *Doctors as patients*, pp. 39–50. Oxford: Radcliffe Publishing.

Klitzman, R. (2008). *When doctors become patients*. Oxford: Oxford University Press.

Lee, F. (1997, December). When the going gets tough, do the tough ask for help? Help seeking and power motivation in organizations. *Organizational Behavior and Human Decision Processes, 72*(3), 336–363.

Miller, L., & Jones, P. (2005). Stigma and discrimination. In P. Jones (Ed.), *Doctors as patients*, pp 61–68. Oxford: Radcliffe Publishing.

Edmondson, A. (1999, June). Psychological safety and learning behavior in work teams. *Administrative Science Quarterly, 44*(2), 350–383.

White, A., Shiralkar, P., Hassan, T., Galbraith, N., & Callaghan, R. (2006). Barriers to mental healthcare for psychiatrists. *Psychiatric Bull, 30*, 382–384.

Women and Equalities Committee. (2020). *Unequal impact? Coronavirus and BAME people*. Third Report of Session 2019–21. House of Commons.

17 Healthcare Professionals Who Have Experienced Trauma and the Role of EMDR Therapy

Dr Shannon Cullerton and Dr Sherry Rehim

The healthcare system is populated by trauma survivors, not only those receiving care but also those providing care. In this chapter we will provide a brief overview of the literature on trauma, the impact of exposure to trauma, and its psychological sequelae as applicable to those providing healthcare. We will explore how for many health professionals, the nature of their own traumatic experiences or 'wounds' (Newcomb et al., 2015) influence their choice to enter a caring profession. These unconscious motives can be a driving force for compassion and commitment, but unresolved traumas may be triggered within an environment with inherent frequent exposure to trauma and potential for re-traumatisation.

Providing staff support in such a challenging context calls for trauma-informed care that is grounded in an understanding of the impact of trauma in the workforce in a way that can recognise and support those with past trauma, while also aiming to prevent or reduce traumatisation and re-traumatisation in the current setting. As such, in the second part of this chapter we focus on how Eye Movement Desensitisation and Reprocessing (EMDR) therapy presents a valuable therapeutic intervention to work with the psychological and emotional consequences of these cumulative events experienced by healthcare workers. We will provide a short summary of EMDR and outline our use of EMDR in treating trauma-related symptoms of past and present experiences in healthcare providers in a busy London Trust. A case example will provide guidance in the application of techniques and protocols used. We aim to show how EMDR can provide an effective, accessible, and short-term framework for working with both historical and recent trauma experiences. We will conclude by thinking more widely about future developments and possibilities using EMDR in these settings, such as groups and rapid response work.

Research findings report increased rates of trauma responses and prevalence of post-traumatic stress disorder (PTSD) among frontline healthcare workers (Gilleen et al., 2021). Therefore, as practitioners in the area of staff wellbeing, it is important to mobilise our psychological understandings of trauma and its impact, to inform our support and interventions. While the established theoretical models have valuable therapeutic implications as they can provide a framework for treatment, we as practitioners must also hold wider context and systems in mind.

As clinical psychologists, we have both worked extensively with people experiencing complex trauma[1] for many years in specialist NHS Trauma Services in London. When taking our current positions supporting staff wellbeing in a major London acute hospital, neither of us realised at the time the direct relevance and value our years working with complex trauma would have in these new roles. We have reflected on how this knowledge and experience has come to play a central role in our work supporting staff wellbeing, some of which we will share in this chapter.

Trauma overview

Originally used in medicine to describe a physical wound, the word 'trauma' has, over the last century, become a dominant term in the psychological understanding of people's responses to highly distressing experiences. Trauma covers a broad spectrum, from Charcot and Freud's exploration of hysteria and neurosis as a product of traumatic life events (Freud, 1966; Micale, 1994), to the examination of the psychological distress manifest from the combat of WWI and II (Kardiner, 1941; Leys, 2000; Rivers, 1919). Since 1980, when the formal diagnosis of the trauma-related PTSD was included in the Diagnostic and Statistical Manual of Mental Disorders (DSM) (American Psychiatric Association, 1980) there has been considerable research and psychological theory developed around the understanding of trauma. In psychology, trauma

---

[1] Rather than single incident trauma, complex trauma refers to multiple traumas in a person's life which tend to have pervasive effects on cognitive development and the capacity to integrate information into a cohesive whole (Briere & Scott, 2006; Cook, et al., 2005). Multiple traumatic events can cause a substantial distortion in autobiographic memory combined with an excessive emotional representation that includes stimuli from different memories. This results in stronger, interconnected activation triggers (Van der Kolk, 2005).

has been defined as an 'inescapably stressful event that overwhelms people's coping mechanisms due to its extreme nature and the acute distress that it causes' (Van der Kolk & Fisler, 1995, p. 505).

Current theories on the psychological processes behind trauma responses are extensive and offer a framework for understanding the ways people may respond. These theories emphasise the fragmented processing of traumatic events and how traumatic memories are stored differently, lacking a clear narrative and contextualisation, alongside negative appraisals of the memories and 'maladaptive'[2] coping strategies (Ehlers & Clark, 2000; Foa & Rothbaum, 1998). Key theories explain how this fragmented memory can result in an immediate sense of threat and intrusive reliving through activation of the memory of the original traumatic event following exposure to current external triggers (Robjant & Fazel, 2010). From a neurophysiological understanding, the massive threat to survivors that characterises traumatic events induces stress effects on the amygdala and hippocampus, which dramatically modulates memory formation and consolidation (Miller & McEwan, 2006). Moreover, sensory interconnections become unusually strong and can later be easily activated and difficult to control. Because of the memory fragmentation they are also 'ungrounded by the narrative and spatiotemporal contextual anchors that tie ordinary experience to reality' (Neuner et al., 2008, p. 649).

The diagnostic category of PTSD is central to the trauma discourse in psychology, where it is understood as the main human response to trauma. In the DSM-5 (American Psychiatric Association (APA), 2013), PTSD is classified as a trauma- and stressor-related 'disorder' that can be severe and disabling. It is aligned with a particular set of 'symptoms': flashbacks, heightened arousal, avoidance, negative mood and/or thoughts that have emerged as a result of experiencing one or more traumatic events (Giaconia et al., 1995). While such effects are common immediately after traumatic events (Yule et al., 2000), for some the effects persist, becoming chronic and interfering with daily functioning (Foa, Hembree & Rothbaum, 2007; Morgan et al., 2003).

It is clear that traumatic events, especially those which induce significant feelings of fear and helplessness, can cause long-standing psychological difficulties. It is also clear that the outlined theories allow important insight into understanding and appropriate interventions and support. However, it must be

---

[2] Throughout this chapter certain terms are used when they represent the language of discourse that is referenced. However, it is recognised that these are problematic concepts, as such inverted commas are used.

recognised that the effects of traumatic events on individuals and communities are complex and differ greatly. Trauma 'symptoms' are a normal response that change over time and one event can be stressful and traumatising for one but not all. There remain questions as to when and how the dominant models can be applied to some of the more varied and complex clinical presentations seen in practice. We find in our work that a trauma-informed lens is valuable in understanding people's thoughts, behaviours, and responses; however, it's important to also be mindful of the wider context and cautious of immediate assumptions.

Psychology's construct of trauma is not without its critics. Although beyond the scope of this chapter, it is pertinent to note that the conceptualisation, diagnosis, and treatment of trauma have never been free of controversy or professional disagreement. Although much research indicates the strengths of the trauma discourse, there is also a strong argument that it inadequately or inappropriately addresses the mental health needs of some individuals and populations (Afuape, 2011; Summerfield, 2000). A number of researchers have criticised the overemphasis on the Western concept of trauma in understanding the impact of violence and abuse and have questioned the diagnostic focus on PTSD (Summerfield, 1995). It has been argued that the attempt to quantify trauma 'symptoms' in an objective and individualistic fashion is not always relevant or beneficial (Bracken, Giller & Summerfield, 1995; Summerfield, 2001). The bio-cognitive focus with trauma means that social and political context (e.g. war and violence against marginalised groups) and systemic past and present factors (e.g. colonialism, patriarchy) are downplayed (Breslau, 2004; Papadopoulos, 2005). Alongside these academics and clinicians, we argue that there needs to be a more contextual and systemic approach in which theories allow for the reality that people construct personal, social, and cultural meanings from their traumatic experiences (Levers, 2012). We advocate taking an approach that is 'multi-factorial, contextualises distress and behaviour, and acknowledges the complexity of the interactions involved in all human experience' (DCP, 2013, p. 4).

Trauma and the healthcare system

Engagement in healthcare, for both patients and staff, is impacted by trauma (Marsac et al., 2016). The healthcare system is a high-stress environment with inherent frequent exposure to trauma and suffering, which can lead to increased vulnerabilities to traumatic stress. Exposure to pain, loss, disability, suffering, disproportionate care or medical futility, and ethical decision-making constitute just some of the trauma dimensions that staff face on a daily basis (Van Mol et al., 2015). This, accompanied with the stressful job demands such as shift work, long working hours, and working a job that carries a high level of visible social responsibility, creates an additional burden on a healthcare worker's ability to cope with traumatic situations.

As we have seen, the healthcare system is populated by survivors of trauma, both those providing and receiving care. The risk of emotional distress implicated in working with traumatised patients is clearly recognised (Van Mol et al., 2015). Likewise, those entering the helping professions also naturally bring their own varied histories, experiences, traumas, and emotions into their working lives. The inherent nature of a caring role can bring forth an individual's own experience of being cared for, historically and currently. Professionals' emotional reactions will be shaped by their own personal history when exposed to workplace traumatic situations and in their interaction with traumatised patients. Under stressful conditions, rather than attending to thoughts and emotions the roles may bring up, there can be a tendency to normalise struggles and remain silent about their own needs. Healthcare professionals commonly feel a great pressure to remain compassionate, attuned, and focused on their patient's wellbeing above their own.

This pressure exists within the context of dealing with often unsustainable workloads and trying to help many patients with problems that cannot easily be treated by the medical interventions available while bearing the distress of their patients. This, together with increasing austerity, repeated restructuring, and marketisation, has left those working in the health service vulnerable in balancing the complex task of caring for their patients and caring for themselves. The pain and overwhelm being felt by NHS staff seems to be reflected in the high rates of bullying, whistleblowing, staff turnover, and sickness.

Secondary traumatic stress, compassion fatigue, and vicarious traumatisation are a few of terms that are used almost interchangeably to describe the 'cost of caring' in healthcare (Dominguez-Gomez & Rutledge, 2009; Meadors & Lamson, 2008; Curtis & Puntillo, 2007). Research conducted prior to COVID-19 found that healthcare workers are at a higher risk of developing PTSD (Skogstad et al., 2013), particularly among critical care nursing (Karanikola, et al., 2015), emergency department (Morrison & Joy, 2016), oncology (Quinal, Harford, & Rutledge, 2009), paediatric nursing (Meadors, Lamson, Swanson, White, & Sira 2010), mental health nursing (Lee, Daffern, Ogloff, & Martin, 2015; Mangoulia, Koukia, Alevizopoulos, Fildissis, & Katostaras, 2015), and midwifery (Beck & Gable, 2012).

Personal and organisational factors contribute to the process of developing secondary traumatic stress in healthcare professionals (Ratrout & Hamdan-Mansour, 2020). Across studies with nurses and medical doctors, personal factors have been shown to include age, gender, years of working experience, education level, amount of trauma training and social support received, personal trauma history, coping strategies, and personality characteristics (Bhugra et al., 2019). Organisational factors include job characteristics, working hours, high work demands in combination with limited autonomy and support (Demerouti et al., 2001), peer and organisational support, and clinical supervision. The risk of emotional distress implicated in working with traumatised patients and in traumatising setting has certainly been recognised.

Undoubtedly, the COVID-19 pandemic has amplified and added to the pressures that were already weighing heavily on healthcare workers. Healthcare workers were initially celebrated as heroes then left feeling abandoned and forgotten during the subsequent waves. The professional challenges increased due to a significantly increased workload, redeployment, higher acuity and death rates, and healthcare workers did not have the time to build progressive skills and psychological protective strategies to face these challenges. There was also pressure on their private lives, as many staff felt under a constant threat of being infected themselves or infecting a loved one. As a result, many isolated themselves from family or had to cope with feelings of guilt on returning home after shifts. Arguably, for all staff, the severity of illness and the level of grief and death they have been exposed to in the pandemic are unlike anything they have ever experienced or expected to experience in their role. When a stressor or sense of threat is temporary or manageable, the threat response system can be efficient and effective. However, when stressors persist and uncertainty continues, the stress response can become 'maladaptive' and lead to more concerning physical and psychological distress (Van der Kolk, 2014).

Providing staff support in such a challenging context calls for trauma-informed care, that is embedded across all levels of the system, organisational, team, and individual, and is grounded in an understanding of the impact of trauma in the workforce in a way that can recognise and support those with past trauma. Also, aiming to prevent or reduce traumatisation and re-traumatisation in the current setting across. Trauma-informed care is discussed further in chapter 2 on Organisational Trauma; in this chapter we will focus on individual and group level staff support interventions.

Trauma interventions

Current UK guidelines for the treatment of trauma-related 'symptoms' promote the use of trauma-focused cognitive behavioural therapy and EMDR (National Institute for Health and Clinical Excellence (NICE), 2018). Although varying in technique, in both approaches the central goal in treatment is reliving the traumatic experience to habituate and reprocess the memory in 'healthier' ways and ameliorate unhelpful thoughts, beliefs, and/or behaviours (Foa, Hembree & Rothbaum, 2007). The clinician's role is to help clients to work through their trauma memories, and situations, people, or objects that have become associated with the trauma, consequently provoking an intense emotional or physical response. In doing so, the unhelpful and distressing emotions and thoughts that relate to the traumatic experience are reprocessed and the associated distress relieved. In our work supporting staff, we have found EMDR has emerged as the central intervention that is valuable in working through the complexities of trauma presentations we see and that it fits well with to the restrictions of this working environment, staff presentations, and system pressures/demands in this setting. We will explore this more here.

EMDR and the healthcare system

From its development in 1989 to resolve traumatic memories (Shapiro, 1989), EMDR has shown its efficacy as a treatment for the impact of trauma experiences as well as showing significant value in wider application (Bisson et al., 2007, 2009; Chen et al., 2014; Cuijpers et al., 2020; Foa, Keane & Friedman, 2009; Lee & Cuijpers, 2013; Smith et al., 2007). The approach is based on activating an individual's information processing in order to help integrate the traumatic event as an adaptive, contextualised memory. To achieve this, people attend to the memory and its associations while their attention is also engaged by bilateral stimulation (BLS: including eye movements, auditory or tactile stimulation) (Shapiro, 2001). Unlike other trauma interventions, clients do not have to put experiences into detailed words as the activation of painful or distressing memories is achieved in the process through accessing associated thoughts and sensations momentarily. EMDR utilises a standard protocol of eight phases (Shapiro, 2001) as described in Table 17.1.

EMDR offers several unique advantages which we have considered particularly useful working in the healthcare setting. Clients are given a high level of control over their treatment and the exposure to feared inner experiences (feel-

TABLE 17.1: Phases of EMDR.

Phases 1–2: History taking and preparation	The first two phases of therapy collect history and ensure preparation for treatment through stabilisation and resource building as well as constructing a list of potential targets (past traumatic experiences) for processing.
Phase 3: Assessment	The client identifies the most distressing moment of a targeted event with the representative image and related cognitive, affective, and somatic components. The client is asked to provide a related rating of disturbance that arises.
Phase 4: Desensitisation	The client focuses on the memory briefly while simultaneously engaging in BLS, after which associative information is elicited. This material typically becomes the target of the next set of BLS. This alternating pattern of focusing on the memory followed by associative links is repeated until all disturbance is eliminated and the rating of disturbance is zero.
Phase 5: Installation	A related positive self-referencing belief is integrated with the traumatic memory.
Phase 6: Body scan	Processing is completed when a body scan evidences no related somatic distress.
Phase 7–8: Closure and re-evaluation	Appropriate steps are taken to end the session (phase 7) and to re-evaluate progress at the beginning of the next session (phase 8). To ensure that all disturbance related to the old traumatic memory is eliminated, the standard protocol also involves addressing all current triggers and concerns about related future events.

ings, sensations, images, and cognitions) can be experienced in relatively short bursts rather than in the more sustained or prolonged manner typical of trauma treatments. Clients are also not required to talk at length about the intolerable or explain why they feel distress, the intention is to help the client stay focused on their internal responses and observe their experiences.[3] This approach directly targets somatic effects of trauma held in the body. Most trauma interventions depend on top-down processing in which the client is taught to use cognitive strategies to manage or inhibit problematic feelings, thoughts, and behaviours. They may learn to notice and manage disturbing body sensations; however, they

---

[3] For further information on EMDR, useful resources can be found at:
https://www.emdr.com/
https://emdrassociation.org.uk/

do not focus on processing and resolving physiological hyperarousal. The focus in EMDR is on emotional and bodily processing (Van der Kolk, 2015).

EMDR is particularly valuable for clients who struggle with self-protective avoidance defence and a core sense of defectiveness, shame, and guilt (Korn, 2009). We have found that this can be the case for healthcare professionals where these emotional experiences are often further complicated and perpetuated by wider problems of institutional and professional stigma regarding mental health illness and the high level of visible social responsibility in healthcare settings. Furthermore, healthcare professional throughout their career have developed defensive structures to deal with the anxiety of working so close to death, despair, disability, and failure. These mechanisms are made up of conscious coping techniques and unconscious defences. They give healthcare professionals the skills and psychological protection to do the work expected of them; it prevents healthcare professionals collapsing into a psychological heap every time they face stressful, painful, and traumatic experiences and gain control over adversity (Missouridou, 2017). For example, we have found that healthcare professionals often intellectualise: shutting down their emotions and approaching a situation solely from a rational standpoint enabling them to think about events in a dispassionate, clinical, problem-solving manner. Also, the physical healthcare context inherently perpetuates the idea that mental health diagnoses are less legitimate than physical problems. The language, environment, and focus are shaped by the medical 'in the body' model. In this way, the psychophysiological approach in EMDR somewhat 'talks the language' of physical healthcare professionals, as delving into feelings too quickly can feel unnatural and unfamiliar.

In EMDR the focus on the 'felt sense' and 'in the body' experience together with less reliance on verbal exchange can help ease common self-protective avoidance and shame defences. However, there is a balance to be struck, and it is crucial that we do not collude in what can be avoidance and dismissive attachments and defensives for too long by keeping things away from the emotional field.

Certainly, some of these defences can be overacted; the scrubs can become a suit of armour, a protection worn to convey power and conceal impotence and fear. It is, therefore, crucial to name the defences operating at both the individual and institutional level. The resource building and stabilisation stage in EMDR offers opportunities to build upon the client's resources and connect healthcare professionals to stories of resilience, competencies, and courage that they undoubtedly have. It is often during this phase of treatment that we encourage clients to connect with their multiple social contexts, for example their cultural beliefs and faith (e.g. prayers).

We also recognise that to continue doing the challenging work in a healthcare setting, some of these functional and protective defences need to remain intact, and reassurance of this is needed even more so as many of our clients attend sessions during the working day. We have found that the high level of control supported through the short bursts of exposure, psychophysiological focus and the autonomy to share as much as feel comfortable can provide important relief, safety, and containment – supporting clients to process traumatic memories without feeling too overwhelmed or destabilised. A more recent development in EMDR called the Flash Technique (FT) has advanced the process of reducing high levels of distress and avoidance impulses. The FT, unlike many conventional trauma therapy interventions, does not require the client to consciously engage with the traumatic memory. This allows the client to process traumatic memories without feeling distress and reduces the disturbance associated with traumatic or other distressing memories, which can help the client move on to the standard EMDR protocol more quickly and with ease (this is discussed in more detail in the case presentation). This technique becomes particularly useful in the NHS, where we are restricted by short treatment times and healthcare professions are required to continue working in challenging environments, sometimes the same environment that triggers their trauma reactions (Manfield et al., 2021).

EMDR and Attachment in healthcare

Particularly relevant for the common presentations we see in healthcare professionals, EMDR places emphasis on identifying client experiences that represent attachment disruptions and failures, neglect and experiences of profound aloneness, and unmet psychological needs, as well as experiences of emotional, physical, and sexual abuse. All caring involves an attachment and when caregivers have a history of disturbing traumatic attachment experiences that remain unresolved, these unelaborated experiences may be reactivated when caring and forming relationships with patients, colleagues, and the wider NHS system. Bowlby (1979) argued that the attachment system is activated throughout the life of all human beings, 'from the cradle to the grave' (p. 129), by experiences of fear, physical or emotional distress, and/or pain, which are inherent experiences in healthcare settings. What is perhaps unique about caring professions is that the roles and experiences involved can give individuals the information and skills to resolve previous conflicts and give to others the care and attention they would have wished for themselves.

This concept is supported by the Woodward et al. (2017) study which explored the reasons junior doctors decide to study medicine, and the most commonly given answer was a desire to help others, driven in part by previous life events. There is also evidence that suggests that staff can be more likely to present with mental health problems when clinical experiences resonate with their earlier conflicts (Gerada, 2020). The unconscious desire to heal a loved one, a sense of responsibility, and the guilt associated with failing to do so can become channelled into a relentless drive to care and do more. These actions are often referred to as the 'wounded healer'. If unchecked, this may not lead to reparation or healing, but repeated failure at attempting to cure the incurable, which further feeds the associated emotional drive to strive for an impossible task. For in 24/7 healthcare settings, how can the work ever be done? For some, this may lead to more difficulties in processing the intense feelings of frustration and powerlessness when patients do not recover, when they are unable to provide care and requests for help feel overwhelming (Coetzee & Klopper, 2010). There may also be sensitivities to feeling 'uncared for' or neglected by the managers, teams, or systems, especially when staff are relentlessly caring for others and working in systems that are not adequately resourced. In responding to attachments in healthcare, unresolved traumatic experiences can surface, consciously or unconsciously, and activate their attachment system together with their caregiving system. If there are no significant others available to soothe and help make sense of these experiences, strong emotions, including fear, anger, shame, and guilt, can be aroused from the activation of the attachment system. Because of the continual re-evaluation of the social learning links between past events and current difficulties and distress inherent in the protocol, EMDR treatment produces an increasingly clear picture of the material most in need of targeting in the processing phase. EMDR contains an inherent feedback loop that allows healthcare professionals in collaboration with the therapist, to increasingly focus in on the experiences (and associated beliefs, behaviours, and affects) that continue to cause distress and challenges. Retaining flexibility is a valuable aspect of EMDR treatment, as a healthcare professional who has a history of complex trauma initially may not remember particular traumatic content, may minimise or deny the connection between current challenges and earlier life experiences, and may be reluctant to disclose certain aspects of their history out of shame or fear (Korn, 2009).

Case presentation

Presenting difficulties

Hannah, aged 29, came to therapy following a period of redeployment to a COVID-19 ward during the pandemic. She had been working as a nurse for five years, and at the time of therapy she was on sick leave due to work-related stress. Her initial presenting problem was anxiety related; however, what seemed to be particularly troubling her was an overwhelming feeling of guilt and responsibility. During redeployment, Hannah felt she lacked the competencies to work on the ward feeling 'useless', 'helpless', 'not good enough', and like an 'extra part'. She spoke of uncertainty and loss of control due to the unpredictability of the virus and the trauma of witnessing patients having to die alone without family. She became numb and withdrawn, further perpetuating feelings of not being able to help. Taking time off work felt shameful and she worried that her colleagues would think she was incompetent. She also had intrusions of distressing situations at work and experienced hyperarousal difficulties including disrupted sleep.

History

Exploring her current thoughts and emotions in the assessment it became clear that these were linked with earlier traumas. Emotional distress in the family home was described as a daily experience and Hannah felt as though her stomach was 'always in a knot' and her head 'feeling very heavy'. At the age of six, Hannah's baby sister died. Her mother become very depressed, and her father had ongoing substance abuse problems. She also experienced her father as having high expectations that she felt she could never meet.

Growing up, her younger brother experienced ongoing mental health difficulties and made several attempts to end his life. Hannah also felt understandably worried for her brother, feeling responsible as his older sister to keep him safe. The siblings are now close, but she noticed that often she feels the urge to avoid her brother as their relationship stirs up difficult feelings of helplessness. Hannah went on to be very studious and was able to become completely absorbed in her studies, which helped block out challenges in her life.

Rationale for EMDR

The assessment phase provided some insight into Hannah's ability to tolerate distressing memories and related avoidance impulses. It became clear that she wanted to 'skip over' certain periods in her life. She often said, 'it's wasn't worth speaking about'. The understandable reluctance to access details of earlier trauma experiences combined with the unavoidable link between past traumas and current work triggers is a common presentation we work with. Due to these factors it was agreed EMDR would be an appropriate model to use in the time frame available, as it allows for minimal discussion of trauma yet still allows for processing of the distressing trauma experiences.

Treatment

Preparation phase: Various relaxations such as the safe place exercise and emotional regulation strategies were taught, and Hannah was encouraged to utilise them between sessions. These exercises are a gentle way to introduce the client to BLS which are used throughout to manage distressing emotions and to close incomplete processing sessions. Central to stabilisation in this early phase is the enhancement of self-belief. Hannah was able to create a few meaningful images of times she had felt competent, for example, running a marathon and a time she supported her friend. She was asked to become aware of related body sensations, that is, what it feels like to be successful/competent.

Developing a target: Once we felt confident that Hannah was able to cope with the intense emotions that may accompany therapy, treatment targets were identified and worked on starting with earlier childhood memories. There were many possibilities for treatment targets. Given the time limit to our therapy and Hannah's goal to return to work we used the float-back technique, to identify which memory was most connected with her present distress. This involved identifying the present-day triggering target (being told to help in an emergency at work by the matron and freezing) and use of EMDR techniques to 'float back' to the earlier association. The earliest memory, often referred to as the 'touchstone memory', was identified, which was of Hannah witnessing her brother attempt to end his life and hiding away in her room feeling helpless.

This memory was very distressing and overwhelming for Hannah to talk about. We, therefore, used the FT to reduce the initial disturbance associated with the trauma memory so that she would not need to dissociate or defend against it in the processing stage. In the healthcare setting, we need to be able to offer quick, accessible interventions to staff who continue to work in the challenging healthcare setting and as discussed, may come to therapy with a number of protective defences reluctant to talk about disturbing memories or dissociate when they do. The task is to offer therapy that is bounded on one side by the need to keep the client within zone of emotional safety and on the other by the need to help the client move towards a healing process, within organisational pressures and time restrictions. The FT has offered a quick process to reduce the initial disturbance associated with trauma memories.

FT involves identifying the overwhelmingly disturbing memory and then instructing the client to access or 'touch on' it for only a brief millisecond. It is beneficial to ask the client not to tell you about the memory in any detail, simply to identify it. The client is then instructed to bring up a positive engaging memory, or person or animal, which evokes a positive feeling and talk it through. Hannah spoke about her dog and her loving and caring relationship with him. BLS was used to strengthen this positive image. During this process the client is asked to blink rapidly three times (i.e. flash) without thinking about the target memory and while maintaining focus and engaged on the positive memory and associated positive feelings. The client is then instructed to 'touch lightly on the target memory', acknowledging that previously you have been asking them to avoid thinking of the memory. This procedure appears to assist clients in titrating the exposure in a way that does not activate a self-protective avoidance impulse. During the process the client is asked 'Does the memory seem different in any way?' and they often report that the target memory seems further away, or the image seems less vivid or upsetting.

Reprocessing phase: Following the use of FT, we returned to reprocessing the disturbing memory or event. The model indicates that images, beliefs, affect, and bodily sensations associated with the experience must be identified for complete reprocessing to occur. Hannah identified a negative cognition 'I should have done more – I'm uncaring' and then a preferred more adaptive, positive cognition, 'I did the best I could'.

After reprocessing this experience, Hannah's distress level (as indicated in the subjective unit of disturbance level – SUD) decreased from 10 to 1, and she was able to realise that she was just a child who was not responsible for her younger brother nor his mental health difficulties. Her SUD level did not reduce below 1 due to the pain and sense of betrayal associated with witnessing her brother's distress and turning away. A certain amount of remorse was appropriate, given the nature of the situation. In EMDR, the aim is to reduce the SUD as low as 0 or 1 before moving on to the installation of the positive cognition. However, there will be understandable and appropriate reasons why residual distress may remain, especially for those with complex and multiple trauma experiences.

Whereas the target memory described was related to responsibility, many of the other key events in Hannah's life were related to her attachment with her parents and the implications on her negative self-concept (e.g. 'I'm not good enough'). While we did not have time to reprocess all these key early memories, the level of disturbance associated with the memories was lower. As the focus of treatment shifted to more recent events, the SUD for these events was also lowered. Therefore, the reprocessing of the more recent event (i.e. the incident at work when she froze and was unable to help) did not take as long. This phenomenon can be explained by the tendency for EMDR's positive effects to generalise to other related events and memories (Shapiro, 2001).

Future template: Subsequent processing addressed present disturbances and future anticipated anxieties (the third prong, for example, return to work). The 'Future Template' involved skill building and mentally rehearsing the process of returning to work. Hannah ran an imaginary movie performing the actions involved in returning to work. When she first did this we noticed unprocessed material and reprocessed any disturbance with (fast) BLS until we ran through the entire 'movie'. The second run through, involved using the most useful/powerful self-referencing positive thought. Hannah said 'I am a competent clinician, our work is a shared responsibility and I am appreciated at work' while she was guided to do more BLS. This process was repeated until Hannah felt emotionally, physically, and cognitively comfortable, as much as possible, with the idea of returning to work. She was able to return soon after the treatment of 14 sessions of 60 minutes each.

Future directions

We see two key areas for developing and utilising EMDR to strengthen the support available for healthcare staff: in groups, and in response to traumatic episodes. Within a large NHS Trust with continued and increasing pressures, yet limited resources, we recognise the importance of reaching wider groups of staff in the system. In our acute hospital setting we have provided numerous reflective and wellbeing-focused group sessions that have been valued by staff and managers. These group sessions have allowed a safe space to normalise and make sense of the impact of the work healthcare professionals undertake. Building on this group offer we see an opportunity in using a structured and evidenced EMDR approach to work with staff groups to process the trauma of individual and shared experiences.

An extension of the EMDR standard protocol is the Group Traumatic Episode Protocol (G-TEP), which provides a valuable structure for the main protocol to be adapted to group work. Allowing the key methods of EMDR to be facilitated in a group has involved the protocol to be designed in a way that works with sensations of calm and strength rather than focusing on the disturbing experience itself. Group forms of BLS are used to ensure participants are able to manage their stress level within the group setting and feel safe and contained. The 'Trauma Episode' is identified individually through writing or drawing simple details to ensure each participant in the group is respected in terms of not needing to share personal information. Most session time is spent identifying and connecting with positive memories, thoughts and sensations, and working to distance the disturbance from the original trauma memory. Like in EMDR's main protocol, the aim is to create distance from the level of disturbance for participants, leading to a sense of increased calm rather than distress when the event is recalled. Using the core EMDR techniques within a safe group framework through a simplified approach provides a visual and engaging way to process in a structured and containing session. It can therefore provide a space to acknowledge and work through trauma experiences within limited resources and time to provide individual staff support for all.

The G-TEP protocol was designed as a group version of the Recent Traumatic Episode Protocol (R-TEP). As the name suggests, R-TEP is designed to be applied to very recent distressing events. This is a significant approach in the context of regular traumatic incidents that staff may have to contend with working in an acute hospital setting. There has been ongoing debate around safe ways to provide staff support in the immediate aftermath of traumatic events (see chapter 18 on debriefs). This adaptation of EMDR has been shown to be safe and effective and therefore offers a valuable opportunity for future development in our healthcare setting as the need for rapid response work is often requested.[4]

Limitations

For the purpose of this chapter, our intention is to demonstrate how useful EMDR can be in the healthcare setting and its future potential. However, we do acknowledge that trauma-focused interventions, including EMDR, are not without their limitations and therefore, we want to briefly acknowledge some of the wider critiques of the model and important cautions when putting it into practice. As EMDR focuses on emotional and bodily processing of trauma,

---

[4] For further information on G-TEP and R-TEP, useful resources can be found on the EMDR foundation website at:
http://emdrfoundation.org/toolkit/gtep.pdf
https://emdrfoundation.org/toolkit/rtep-manual.pdf

this means that therapists must be mindful that trauma experiences are not decontextualised; that time and attention is given to understand the wider context in which trauma occurs. For example, the social-political context of adversity and government cuts in the UK have direct and significant implications on the experiences of healthcare professionals within the NHS. Similarly, while EMDR does incorporate skill and resource enhancements, there are other approaches (e.g. working with trauma using narrative therapy) which centre a strength-based approach. We consider this aspect of therapy to be crucial when working with trauma to ensure that the message conveyed is as follows: 'the problem is not located within you' and to give our clients an opportunity to reconnect with a positive sense of self. We have also learned that given its unique and unconventional techniques (i.e. the BLS finger or tapping movement) EMDR can be assumed to be unusual until it is experienced. We have found it helpful to give our clients an experience as early as possible in therapy in a gradual approach (e.g. doing BLS during the safe place exercise).

Conclusion

With the backdrop of the pandemic and increasing demand of the healthcare setting, there is a crucial need to offer an accessible and responsive approach to address the complexity and depth of trauma that healthcare professionals experience. The pandemic certainly accelerated the need for psychological responsiveness to trauma, and we have witnessed the psychological and emotional consequences of cumulative events experienced by healthcare workers affecting their current distress. Healthcare services must develop sustainable staff support provision while also managing the ongoing challenges of limited resources; EMDR provides a valuable trauma-informed approach to meet this challenge and the needs of our 'in need' workforce.

References

Afuape, T. (2011). *Power, resistance and liberation in therapy with survivors of trauma: To have our hearts broken*. East Sussex: Routledge.

American Psychiatric Association (APA). (1980). *Diagnostic and statistical manual of mental health disorders (3rd edition)*. Washington, DC: American Psychiatric Publishing.

American Psychiatric Association (APA). (2013). *Diagnostic and statistical manual of mental health disorders (5th edition)*. Washington, DC: American Psychiatric Publishing.

Beck, C. T. and Gable, R. K. (2012). A mixed methods study of secondary traumatic stress in labor and delivery nurses. *Journal of Obstetric, Gynecologic & Neonatal Nursing*, 41(6), 747–760.

Bhugra, D., Sauerteig, S. O., Bland, D., Lloyd-Kendall, A., Wijesuriya, J., Singh, G., Kochhar, A., Molodynski, A. and Ventriglio, A. (2019). A descriptive study of mental health and wellbeing of doctors and medical students in the UK. *International Review of Psychiatry*, *31*(7–8), 563–568.

Bisson, J. I., Ehlers, A., Matthews, R., Pilling, S., Richards, D. and Turner, S. (2007). Psychological treatments for chronic post-traumatic stress disorder: Systematic review and meta-analysis. *The British Journal of Psychiatry*, *190*, 97–104.

Bisson, J. M., and Andrew, M. (2009). Psychological treatment of post-traumatic stress disorder (PTSD) (Review). The Cochrane collaboration. Available at: http://summaries.cochrane.org/CD003388/psychological-treatment-of-posttraumatic-stress-disorder-ptsd.

Bowlby, J. (1979). The bowlby-ainsworth attachment theory. *Behavioral and Brain Sciences*, *2*(4), 637–638.

Bracken, P. J., Giller, J. E. and Summerfield, D. (1995). Psychological responses to war and atrocity: The limitations of current concepts. *Social Science & Medicine*, *40*(8), 1073–1082.

Breslau, J. (2004). Introduction: Cultures of trauma: Anthropological views of posttraumatic stress disorder in international health. *Culture, Medicine and Psychiatry*, *28*(2), 113–126.

Chen, Y. R., Hung, K.-W., Tsai, J. C., Chur, H., Chung, M. H., Chen, S. R., Liao, Y. M., Ou, K. L., Chang, Y. C., and Chou, K. R. (2014). Efficacy of eye-movement desensitization and reprocessing for patients with posttraumatic-stress disorder: A meta-analysis of randomized controlled trials. *PLOS One*. Published online Aug 7; *9*(8):e103676, doi: 10.1371/journal.pone.0103676.

Coetzee, S. K. and Klopper, H. C. (2010). Compassion fatigue within nursing practice: A concept analysis. *Nursing & Health Sciences*, *12*(2), 235–243.

Cuijpers, P., Noma, H., Karyotaki, E., Vinkers, C. H., Cipriani, A. and Furukawa, T. A. (2020). A network meta-analysis of the effects of psychotherapies, pharmacotherapies and their combination in the treatment of adult depression. *World Psychiatry*, *19*(1), 92–107.

Curtis, J. R. and Puntillo, K. (2007). Is there an epidemic of burnout and post-traumatic stress in critical care clinicians? *American Journal of Respiratory and Critical Care Medicine*, *175*(7), 634–636.

DCP. (2013). *Classification of behaviour and experience in relation to functional psychiatric diagnoses: Time for a paradigm shift: Division of clinical psychology position statement*. Retrieved from http://dcp.bps.org.uk/dcp/the_dcp/news/dcp-position-statement-on-classification.cfm

Ehlers, A. and Clark, D. M. (2000). A cognitive model of posttraumatic stress disorder. *Behavioural Research and Therapy*, *38*(4), 319–345.

Demerouti, E., Bakker, A. B., De Jonge, J., Janssen, P. P. and Schaufeli, W. B. (2001). Burnout and engagement at work as a function of demands and control. *Scandinavian Journal of Work, Environment & Health*, 27 (4), 279–286.

Dominguez-Gomez, E. and Rutledge, D. N. (2009). Prevalence of secondary traumatic stress among emergency nurses. *Journal of Emergency Nursing*, *35*(3), 199–204.

Foa, E. B., Hembree, E. A. and Rothbaum, B. O. (2007). *Prolonged exposure therapy for PTSD: Emotional processing of traumatic experiences therapist guide*. New York: Oxford University Press.

Foa, E. B., Keane, T. M. and Friedman, M. J. (2009). *Effective treatments for PTSD: Practice guidelines from the international society for traumatic stress studies (2nd edition)*. New York: Guilford Press.

Foa, E. B. and Rothbaum, B. O. (1998). Treating the trauma of rape: Cognitive behavioural therapy for PTSD. In *Treatment manuals for practitioners*. New York: Guildford Press.

Freud, S. (1966). *The complete introductory lectures on psychoanalysis* (J. Strachey, Trans.). New York: W. W. Norton.

Gerada, C. (Ed.). (2020). *Beneath the white coat: Doctors, their minds and mental health*. London: Routledge.

Giaconia, R. M., Reinherz, H. Z., Silverman, A. B., Pakiz, B., Frost, A. K. and Cohen, E. (1995). Traumas and posttraumatic stress disorder in a community population of older adolescents. *Journal of the American Academy of Child and Adolescent Psychiatry, 34*(10), 1369–1380.

Karanikola, M., Giannakopoulou, M., Mpouzika, M., Kaite, C. P., Tsiaousis, G. Z. and Papathanassoglou, E. D. (2015). Dysfunctional psychological responses among intensive care unit nurses: A systematic review of the literature. *Revista da Escola de Enfermagem da USP, 49*, 0847–0857.

Kardiner, A. (1941). *The traumatic neurosis of war*. Washington, DC: National Research Council.

Korn, D. L. (2009). EMDR and the treatment of complex PTSD: A review. *Journal of EMDR Practice and Research, 3*(4), 264–278.

Lee, C. W. and Cuijpers, P. (2013). A meta-analysis of the contribution of eye movements in processing emotional memories. *Journal of Behaviour Therapy and Experimental Psychiatry, 44*(2), 231–239.

Lee, J., Daffern, M., Ogloff, J. R. and Martin, T. (2015). Towards a model for understanding the development of post-traumatic stress and general distress in mental health nurses. *International Journal of Mental Health Nursing, 24*(1), 49–58.

Levers, L. L. (2012). *Trauma counseling: Theories and interventions*. New York: Springer Publishing Company.

Leys, R. (2000). *Trauma: A genealogy*. Chicago: The University of Chicago Press.

Gilleen, J., Santaolalla, A., Valdearenas, L., Salice, C. and Fuste, M. (2021). Impact of the Covid 19 pandemic on the mental health and well-being of UK healthcare workers. Cambridge University Press (online), 29 April 2021.

Manfield, P. E., Engel, L., Greenwald, R. and Bullard, D. G. (2021). The flash technique in a low-intensity group trauma intervention for healthcare providers impacted by COVID-19 patients. *Journal of EMDR Practice and Research*. 10.

Mangoulia, P., Koukia, E., Alevizopoulos, G., Fildissis, G. and Katostaras, T. (2015). Prevalence of secondary traumatic stress among psychiatric nurses in Greece. *Archives of Psychiatric Nursing, 29*(5), 333–338.

Marsac, M. L., Kassam-Adams, N., Hildenbrand, A. K., Nicholls, E., Winston, F. K., Leff, S. S. and Fein, J. (2016). Implementing a trauma-informed approach in pediatric health care networks. *JAMA Pediatrics, 170*(1), 70–77.

McEwen, B. S. (2007). Physiology and neurobiology of stress and adaptation: Central role of the brain. *Physiological Reviews, 87*(3), 873–904.

Meadors, P. and Lamson, A. (2008). Compassion fatigue and secondary traumatization: Provider self care on intensive care units for children. *Journal of Pediatric Health Care, 22*(1), 24–34.

Meadors, P., Lamson, A., Swanson, M., White, M. and Sira, N. (2010). Secondary traumatization in pediatric healthcare providers: Compassion fatigue, burnout, and secondary traumatic stress. *OMEGA-Journal of Death and Dying, 60*(2), 103–128.

Micale, M. S. (1994). Charcot and les neuroses traumatiques: Scientific and historical reflections. *Revue Neurologique, 150*(8–9), 498–505.

Miller, M. M. and McEwan, B. S. (2006). Establishing an agenda for translational research on PTSD. *Annals of the New York Academy of Sciences, 1071*, 294–312.

Missouridou, E. (2017). Secondary posttraumatic stress and nurses' emotional responses to patient's trauma. *Journal of Trauma Nursing|JTN, 24*(2), 110–115.

Morgan, L., Scourfield, J., Williams, D., Jasper, A. and Lewis, G. (2003). The Aberfan disaster: 33-year follow-up of survivors. *British Journal of Psychiatry*, 182, 532–536.

Morrison, L. E. and Joy, J. P. (2016). Secondary traumatic stress in the emergency department. *Journal of Advanced Nursing*, 72(11), 2894–2906.

Neuner, F., Catani, C., Ruf, M., Schauer, E., Schauer, M. and Elbert, T. (2008). Narrative exposure therapy for the treatment of traumatised children and adolescents (KidNET): From neurocognitive theory to field intervention. *Child and Adolescent Psychiatric Clinics of North America*, 17(3), 641–664.

Newcomb, T. M., Turner, R. H. and Converse, P. E. (2015). *Social psychology: The study of human interaction*. New York: Psychology Press.

Papadopoulos, R. K. (2005). *Therapeutic care for refugees: No place like home*. London: Karnac.

Quinal, L., Harford, S. and Rutledge, D. N. (2009). Secondary traumatic stress in oncology staff. *Cancer Nursing*, 32(4), E1–E7.

Ratrout, H. F. and Hamdan-Mansour, A. M. (2020). Secondary traumatic stress among emergency nurses: Prevalence, predictors, and consequences. *International Journal of Nursing Practice*, 26(1), e12767.

Rivers, W. H. R. (1919). Psychiatry and the war. *Science*, New Series, 49(1268), 367–369.

Robjant, K. and Fazel, M. (2010). The emerging evidence for narrative exposure therapy: A review. *Clinical Psychology Review*, 30(8), 1030–1039.

Shapiro, F. (1989). Efficacy of the eye movement desensitization procedure in the treatment of traumatic memories. *Journal of Traumatic Stress,* 2(2), 199–223.

Skogstad, M., Skorstad, M., Lie, A., Conradi, H. S., Heir, T. and Weisæth, L. (2013). Work-related post-traumatic stress disorder. *Occupational Medicine*, 63(3), 175–182.

Smith, P, Yule, W., Perrin, S., Tranah, T., Dalgleish, T. and Clark, D. M. (2007). Cognitive-behavioural therapy for PTSD in children and adolescents: A preliminary randomized controlled trial. *Journal of the American Academy of Child and Adolescent Psychiatry*, 46(8), 1051–1061.

Summerfield, D. (1995). Addressing human response to war and atrocity: Major challenges in research and practices and the limitations of western psychiatric models. In C. R. Kleber and B. P. Gersons (Eds.), *Beyond trauma*. New York: Plenum Press, 17–30.

Summerfield, D. (2000). War and mental health: A brief overview. *BMJ*, 321(7255), 232–235.

Summerfield, D. (2001). The invention of post-traumatic stress disorder and the social usefulness of a psychiatric category. *BMJ*, 322, 95–98.

Van der Kolk, B. (2014). *The body keeps the score: Mind, brain and body in the transformation of trauma*. London: Penguin UK.

Van der Kolk, B. A. and Fisler, R. (1995). Dissociation and the fragmentary nature of traumatic memories: Overview and exploratory study. *Journal of Traumatic Stress*, 8(4), 505–525.

Van Mol, M. M., Kompanje, E. J., Benoit, D. D., Bakker, J. and Nijkamp, M. D. (2015). The prevalence of compassion fatigue and burnout among healthcare professionals in intensive care units: A systematic review. *PloS ONE*, 10(8), e0136955.

Woodward, A., Thomas, S., Jalloh, M. B., Rees, J. and Leather, A. (2017). Reasons to pursue a career in medicine: A qualitative study in Sierra Leone. *Global Health Research and Policy*, 2(1), 1–11.

Yule, W., Bolton, D., Udwin, O., Boyle, S., O'Ryan, D. and Nurrish, J. (2000). The long-term psychological effects of a disaster experienced in adolescence: I: The incidence and course of PTSD. *Journal of Child Psychology and Psychiatry*, 41(4), 503–511.

18 Debriefs?
Offering Group Interventions in Response to Difficult Events

Dr Sadie Thomas-Unsworth, Dr Harriet Conniff, Dr Zoe Berger, and Dr Joanna Farrington-Exley

There is an almost dazzling array of off-the-shelf interventions for teams that have been involved in potentially traumatic or distressing events,[1] and the recent pandemic has seen an unparalleled amount of attention given to the psychological wellbeing of healthcare staff. However, the area has also been dominated with controversy, in particular around the role of psychological debriefing. This has led many psychologists to feel uncertain about what they can or should offer teams. This chapter outlines some of the current evidence and provides pointers for ways in which practitioner psychologists can use their skills to work with teams and staff groups following difficult events.

We know that being involved in distressing or potentially traumatic events at work can have a profound effect on wellbeing. While most will not develop a mental health disorder such as post-traumatic stress disorder (PTSD), anxiety, or depression, many can suffer from temporary acute distress, and some may develop work-related stress. Such ongoing effects on psychological wellbeing may manifest in work performance and sickness absence which are challenging for both individuals and organisations. Sickness absence in the NHS is higher than in any other part of the UK workforce and problems with psychological wellbeing account for more than a quarter of the reason for absence (The King's Fund, 2019). Several recent publications and reviews of the impact of pandemics on the psychological wellbeing of healthcare workers have indicated that healthcare staff are at increased risk of psychological distress in a variety of

---

[1] For instance, Mental Health First Aid, Trauma Risk Management, and Critical Incident stress debriefing.

forms, with a particular focus on the risk of trauma responses, moral distress,[2] and burnout[3] (see Bashar and Bammidi, 2020; Preti et al., 2020; Billings et al., 2020, Roberts et al., 2020). Alongside this, there is a body of research indicating that even outside the pandemic, certain staff groups, such as those working in Emergency Departments and Intensive Care Units, alongside first responders, are more likely to experience a number of different forms of distress (McKinley et al., 2020, Colville et al., 2018). Within this, being involved in traumatic incidents plays a part.

Introduction to debriefs – definitions and the role of post-event group interventions

Perhaps one of the most talked-about and controversial group interventions following potentially traumatic events or distressing events is debriefs. Evaluation of the evidence base and clinical practice has been hampered by the term being used interchangeably to refer to different processes and meetings after challenging events which might be delivered by different kinds of healthcare staff. We have come across the following meetings that are sometimes called debriefs by healthcare staff: Wellbeing check ins, 'Hot' debriefs, morbidity and mortality meetings, feedback sessions from Root Cause Analyses, Child Death Reviews, and Simulation Training debriefing. Oh, and of course, going to the pub. While many of these are not included in formal evaluation of debriefs within the evidence base, referring to them as debriefs muddies the waters.[4] These kinds of meetings are all run quite differently and have different purposes and psychological debriefs are different again.

Within the psychological world, things are not much clearer. The following fall under the debrief umbrella: critical incident stress debriefing, bereavement debriefs, and psychological debriefs. All of these interventions are frequently grouped under the broader category 'psychological debriefs' and yet they are often delivered with different purposes, in very different contexts and using varying frameworks. This is important as it seems likely that interventions that are appropriate for teams following a potentially traumatic event may differ

---

[2] The experience of feeling as though the care you give contravenes what you believe to be right.
[3] Burnout is typically characterized by a loss of enthusiasm for work (emotional exhaustion), feelings of cynicism (depersonalisation), and a loss of perspective that work is meaningful (low sense of personal accomplishment).
[4] It is certainly our experience that hospital staff often state they have attended a debrief which has not been offered by (staff support) psychologists and the format is not clear.

from those required following a distressing one (e.g. a sad, but not traumatic event).

So, what do we actually mean by offering a debrief? What images or ideas get conjured up for you when we use this term? Our experience shows us that staff (and psychologists!) have very different emotional reactions to the term. It is not uncommon for us to be greeted with a mixture of dread and hope in relation to talking about this. We would argue that because of the lack of clarity around what we mean when we use the term, the evidence about their use and efficacy has been mixed, and it has become a contentious term. And because the definition has been unclear, the domain of who delivers or offers these has also become muddied. We hope to provide some clarity in this chapter by presenting a model of psychological debriefs built on the latest evidence and clinical practice. The model presented here is for debriefs in acute hospital settings but could be applied to other settings too.

The evidence base

Early research in the 1980s tended to focus on the use of 'debriefing' as a tool to prevent PTSD. Indeed, debriefs in various guises continue to be a frequently used approach to support staff involved in potentially traumatising events. However, the Cochrane review in 2002 concluded that the use of individual and group psychological debriefing in the prevention of PTSD was contraindicated (Rose et al., 2002). The review found a failure to show benefit in terms of preventing PTSD and some indicated an increased risk of psychological harm. Since then, it has emerged that the evidence base the Cochrane review looked at was of poor quality and only three studies looked at group interventions; one of these studies brought together individuals involved in road traffic accidents for group debriefing and, not unsurprisingly, people were retraumatised. Finally, while this review sought to address the role of debriefing in the prevention of PTSD, it did not seek to evaluate its other potential uses (enhancing peer support or team-based working). The impact of the Cochrane review and subsequent NICE guidance (2005) have been far-reaching, and we are regularly asked (by colleagues from within psychology and beyond) about concerns people have about the perceived detrimental effect of debriefs and fears around causing harm. It has meant that psychological professionals have faced a challenging dilemma aptly summed up by the title of this article 'To debrief or not to debrief our heroes: That is the question' (Hawker & Hawker, 2010).

More recent reviews have suggested that there may be a role for group interventions for staff working in highly demanding contexts and after difficult events (Richins et al., 2019). It is well established that social and peer support is protective of psychological wellbeing, particularly in a trauma context (Brewin et al., 2000; Trickey et al., 2012). International studies of responses to mass trauma events have indicated that supporting staff to feel connected with each other, understand decision-making processes, engage in peer-to-peer support, connect with their values, and find meaning in what they do can all help boost workplace resilience and decrease the impact of moral distress and risk of burnout (Hobfoll, et al., 2007). In health contexts, staff commonly experience challenging events as a group because they work in teams (i.e. when attending a crash call or when a palliative long-stay child dies on the ward). Therefore, the benefits of coming together as a group are likely to be very different to those group-based interventions offered to people involved in separate traumatic events described in the Cochrane review (Rose et al., 2002).

We present a model for group psychological input following difficult events allowing staff working in health contexts to gain support from their peers. The purpose of this approach is not to prevent PTSD but to bring professionals together to build a sense of shared connection driven by the recognition of shared experiences and values. This is in line with the latest guidance during the pandemic (COVID Trauma Response Group, 2020) and with broader guidance for interventions following mass trauma (Hobfoll et al., 2007). This can be used after a specific event or at any time a staff team identify a need to come together and consider the impact of their shared experiences on one another.

A model of psychology-led debriefs within a pathway and part of a system of staff support[5]

We propose that psychology-led debriefs must be part of a comprehensive system of staff support and wellbeing which takes more practical and preventative forms. Many aspects of which do not need to be delivered by psychologists but may benefit from the involvement of psychologists when considering how we support the supporters and ensure the interventions fit together in a theoretically considered and psychologically safe way. In terms of the more preventative, ongoing spaces that psychologists would be involved

---

[5] This model was first described in Thomas-Unsworth et al. (2021).

in, we thought it useful to briefly differentiate them from psychology-led debriefs. We define a psychology-led debrief very generally as a meeting after a significant event (such as an unexpected death, difficult situation, critical incident) where the focus is on social connection, individual and team coping and, often, to build a broad shared narrative of what happened. Therefore, the focus is not of driving learning but rather enhancing connection and meaning-making. Reflective practice, on the other hand, is something we might broadly define as an intervention that is ongoing, preventative, and may well be scheduled regularly. The focal point of reflective practice could be on the impact of the work, an opportunity to discuss cases and themes in the work, and think about ways forward.

An additional intervention we have found ourselves offering in acute healthcare is a 'pre-brief' which sits between reflective practice and psychology-led debriefs. These are meetings before a significant event happens (if indeed it does happen), but the situation is already causing significant staff distress. Reasons for running these usually fall under two main areas in our clinical experience. Firstly, when there is a deteriorating patient that is expected to die who is well known to the team. Or secondly, when there is a long stay patient with complex physical health problems with multiple teams involved, possibly ethical and moral issues and additionally there may be complaints and/or litigation contexts. We have found that offering pre-briefs (which are run in a similar way to psychology-led debriefs as described below) can help staff prepare for the emotional impact on them and clarify the medical plan. Subsequently, after having delivered a pre-brief (or sometimes a series of them in complex situations), we have found that there is often not a request for a psychology-led debrief, and staff describe that being prepared renegaded the need for this.

Debrief pathways

We would recommend that psychological debriefs sit within a pathway where first there is a meeting in the immediate aftermath of an event (without psychology present). These are often called 'hot debriefs' or in some of our practice 'Time out' (Cooper, Winton, & Farrington-Exley, 2019) or an 'immediate huddle' (Macaulay & Conniff, 2020). They tend to be shorter than psychological debriefs in length, for example 20 minutes. Box 18.1 outlines some recommendations as to how to run immediate huddles (or hot debriefs). Secondly, there should be some sort of follow-up check in by managers/supervisors, thirdly followed at a later point by psychology-led debriefs if needed. We will briefly run through some ideas about holding these immediate meetings before turning to psychological debriefs. All the authors of this chapter have been involved in developing debrief pathways in our places of work.

These initial meetings (hot debriefs) are not usually attended by psychologists and just for those directly involved in an incident or event, following the principles described earlier of peer support, connectivity, and normalising responses as being useful in recovery. If we (practitioner psychologists) do see teams/individuals in the immediate aftermath, we would only do so in a 'containing-of-anxiety role', for example, to run through the process of the debrief pathway – what to expect and when, give details about what we can offer, normalise responses and provide some basic psychoeducation and, possibly, resources.

In terms of the timing of when to hold these types of meetings, there are various possibilities: directly after the event, the end of shift, or the next day. Feedback from clinicians tells us that it is usually best to hold it as soon after the event as possible, because otherwise staff get drawn back to their home areas (e.g. the crash team) and get pulled into the rest of their busy shift. Our clinical colleagues have learnt that leaving it any later than 48 hours after the event can also mean that the meeting takes on a different nature; staff will have had longer to process the event, be more able to articulate and identify their feelings and thoughts about the event – meaning a longer meeting is needed and requires the facilitation to be led by a differently skilled professional (such as a practitioner psychologist).

Additionally, clinicians report that the potential location of the immediate meeting is impacted by the timing of the difficult event (e.g. resuscitation) and busyness in the clinical area which obviously affects finding a space to hold it. Where possible, it is key to find a space away from the area where the incident occurred.

We have learnt that senior clinicians (consultants, senior nurses, site practitioners) are best placed to run these immediate meetings. Sometimes senior clinicians may not have been part of the trigger event and may be involved at the end (e.g. to call the time of death) and so in these instances, find it easier to stand back and lead the immediate meeting. If a senior clinician was directly involved in the incident, they may feel too close to the event to be able to facilitate the immediate meeting. In that situation, they may ask a colleague to facilitate it. A lot of the work of these immediate meetings is emotional containment for staff which can also take its toll on the facilitator so they need to be prepared for this and be aware of follow-up for themselves should they need it.

Box 18.1: Running immediate huddles (hot debriefs)

Meet

- Invite all involved to meet in an appropriate location
- Attendance not compulsory
- Consider those who may have witnessed the event and offer support independently, for example, patients, relatives, and other staff especially non-clinical staff who can get forgotten
- Decide who will lead the huddle
- Document all names of staff involved – have a paper sign in sheet.

Explain the purpose

- To check in with everyone to see if they are okay in response to the event and okay to continue working
- To pause and acknowledge what has happened
- To allow staff to recharge
- To briefly clarify the events as a team immediately after the event
- To focus on factual information
- To avoid discussion of performance, opinion, and/or analysis.

Discuss

- Do not go around the group – contributions (speaking) should be voluntary
- Briefly describe the events that occurred as a group
- Any burning issues or questions staff involved may have
- What went well?
- Are there any immediate concerns to be addressed or issues that need to be followed up?
- Clarify roles and responsibilities going forward
- Does any documentation need completing and do staff need support with this?

Next steps

- Consider making supervisors/line managers, for example, consultant on service, educational supervisors, nurse in charge, or ward manager, aware of those involved in an incident so everyone can be offered future support as part of the debrief pathway
- Contact psychology team about running a psychology-led debrief if needed.

With regard to following up after a challenging event, it is useful if this can happen within 48 hours. Ideally this should be done by a line manager or supervisor, or another senior clinician. This can range from a simple check-in – 'how are you doing after yesterday?' to a sit-down discussion about wellbeing and whether the staff member needs to take time off and/or needs any additional supports.

Psychology-led debriefs for staff

Who should deliver them? The extent to which healthcare staff who witness distressing or potentially traumatic events are at risk of developing PTSD is unclear. However, the idea that their wellbeing is likely to be impacted is not. To ensure the risk of re-traumatising participants is monitored appropriately, we recommend that at least one member of staff is a qualified mental health professional with knowledge of risk factors for PTSD and familiar with delivering psychological interventions with groups. It is also suggested that post-event group interventions of this nature are facilitated by two facilitators so that one staff member can monitor the 'emotional temperature' of the room and if required follow up with anyone should they choose to step out.

Psychological interventions for staff teams should ideally be delivered by professionals who have a working knowledge of the local context, understand, and know the team or service and be based on a thorough assessment of need. Where this is not possible, and facilitation is sought from external sources, interventions must not be delivered in isolation and care should be taken to ensure they work alongside other locally available packages of support, for instance, Trauma Risk Management or Occupational Health Services. We highlight a model here with stages for the benefit of the reader. While psychological debriefs we run do tend to follow this process, in our experience the stages are rarely clear cut. Staff may move around between stages, and sometimes we may spend a lot of time in one stage and less in another. Key aspects to consider when running psychological debriefs are presented in Box 18.2.

Introduction to the session

It is important to try to make the session feel as psychologically safe as possible by discussing the boundaries of the meeting at the start, for example, confidentiality, timings, and ground rules. Much of this information should be sent to staff prior to attending the intervention so they are able to meaningfully opt in. Staff may need time to adjust to the mental 'change in gear' that is required for a reflective space. Inviting participation in a brief grounding exercise may help (e.g. five senses grounding exercise). This stage of the debrief along with other stages of the process are highlighted in Box 18.3.

> **Box 18.2: Key considerations when delivering a psychological debrief**
>
> - It is critical that holding a psychological group session is recognised as being only one element of a support package for staff (Macaulay & Conniff, 2020; Richins et al., 2019).
> - Attendance at the meeting is voluntary; staff should be able to choose whether to attend. It is important that staff are able to use their own natural coping strategies, which may or may not include talking to colleagues about how they are feeling in relation to the crisis/specific event/period of time.
> - For many, access to other interventions such as 1:1s, rest, space to relax and unwind away from the busyness of the ward, and time with colleagues will be more appropriate.
> - Before delivering a psychological debrief, assess whether the difficulty can be safely discussed in a group setting. This is discussed in more detail below.
> - Psychological group sessions are most effective when attendance is explicitly supported by senior members of the team. Wherever possible, this should include cover being provided so staff can attend in work time. This signals an important message about how we value staff.
> - It may be useful to keep an attendance list of staff who attended the meeting and their role. It is however not essential to keep notes of the content of the meeting, although key themes may be useful in offering feedback or in follow-up. Confidentiality is an important aspect of the interventions, and it must be agreed with the group what, if any, information is to be taken out of the meeting, for example, actions or learning points and where it will be shared (e.g. leadership team).
> - All staff should have access to further follow-up if needed and can therefore be signposted to further sources of support.

Setting the scene

Where relevant, lead clinicians are invited to share briefly what led to the psychological session being requested and their hopes for the discussion. Depending on the reason for the psychological session, it may be helpful to spend most of the session supporting staff to tell the story of the event, taking care not to encourage reprocessing (a detailed description of the felt experience of the event) but rather support staff to build a shared narrative of what happened. Often this involves a senior clinician giving a summary of the event where there is then an opportunity for staff to ask brief questions about something which may be causing them distress (e.g. I was busy on the ward, so the patient's medications were 10 minutes late did this cause them to deteriorate?). For many staff, this is a hugely beneficial experience as worries about not knowing what happened or if they did something wrong may be the root of their distress rather than the incident per se. There are some specific circumstances when we would urge caution around retelling in detail the story of the event. These include when any of the team were likely to have felt their personal safety was at risk (e.g. in incidents of threat or violence) and/or if the event itself was particularly traumatic to witness (e.g. a very difficult end of life). In these circumstances it may be more appropriate to focus on a more general guided reflection recognising that not all staff attending will want to hear the details itself.

Facilitating the storytelling

At this stage, we encourage staff to build on the story of what happened from their perspective. Later we move into reflecting on the impact of the event on staff and how they coped as individuals and as a team. The facilitator gently supports the storytelling, taking care not to invite detailed sensory descriptions but focus on what happened, and putting the pieces together. Care should be taken not to *require* staff to recall or share specific thoughts or feelings during the event. Staff support and psychological debriefs, while therapeutic, are different to psychological therapy. A psychological debrief addresses people's experience in a different and less direct way than if it was individual or group therapy where, as clinicians, we are trained to ask for detail to deconstruct words to help bring about alternative meaning. While we draw on this Socratic open questioning in psychological debriefs and it may well be that staff do share how they felt or what stood out to them about an incident, we don't ask for the individual detail of people's experiences.

Guided group reflection

Attendees are invited to reflect on the impact of the event and share some of their responses *if they wish to*. In reality, these 'stages' of a debrief are generally not clear cut; for example, people have often talked about their response to the event in building a shared narrative. It must be remembered that all contributions should be voluntary, and staff should never be pressured to speak. It can be useful to offer brief psychoeducation about common responses to anxiety and trauma. During this part, we support the group to make sense of their distress and think about why their buttons may have been pushed. It may be because what happened goes against their primary task 'I felt I could not help the family and I am trained to help', the event could have taken place in an unusual setting where deaths or crash calls don't usually happen or it could be to do with the unexpected nature of the event, 'we normally work with sedated children'.

Connecting with values, coping and each other

During the meeting, staff are encouraged to reflect on their strengths and resources as individuals and as a team, their values, what they were most proud of and self-care/coping strategies. We might explore what mattered to them the most and what was important to them during and after the event. We might ask how people managed despite the difficult situation, what helped, what skills and values they drew upon and think together about individual and group self-care.

Learning

Eliciting learning points is not the aim of the meeting; however, sometimes the group may decide on actions that need to be taken out of the meeting. For some staff, it appears to aid their emotional recovery when they have concrete learning points to take forward, especially if they are actively changing clinical practice personally and in their teams with the aim to prevent the event/error happening again. A psychological debrief does not replace any other meetings or governance processes required by the hospital system such as root cause analyses or other learning and improvement meetings.

> **Box 18.3: Suggested process for running psychological debriefs**
>
> 1. List of attendees – state for own clinical governance and would only be revealed to managers to demonstrate a staff member was offered support. If general themes are to be shared, stress that they will not be attached to who said what.
> 2. Introduce selves name and role – It may be helpful to invite staff to share their role in the event, but this will depend on the size of the group and the context of the debrief.
> 3. Ground rules – what do we need to agree to make this talking comfortable/safe? (Confidentiality, create equal opportunity to speak/do not have to speak, can be normal to get upset – that's okay). State plan if someone leaves the room and is upset, another staff member will go find them 5 minutes later (check everyone has contact details for each other if online).
> 4. What is useful to cover? Try to bring out different ideas and voices (usually people after a critical incident ask for medical update/medical questions answered plus space to talk about feelings that arose).
> 5. Senior clinician (whoever feels best placed to do this) outlines what happened (with others chipping in).
> 6. Opportunity for people to ask questions and add to the story.
> 7. Normalise distress – psychoeducation about fight and flight, trauma, and common reactions to traumatic events.
> 8. Do not encourage detailed sensory descriptions of the event.
> 9. Conceptualise distress – group generate possible reasons they may feel like they do.
> 10. Pull out coping as individuals and as a team.
> 11. Summarise, what needs to be taken forward and by whom.
> 12. Evaluation.

Psychological facilitation skills required

Throughout the above, facilitators will use their psychological training to draw out narratives of hope, connectivity to one another, and working in accordance with individual, team, and organisational values. It is also the role of the facilitators to manage dominant voices or difficult group dynamics that may be impacting on the psychological safety of the space. Psychologist facilitators are also trained to work with high levels of distress and to recognise when signposting on to specialised support may be needed. It may be easy to fall into the trap of prematurely reassuring teams or offering praise and congratulations to staff who have faced a challenging incident. Box 18.4 suggests some 'do's' and 'don'ts' for facilitators of psychological debriefs. It is important to ensure there has been sufficient space for staff to talk about the aspects of the event that were more difficult or have left them grappling with how they feel about work or their role in the event. We have often seen our colleagues fall into this trap and while some in the group will be grateful of the appreciation and thanks bestowed upon them in that situation, we know of others who find this experience devaluing and undermining of their own struggle. Being able to sit with and tolerate the sometimes messy emotional landscape for staff and offer reflections and shared hypotheses about why something might be particularly challenging is often necessary.

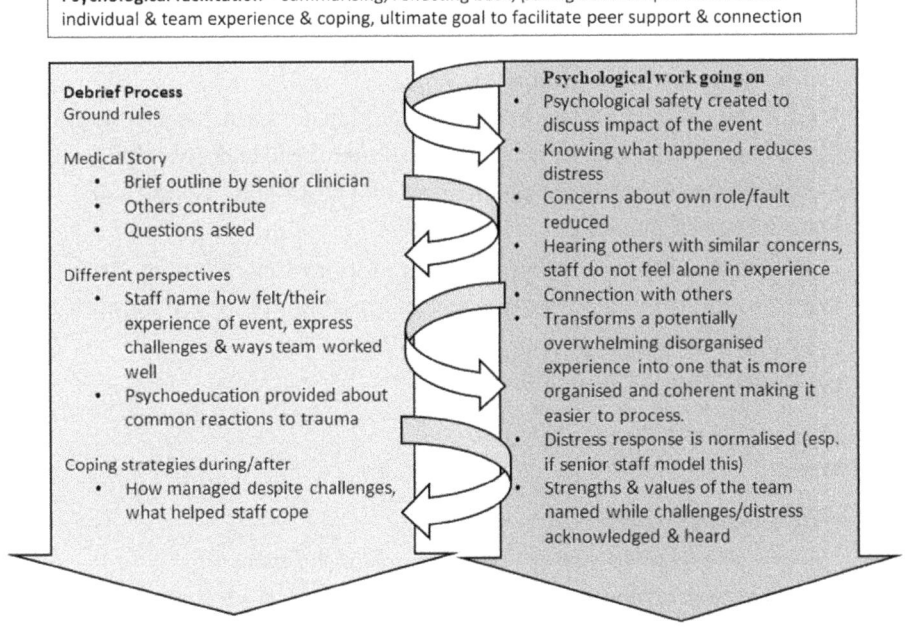

FIGURE 18.1: The psychological debrief structure and underpinning psychological processes.

Box 18.4: Do's and don'ts for facilitators

Do

- Set up the session well, for example, meet with and prepare the lead clinician ensuring they know what to expect, their role and rationale for the intervention
- Ensure detailed information has been sent out to all invitees so they know what to expect and can make an informed choice regarding whether to attend
- Be clear about the boundaries of the meeting, for example, confidentiality
- Use active listening skills
- Encourage discussion
- Listen out for and highlight the resources and strengths within the team and individuals while also allowing time for expression of emotions, for example, sadness, guilt, distress
- Pay attention to strong feelings in the room responding with empathy and compassion so that the speaker feels heard
- Think about power in medical hierarchies and possible discrimination of certain staff groups and how this may impact on safety to speak/be in groups
- Consider other contexts that may be at play, for example, ethnicity, class, age, sexuality, and gender of staff members, and how this relates not only to their participation in a group but also to their experience of the event
- Challenge colleagues if they are being disrespectful, blaming, or critical, for example, by reminding group of ground rules, request the discussion is taken outside the meeting
- Offer signposting to follow up support.

Don't

- Pressure staff to attend
- Encourage detailed sensory descriptions of the event
- Pressure staff to speak during the meeting or go around the room.

Common challenges and dilemmas

Deciding if a debrief is appropriate

It is crucial to consider if a debrief is the right intervention to offer and to assess the appropriateness of delivering one. This requires a thorough assessment of need and reflection on the considerations mentioned. In addition, clinicians should assess:

What is the primary psychological need for the staff group at this time?

Staff can have a diverse range of needs after being involved in a potentially traumatic event, and it should not be presumed that a group psychology-led debrief is the only or most appropriate intervention. Staff may need time and space, informal peer support, more formal 1:1 support with a peer, 1:1 support with an embedded professional, or external profession 1:1 support. To assist with identifying the need, you should specifically consider:

The nature of the event and the likely psychological impact

It is necessary to consider specifically the nature of the event and the context within which it occurred so that we can understand the likely meaning and impact it may have had on the team. This is a crucial first consideration. Particular consideration should be given as to whether, during the course of the event, staff were at risk of (or the victim of) violence or aggression themselves or whether they witnessed anyone else who was. This is important given the link between these types of events and the risk of developing PTSD. In these circumstances, attention should be given to whether a group intervention is the most appropriate, when it is offered and what is covered, with extreme caution being taken around any description of the event. It is then important to consider again specifically what it is about this event that made it so distressing and/or highly traumatic. Was it expected or unexpected? Did the staff feel proud of the care they delivered or are they concerned about it? Is the primary experience shock, grief, horror, sadness, or a mixture of them all?

What is the purpose of bringing staff together in a facilitated space at this point?

Once you have an understanding of the nature of the event itself and the likely psychological impact, you can consider what purpose bringing staff together might have and then specifically what a psychology-led debrief might offer. As outlined earlier, we know that after involvement in potentially traumatic events people benefit from being supported to feel safe, calm, connected, effective individually and collectively, and to hold a sense of hope. Bringing staff together as peers can help them to feel connected, calm, and safe but skilful facilitation can also help draw these narratives out more directly as well as fostering more explicitly a sense of self and collective efficacy and hope. It can also ensure that qualified staff get early eyes on their colleagues so that staff showing high levels of distress can be picked up quickly and signposted appropriately.

When

Careful thought should be given to the timing of the event. While teams may seek facilitation very rapidly, it is important to be clear about what this can and cannot achieve. If the primary purpose is around fostering connection, hope, and meaning-making, it is likely that teams will be best served by having a little more time between the event and the facilitated debrief itself.

Evaluation, themes, and learning: What works

It is essential to collect staff experience evaluation data. It is recognised that this is new and emerging area and in the absence of a robustly evaluated evidence base it is particularly important that teams monitor the acceptability and perceived effectiveness of the interventions. We will share here some of the main themes from unpublished data collected by the authors using self-reported semi-structured questionnaires evaluating the usefulness of debriefs and asking about the impact of them on staff's work.

Staff routinely describe that it is helpful to talk openly in safe space and express their thoughts, feelings, and views. Being released from duties to attend in this protected time makes staff feel cared for by senior colleagues and the organisation. They have told us that debriefs help them to realise what is working and what existing support there is in their team as well as making them aware of more formal staff and wellbeing supports. Staff also report the value in listening to others talk about their experience which supports them to not feel alone in their emotional response. Importantly, individuals have told us directly and through feedback surveys that debriefs help them remain in work or return to work after an incident. Additionally, staff have told us debriefs improve multidisciplinary working and clinical learning through supporting emotional expression and reflective communication. Overall, our data and clinical experience consistently indicate that our debrief format is well received and beneficial to participants. Formal research is now required.

Conclusion

The authors of this chapter all developed debrief offers in relation to their work in paediatric hospitals with a focus initially on supporting staff in a paediatric context. However, over time requests have increased, and the model has been developed to be applicable following a range of events including incidents of violence and aggression and complex situations involving long-stay cases where challenges have developed over time. We have observed the different functions of debriefs contrasting when they are being delivered to support a team following the loss of a patient known well versus after a complex safeguarding case or incidence of aggression against staff.

There is huge power in bringing staff together to share stories of an event. But it is also an incredibly delicate process that requires skills and strength in facilitation. The value, where possible, in shadowing a more experienced colleague and observing how they navigate the inevitable challenges cannot be emphasised enough. The facilitator needs to do two important things in parallel: maintain the psychological safety of the space through the construction and maintenance of clear boundaries and hold the space gently and lightly so that the focus is on harnessing the team's own resources to support themselves and one another. As one member of staff commented in their evaluation form: 'The facilitation was excellent, almost like a conductor, guiding us through the process whilst we had control of our contribution.'

It is also our experience that debriefs can take many forms and still be of enormous benefit to those who attend. We have facilitated debriefs that have become very focused on medical details or alternatively not described the trigger event at all, and both have had huge merit. It can be really hard to judge as facilitators how useful the space is, so getting feedback is essential. What does a good debrief look like after all? Does everyone need to cry? Does everyone need to talk? Should they arrive sad but leave happy? The best debriefs for us are when staff get to share their individual part of a story to build a collective story and in doing so, they feel heard, less alone, and connected. Sometimes, through gentle questioning by the facilitator, they may also develop new ways of looking at things – perhaps considering more their intention than the outcome of an event or the way in which they wish to grow or develop on the back of it.

In this work, it is vital to consider your own needs as a clinician and the psychological impact of delivering debriefs. We often find we feel extraordinarily drained after facilitating these spaces both because of the emotional content but also the high levels of concentration required. We now therefore try to ensure we do not have to go straight onto anything else after and avoid facilitating two in one day. We also find it helpful to ground ourselves at the start (either with the group or individually) as well as consciously setting our intention before we join the call or walk in the room. So much exists in the space between us ensuring we show up knowing how we want to be and what we want to communicate verbally and otherwise feels hugely important.

Between us we have delivered hundreds of debriefs over the past decade. They remain one of the most challenging and fulfilling aspects of our staff support work. Our work and that of others are developing all the time. We have described a broad framework that can be used to facilitate staff teams to come together after challenging events to support each other, build a shared narrative of the event, and reconnect with their individual and team values and ways they usually cope. This is not meant to be a blueprint or formula however, as every situation and staff team (and what their needs might be) are very different. It is more of a guide, with important factors to consider, to facilitating a space for healthcare staff to connect, support, and find solace in each other as a team.

References and suggested reading

Bashar, M. A., & Bammidi, R. (2020). Psychological impact of COVID-19 pandemic on health care professionals and workers. *Industrial Psychiatry Journal, 29*(1), 176–179. https://doi.org/10.4103/ipj.ipj_99_20.

British Psychological Society. (2015). Early interventions for trauma. Available at: www.bps.org.uk

British Psychological Society Covid 19 Staff Wellbeing Group. (2020). The psychological needs of healthcare staff as a result of the Coronavirus pandemic. *British Psychological Society*. Available at: www.bps.org.uk

Brewin, C. R., Andrews, B., & Valentine, J. D. (2000). Meta-analysis of risk factors for posttraumatic stress disorder in trauma exposed adults. *Journal of Consulting & Clinical Psychology, 68*, 748–766.

Colville, G. A., Dawson, D., Rabinthiran, S., Chaudry-Daley, Z., and Perkins-Porras, L. (2018). A survey of moral distress in staff working in intensive care in the UK. *Journal of the Intensive Care Society*, 20, 196–203.

Cooper, S., Winton, M., & Farrington-Exley, J. (2019). Fifteen-minute consultation: Time Out as an alternative to toxic debrief. *Archives of Disease in Childhood Education & Practice Edition*, 105, 1–6.

Covid trauma response working group rapid guidance version 3 – 7th April 2020 guidance for planners of the psychosocial response to stress experienced by hospital staff associated with COVID: Early interventions. Available at: www.kingsfund.org.uk

Davidson, S. (2010). The development of the British red cross' psychosocial framework: "Calmer". *Journal of Social Work Practice*, 24, 29–42.

Hallam, R. (2019). Mental health & discrimination at work. *Clinical Psychology Forum*, Vol 315, 7–10.

Hawker, D. M., Durkin, J., & Hawker, D. S. J. (2010). To debrief or not to debrief our heroes: That is the question. *Clinical Psychology and Psychotherapy*, 18(6), 453–463.

Health & Safety Executive. (2020). Work-related stress, anxiety or depression statistics in Great Britain, 2020. [Internet]. https://www.hse.gov.uk/statistics/causdis/stress.pdf (accessed 20 October 2021).

Hobfoll, S. E., Watson, P. Bell, C. C., Bryant, R. A., Brymer, M. J., Friedman, M. J., Friedman, M., Gersons, B. P. R., de Jong, J. T. V. M., Layne, C. M., Maguen, S., Neria, Y., Norwood, A. E., Pynoos, R. S., Reissman, D. Ruzek, J. I., Shalev, A. Y., Solomon, Z. Steinberg, A. M. and Ursano, R. J. (2007). Five essential elements of immediate and mid-term mass trauma intervention: Empirical evidence. *Psychiatry*, 70, 316–69

King's Fund. (2019). NHS Sickness absence: Let's talk about mental health. [Internet] https://www.kingsfund.org.uk/blog/2019/10/nhs-sickness-absence (accessed 20 October 2021).

Macaulay, C., & Conniff, H. (2020). Developing a programme of staff support in a children's hospital. *Archives of Disease in Childhood British Medical Journal*, June, 106, 1–2.

McKinley, N., McCain, R. S., & Convie, L., Clarke, M., Dempster, M. Campbell, W. J. and Kirk, S. J. (2020). Resilience, burnout and coping mechanisms in UK doctors: A cross-sectional study. *BMJ Open*, 10, e031765.

National Institute for Health and Care Excellence (NICE). (2005). *Post-traumatic stress disorder (PTSD): The management of PTSD in adults and children in primary and secondary care.* Clinical Guideline 26. 2005.

Preti, E., Di Mattei, V., Perego, G., Ferrari, F., Mazzetti, M., Taranto, P., Di Piero, Rossella, Madeddu, F. and Calati, R. (2020). The psychological impact of epidemic and pandemic outbreaks on healthcare workers: Rapid review of the evidence. *Current Psychiatry Reports*. Vol 22.

Rose, S. C., Bisson, J., Churchill, R., & Wessely, S. (2002). Psychological debriefing for preventing post traumatic stress disorder (PTSD). *Cochrane Database of Systematic Reviews, 2002*(2), CD000560. https://doi.org/10.1002/14651858.CD000560.

Richins, M. T., Gauntlett, L., Tehrani, N., Hesketh, I., Weston, D., Carter, H., & Amlôt, R. (2019). Public health England, British psychological society & royal college of policing scoping review: Post-trauma interventions in organisations final report. Available at: www.bps.org.uk

Roberts, T., Daniels, J., & Hulme, W. (2021). Psychological distress during the acceleration phase of the COVID-19 pandemic: A survey of doctors practising in emergency medicine, anaesthesia and intensive care medicine in the UK and Ireland. *Emergency Medicine Journal*, 2021, 450–459.

Thomas-Unsworth, S., Berger, Z., Conniff, H., & Farrington-Exley, J. (2021). What can psychologists offer teams after difficult events?. *Clinical Psychology Forum*, 344, 60–64.

Trickey, D., Siddaway, A. D., Meiser-Stedman, R., Serpell, L., & Field, A. P. (2012). A meta-analysis of risk factors for post-traumatic stress disorder in children and adolescents. *Clinical Psychology Review*, 32, 122–138.

UK Psychological Trauma Society. (2014). Traumatic Stress Management Guidance: For organisations whose staff work in high-risk environments. Available at: www.ukpts.org.uk

Gathering Our Thoughts

Dr Harriet Conniff

The wealth of chapters presented here cover an impressive variety of ways we can support healthcare staff psychologically. We have seen how psychological staff support operates at different levels and is different to traditional clinical work or therapy with clients. We have also seen how supporting staff psychologically works best when within a system of staff wellbeing that attends to practical and spiritual aspects and to working conditions, and to bring this all about we need organisational backup. Building relationships is central to the work and creating conditions for connection and peer support is vital. *Connection, belonging, compassion, relationships* – these words seem important. However, as Raselle Miller noted in chapter 1, words change their meaning and relevance over time. We have also seen it is *how* organisations and leaders make use of words like resilience, compassion, and EDI that impacts staff on the ground so if deployed as tick-box buzzwords they become empty concepts, lose meaning, and can negatively affect wellbeing. I wonder what words will be important to us, our colleagues and in staff wellbeing generally, going forward?

As many authors have commented, what we do may not fit into a neat box. It can be difficult to quantify our activity. In my own practice, I do 'walk and talks' with individual staff for support, supervision or meetings, and 'morale check-ins' with clinical leads. Both of these can take different forms again depending on what arises when working with team culture. Distinguishing between types of staff support work can be hard: for instance, there may be overlap between group supervision and reflective practice and a training session may become more focused on reflection. The work requires agility, something that many who work in health are accustomed to, and typically involves snatched corridor conversations about setting up work. It can be complex to navigate this, but the flexibility of the work is also appealing.

Future directions

There is obviously so much more that could be covered in this book. I recognise that there are other practitioners whom I could have included. It would have been wonderful to bring in more international authors and share more collaborations across the globe and across (professional) roles. We have been presented with a range of compassion practices useful in staff support. We have seen the role of staff support chaplains and the importance of weaving spirituality and faith into our conversations with staff, and in designing psychological staff support input. Wright (2021, p. 257) argues that we need to consider spiritual issues more in thinking about burnout and comments on how it has been a neglected issue:

> *Spirituality and its impact upon health has only recently been given more attention. It inevitably gets caught up in reservations associated either with fluffy, touchy-feely therapy or hard-boiled religiosity.*

As we have discovered, many adaptations of traditional psychological approaches are being used in staff support. And yet, given more time and space, other ideas and interventions potentially warrant chapters, such as Solution-Focused working, Acceptance and Commitment Therapy, coaching, and Ecotherapy to name a few. Perhaps readers will take the baton on. Future publications on psychological staff support could explore further the breadth of cross-working with colleagues in organisational development, human resources, chaplaincy, and occupational health, as well as with leaders, clinicians, and non-clinical staff who champion staff wellbeing.

Even in a system of staff support with a variety of offerings, we know that no amount of staff wellbeing resources and professionals alone can address broader issues such as healthcare funding, resource, and staff shortage which (and of course fundamentally) affect the wellbeing of staff: "The burnout of individual workers says more about workplace conditions than it does about that person" (Highfield and Neal, chapter 15). Siddharth Shah's remarks[1] are pertinent here about the need to change the system:

> *While helping individuals cope is worthy of time and attention, health professionals must put more focus on changing the system itself [which] seems to be getting off easy and deserves more heat. (Global Forum, 2019, p. 51)*

---

[1] When he summarised discussions between healthcare leaders at an international conference

Subsequently, we need to be mindful about causing unintentional harm in doing psychological staff support. We must be wary of contributing to programmes that are only top down, introduced enthusiastically by leadership based on what 'the experts say is needed', but which leave the system, teams, and staff members feeling 'done to', however well intentioned. In the context of COVID-19 recovery, Greenberg (2020, p. 1) flags the danger of a "poorly implemented post-COVID-19 plan, leading to seemingly false promises of support or … managers making high work demands on staff who have been working 'flat out' [which] has the potential to derail staff support efforts to date and to cause serious psychological harm". We need to remember that talking in psychological ways is not for everyone. Additionally, ignoring the context of where staff work or not having proper structures in place (such as employing mental health first aiders without any clinical governance or support in place for them) can be detrimental to employee mental health (Rhodes, 2021).

Managing the challenges of psychological staff support

We have learnt that how the work is approached is key. A strong message from our authors is that we should approach the work with compassion for ourselves and those we support, and also with a readiness to ask questions and effect change where needed. This is no easy task. Throughout this book we have seen how we are often asked to come in and respond to the distressing elements of healthcare work, for example supporting staff around a gruelling crash call, death of a child, intensive care and emergency department working, conflict with patients and families, court cases, risk, and safeguarding. We may also be providing staff support within the following difficult contexts: death of colleagues, investigations, bullying and discrimination, and working in systems where we may disagree with processes and practices.

The chapters here cover the variety of roles psychologists providing staff support might find themselves in, such as facilitator, listener, space holder, advocate, assessor of mental health, mediator, messenger, and communicator. Moving between different roles can be taxing while carrying out some roles may pose challenges; for example, in delivering themed feedback from staff groups, we become messengers who get shot down. We might also be portrayed as fixers or miracle workers who can simply deliver a one-off group session which will solve problematic team dynamics. Alternatively, we may be charged with solving big issues, such as racism in a department without system buy-in or back-up.

How might we navigate these demanding contexts and being positioned in these ways? The wisdom across the book suggests how to do this. Collaboration is clearly essential, and it is worthwhile to work alongside or jointly with other wellbeing colleagues as we have seen. We always need to reflect on whether psychologists are the best people or best placed in organisations to deliver staff support and wellbeing. Again, we return to how we approach the work; *how* we offer and *be with* people is crucial. A stance of cultural humility and curiosity is important and can assist with tackling barriers to help-seeking. I am drawn to the concept of 'reaching in' rather than always expecting others to reach out (Smith, 2021, p. 26). We can apply this to ourselves too in working in psychological staff support.

Looking after ourselves: Pulling off the superhero's mask?

Successive British Psychological Society surveys of the psychology workforce since 2014 have consistently demonstrated that psychologists report lower general wellbeing than the general population (Rao & Clarke, 2022). While these findings match surveys of NHS staff generally, there are some indications that reduced wellbeing, work-related stress, and distress in psychologists may take a particular form. For instance, psychologists have described feeling undervalued, being viewed as non-essential, and doing work which is emotionally exhausting. It may be that this is contributing to psychologists reducing their hours or even leaving the profession (Tolland & Drysdale, 2022), but more detailed exploration is needed.

Clearly our profession needs to do more to look after its workforce. With the rise in psychological staff support posts, we need to think about the peculiarities of this role too. We have seen how for staff psychologists the pandemic exaggerated the fact that when working we may experience similar issues as the staff we support at work or home. Many of us have had experiences of being 'on the other side' of healthcare as patients or relatives. More research is required into the wellbeing of psychologists and other professionals involved in delivering psychological staff support, and as Rao and Clarke (2022, p. 2) point out:

> *[the] needs of psychologists offering wellbeing support to wider health & social care staff require attention.*

We're all probably fairly good at looking after ourselves following a particularly challenging day or event; however, we need to think about how we sustain ourselves on the okay or good days too. What makes a 'good' or 'bad' day can be down to chance and sometimes we forget to appreciate how much energy can go into work on any average day. Much has been said about the superhero narrative as being unhelpful for healthcare staff as it loads unrealistic expectations on them and pressurises them to always be okay and cope like 'superheroes' helping others. It can make staff feel like they cannot have an off day and reach out for support. Quite a few chapters include comments on psychologists' own help-seeking and our narratives about coping. It is almost as if psychologists and wellbeing professionals are meant to be invincible too. Consequently, for those of us working in staff support, it could be said that we are positioned as the superhero's superhero. So, with these narratives and practices surrounding us, how might we receive offers of help and support? Who will reach in for us?

How *do* we make space to sustain us and think about how we cope doing this work? We can start perhaps by reframing the superhero narrative, taking a leaf out of Dr Janina Scarlet's (comic) book. She developed superhero therapy on the basis that superheroes are in reality flawed; they all have origin stories with tragic events and weaknesses, as well as having superpowers (Scarlet, 2021). A reframe for us could be that we allow ourselves to be human, be open about life and work impacting on us, and accept that this is normal and okay. In other words, we should practise what we preach.

The danger is that we end up replicating an individual focus in thinking about support for ourselves as psychologists (and others in staff wellbeing). This is where we can learn more from organisational psychology about considering self-care at a group level, as Alex Haslam (2021, p. 33), professor of social and organisational psychology, reflects:

And self-care – what does collective self-care mean? Is my group looking after itself, am I looking after my group, is my group looking after me? That leads to all sorts of productive possibilities because lots of problems around resilience and mental health become pretty intractable if you only look at them at the individual level. Open your eyes to collective dimensions of these phenomena and you'll be surprised what you find.

We might make use of some of the collective offerings discussed in this book as well as more established ways of supporting supporters such as the British Red Cross working (chapter 7). We can look to the pioneering work of psychologists who work hard to destigmatise lived experience of mental health difficulties in mental health professionals (Kemp, 2022). Other possibilities are peer supervision, accessing professional networks and group supervision with an external facilitator. And we can informally join with others in a similar role to learn from each other and provide mutual support, as described in chapter 13:

> *We call it self-relational-community care so we can include all aspects. You can take a warm bath ... but relational care is about connecting with others – those who are your chosen community ... and community care is about taking care of others in your community. (Uma Millner, INDEAR Listening circles)*

Summing up

Psychological staff support is a key aspect of staff wellbeing and can take many forms and exist at varied levels in healthcare organisations. Some of the work outlined here has a formula for interventions; those with a set structure can be incredibly effective and useful – not least to contain staff (and facilitators') anxieties and manage boundaries. Yet sometimes the main work is done in setting up and talking about the work. Then again, the work can be more fluid, pared down to the basics of connection, listening, and being with.

The staff support role is a tricky one and we must think about our values and motivations in taking it on. Ultimately, this work is messy. Often despite the best setting up conversations, the task or focus can change when we are in the middle of it. It is not always neatly separated into individual, team or organisational level or by name of intervention, like these chapters are laid out here. This is for me part of the appeal; it makes you work hard, think on your feet, and every day is truly different. Nurturing and sustaining each other is fundamental to doing this work while maintaining our joy for it (Walrond, 2021).

When the pandemic hit, the profile of staff health and wellbeing shot through the roof. Suddenly it was sexy, and everybody was talking about it. There has been lots of funding for roles in staff health and wellbeing, and new initiatives and resources being rolled out. This is clearly brilliant, but it is sad that it's taken a pandemic to do this. I am hopeful that the legacy of this will continue. We need to build on this legacy by consolidating what exists and supporting ongoing preventative ways of working and decent working conditions that treat staff well. This is the right thing to do for healthcare staff, and it means that people can thrive in their jobs to deliver compassionate care to patients. Let us hope that the importance of looking after staff continues to be recognised and becomes part of the fabric of working in healthcare.

References

Haslam, A. (2021). 'Open your eyes to collective dimensions'. *The Psychologist*, November 2021, 34, 33–35.

Greenberg, N. (2020). '"Going for growth" an outline NHS staff recovery plan post-COVID19 (outbreak 1)'. The Royal College of Psychiatrists (May 2020).

Kemp, N. (2022). https://www.in2gr8mentalhealth.com. Accessed on 12/03/2022.

Rao, A. S., & Clarke, J. (2022). *Psychological professionals wellbeing survey summary 2021*. Produced by the DCP & New Savoy Conference Re-setting the Balance – Workplace Wellbeing Project Steering Group.

Rhodes, E. (2021). 'Interview piece on Emma Donaldson-Feilder & Joanna Wilde's work for the health & safety executive's review of the evidence into workplace interventions to improve psychological wellbeing'. *The Psychologist*, September 2021, 34, 16–17.

Scarlet, J. (2021). 'Superhero-therapy online training'. September 2021. http://www.superhero-therapy.com.

Smith, J. (2021). *Nurturing maternity staff: How to tackle trauma, stress and burnout to create a positive working culture in the NHS*. London: Pinter & Martin.

Tolland, H., & Drysdale, E. (2022). 'Exploring the prevalence and reasons for clinical psychologists leaving the NHS in one health board'. *Clinical Psychology Forum*, 351, March 2022, 33–38.

Walrond, K. (2021). *The lightmaker's manifesto: How to work for change without losing your joy*. Minneapolis: Broadleaf Books.

Wright, S. G. (2021). 'Burnout: A spiritual crisis, from trauma to transformation'. In: Aris, S., Garraway, H., & Gilbert, H. (Eds.), *Mental health, spirituality and wellbeing*. Hove: Pavilion, 253–264.

Acknowledgements

In the first place, thanks go to all the remarkable contributors to this book who gave their precious time when it was already stretched by clinical demands (and then some by the pandemic). Huge thanks go to Dr Arabella Kurtz as consultant editor for cultivating the initial idea and then growing this book with me. Also, to Jenny Vohlic the development editor from Sequoia books whose input has been invaluable and thoughtful. I would like to thank Andrew Peart, publisher at Sequoia for his support and getting stuff done without needless bureaucracy and Jayanthi Chander and her copy-editing team for their tireless work. I am grateful to ACP-UK for this opportunity and for all their support and encouragement throughout.

I would also like to thank those people that have helped develop my thinking and encouraged me in the task of producing a book who include GSTT psychologists, the staff psychology team and those I have previously worked alongside in other hospitals. Above all I have learnt (and continue to learn) from all the staff I have been privileged to work with. Together we have co-produced initiatives and advocated for staff by bringing issues to the attention of organisations and management.

In the realm of staff support working, we cannot do this without leadership back up; I have been privileged to have huge support from these great women in first developing a system of staff support in our children's hospital before the pandemic: Sara Hanna (Medical Director), Chloe Macaulay (Paediatrician), Kirsteen McCullough (then Head of Nursing for Theatres, Surgery & intensive care), and Melinda Edwards (then Paediatric Psychology Lead). Numerous others have supported the work (and me) since and particularly include Debbie Komaromy, Claire Lemer, James O'Brien, Neil Rees, Debbie Ford, Amanda Mwale, Raselle Miller, Amelia Carton, Kate Le Marechal, Deborah Woodman and Lisa Barkley. I am also grateful to Ali Hashtroudi and Helen Kay, GSTT Occupational Health leads, for their vital support and the GSTT charity for their backing of the wider staff wellbeing work in our Trust, especially for funding staff psychology posts.

Last, but by no means least, come my loved ones. Immense gratitude to my family and friends for nourishing me in different ways. For kindly reading drafts

ACKNOWLEDGEMENTS

and boosting my confidence in writing, thank you Jon. Special thanks to Hannah for her wisdom and our replenishing walks. Loving thanks to my mum and (of course) to Jasmine, my incredible daughter, both of whom really kept me going during some tough moments.

This book is dedicated to the memory of Desmond Fawcett (or Bappy) without whom I would never have found clinical psychology.

Dr Harriet Conniff, Summer 2022

Contributor Biographies

Paula Aredez Arriazu CPsychol (she/her) is a counselling psychologist. She works at the British Red Cross offering reflective practice, supervision groups and 1:1 support to Refugee and Anti-trafficking services in London. She also works as a Senior Trauma Specialist at the NHS Grenfell Health and Wellbeing Service supporting children and young people suffering from trauma and offers consultation services to international humanitarian organisations. Her background includes working in emergency settings and with survivors of gender-based violence, human rights abuse, and various trauma presentations across the lifespan.

Professor Poornima Bhola is a psychotherapist, teacher, supervisor and researcher and is currently professor, Department of Clinical Psychology, National Institute of Mental Health and Neurosciences (NIMHANS), Bangalore, India, where she completed her M.Phil. and Ph.D. degrees. She works with adults to foster emotional and relational growth and towards psychosocial rehabilitation of persons with severe mental illnesses. What Poornima most enjoys is the process of training and supervision, and she is currently the Coordinator of the psychotherapy training programme in the department.

Poornima has conducted numerous workshops on reflective practice, ethics and youth mental health for counsellors and psychotherapists and on workplace mental health for several organisations. She is on several research, editorial and ethics committees and is a member of the consultative committee on transgender rights.

Her research interests include psychotherapy processes, training and development, youth mental health and personality dimensions. She has authored a book on Reflective Practice and Professional Development in Psychotherapy (Sage Publications, 2022), in collaboration with Dr Chetna Duggal and Dr Rathna Isaac. She has also co-edited a book, *Ethical Issues in Counselling and Psychotherapy Practice* (Springer, 2016, with Prof. Ahalya Raguram).

CONTRIBUTOR BIOGRAPHIES

Andy Bradley is the originator of the 60-minute Compassion Circle, the original of the Compassion Practices shared at CompassionPractices.net; Andy is the catalyst who connected the co-founders of CompassionPractices.net.

Andy's belief is that when we are vulnerable we should be met with consistent kindness and that we must 'elevate the status of care giving'. Andy was a care home manager in the 1990s and early 2000s when he became uncomfortable with the culture and working practices he saw in many care settings. Having grown up in a compassionate care home run by his parents in Herefordshire, Andy knew that better was possible, so he set out on a 15-year journey to try to bring more compassion to the health and social care sectors in practical ways. Andy went on to give hands-on support to people with profound learning disabilities and older people and went on to fill a range of leadership positions.

Andy founded Frameworks4Change in 2004, built a reputation as a leading thinker and practitioner in compassionate cultures, and was recognised by the Observer and NESTA (the National Endowment for Science, Technology and the Arts) in 2012 as one of the UK's New Radicals. The habit-building programmes that Andy designed and facilitated with the team at Frameworks 4 Change saw dramatic results with continuous improvements to care and staff teams feeling valued and appreciated. Andy worked with the NHS, Local Authorities and a range of care provider organisations and has advised organisations internationally.

Dr Penelope Cream holds dual qualifications as a clinical and a health psychologist. She has worked in the fields of the psychology of complex medical conditions, long-term health problems, experiences of hospital treatment and healthcare delivery in many of London's large teaching hospitals since 2001.

Penelope has taught in hospitals, clinics and medical schools and has supervised clinical psychologists, medical students and junior doctors undertaking research. She has worked in and managed psychology services across many different medical specialties, including intensive care, pain management, general medicine and endocrinology. For several years Penelope was the clinical psychologist for complex diabetes and pancreatic islet transplantation at The Royal Free Hospital. In 2011 she set up the psychology service for sickle cell and thalassaemia at St George's Hospital and was part of a national team establishing policy and psychology standards for haemoglobinopathies treatment across the United Kingdom and Ireland. She is the Lead for the Association of Clinical Psychologists' COVID-19 three staff support schemes and is currently the director of Operations for ACP-UK.

Dr Shannon Cullerton is a clinical psychologist currently in the role of Lead Psychologist for Staff Wellbeing on COVID-19 Wards at Guy's and St Thomas' NHS Foundation Trust. She comes to this position after previously working in specialist services within the NHS that work with people who have experienced complex trauma. Prior to her career in the NHS she worked for a number of well-known Human Rights organisations for over a decade. Her current role was created in the context of a rapid COVID-19 response. In her current role she has been informed by traditional psychological thinking on responses to the impact of crisis and traumatic incidents as well as drawing on her interest and experience in systemic, narrative and community psychology approaches to meet the diverse needs of the staff and ensure the offer of support is as accessible and meaningful to as many as possible.

Dr Sarah Davidson, MBE, is the head of Psychosocial and Mental Health at the British Red Cross. In this role she leads on strategy, programme delivery and development of mental health and psychosocial support. She is also the co-chair of the International Federation of Red Cross and Red Crescent's Research Network on mental health and psychosocial support and is co-chair in the Red Cross and Red Crescent Movement wide initiative to guarantee a basic level of psychosocial training for all staff and volunteers and ensure the integration of mental health and psychosocial support in all the Movement's services globally. She is a consultant clinical psychologist who worked for 15 years as such in a specialist, national NHS service and initially trained as a nurse. She has been involved in developing and delivering staff support for the last 30 years across a range of sectors.

Dr Chetna Duggal is a clinical psychologist and associate professor at the School of Human Ecology, Tata Institute of Social Sciences, Mumbai. She completed her M. Phil (Clinical Psychology) from the National Institute of Mental Health and Neurosciences (NIMHANS), Bangalore, and PhD from the Tata Institute of Social Sciences (TISS), Mumbai. Her research interests include psychotherapy practice, training and supervision, and adolescent and youth mental health. She has been in psychotherapy practice for over 15 years. In recent years, she has launched the School Initiative for Mental Health Advocacy (SIMHA), and Rahbar, an initiative for supervision.

Dr Joanna Farrington-Exley is a principal clinical psychologist and lead for Staff Wellbeing at Leeds Children's Hospital within Leeds Teaching Hospitals

NHS Trust. She also leads the Schwartz Round programme in Leeds Children's Hospital. For the first 10 years of her qualified life, Joanna worked in Child and Adolescent Mental Health Services across the North of England. Joanna moved into the area of workforce well-being in 2017. She has a long-term interest in supporting colleagues and a particular curiosity about how we can sustain ourselves and each other as healthcare providers, through compassionate cultures and systems.

Dr Julie Fraser is a clinical psychologist and systemic family therapist. She has been working with families and service users in community mental health teams, acute wards, and rehabilitation wards since 2003. Dr Fraser trained as a systemic supervisor, and is also a clinical supervisor for the Kings MSc Family Therapy training. Dr Fraser first became inspired by the Tree of Life in 2011 and the work of Angela Byrne in East London using Ncube's (2006) model. In 2012, her team were awarded funding from Maudsley Charity to design, develop and implement 'service user/peer co-produced tree of life workshops' across the adult acute wards in SLAM. As a result of the success of this work, co-produced Tree of Life is now an integrated part of the acute psychology model of care and won a national mental health award for 'Promoting Equality and Diversity in Service Provision'. Dr Fraser has been involved in numerous Tree of Life projects in SLAM and developed a training package for using Tree of Life as a co-produced model in the NHS. She also created a group couple Tree of Life programme for couples in the perinatal period and continues to use the Professional Tree in my systemic therapy training clinics as a tool for supervision and professional development.

Dr Julie Highfield is a consultant clinical psychologist and Lead for Organisational Health in Adult and Paediatric Critical Care, Cardiff. She is the National Project Director for Wellbeing in the Intensive Care Society. She has a long experience of working as a psychologist in medical and healthcare settings and works closely with staff in their experience of working in healthcare, as well as advising managers on matters of workforce well-being. She has previously been the Associate Clinical Director for Wales's largest ICU, a position traditional held by a medic. Julie has worked with the British Psychological Society (BPS) and its Division of Clinical Psychology in Wales. She led the BPS team writing the National Guidance for Staff in the Coronavirus Pandemic. Julie has worked with Welsh Assembly Government in various projects, including as the lead for Critical Care Workforce in the 2018-19 Task and Finish Group, Modelling for

Rehabilitation for patients post COVID-19, and the Wellbeing Conversation Tool.

Dr Matthew Hotton is a clinical psychologist in the Spires Cleft Service, Oxford University Hospitals NHS Foundation Trust, and is a Research Tutor at the Oxford Institute for Clinical Psychology Training and Research at the University of Oxford. He led on evaluating the Oxford University Hospitals NHS Foundation Trust staff support initiative during the first wave of the COVID-19 pandemic and helped establish the ACP-UK Member Network for Staff Health and Wellbeing. He also is a founding member of the Surgical Psychology and Performance group – a collaboration between psychologists and surgeons regarding the psychological factors influencing surgical well-being and performance.

Dr Rathna Isaac is a clinical psychologist who completed her training in NIMHANS in 2005 and is a private practitioner and supervisor with 20 years of experience. She is an external consultant and supervisor for the Couple and Family Therapy Programme at Parivarthan Counselling, Training and Research Centre. She has created and conducted both basic and advanced training programmes on couple therapy and provides ongoing group supervision for couple counsellors. She has conducted several training workshops for counsellors and psychotherapists at all levels and is deeply interested in the psychotherapy process.

Arabella Kurtz is a consultant clinical psychologist and a psychoanalytic psychotherapist. She studied English Literature at University before training as a clinical psychologist and is interested in the interface between psychology and the arts, and creative ways of approaching clinical practice and the development of services. Arabella has held posts in NHS adult and forensic mental health services, and worked for many years on the University of Leicester training course, coordinating the reflective practice seminar programme, carrying out research on the needs of staff and developing teaching focused on the understanding of organisational culture. She is now clinical lead for the Staff Health and Wellbeing Service in Northamptonshire. Arabella enjoys writing and has produced two books: The Good Story: Exchanges on Truth, Fiction and Psychotherapy (co-authored with the novelist JM Coetzee and published by Vintage in 2016) and How to Run Reflective Practice Groups: A Guide for Healthcare Professionals (published by Routledge in 2020).

CONTRIBUTOR BIOGRAPHIES

Charlie Jones is a consultant clinical psychologist at North Bristol NHS Trust. He has a passion for systemic and relational approaches to working in healthcare, and how we can create sustainable conditions for safe, honest conversations. He's a dad with two lively boys.

Dr Louise Johnson is a principal clinical psychologist at Leeds Teaching Hospitals NHS Trust. Dr Johnson provides clinical psychology input to children and adults within Leeds Major Trauma Centre, Orthopaedics and Plastic surgery departments. Her current research interests include predictors of psychological distress following major trauma, quality of life and psychological functioning following limb reconstruction, and the emotional well-being of major trauma clinicians. Dr Johnson is the current Chair of the National Major Trauma Psychology Network. She is also a Trustee for Day One Trauma Support charity. During the first wave of the COVID-19 pandemic, Dr Johnson was involved in leading the evaluation of the staff support service delivered by the Department of Clinical and Health Psychology, Leeds Teaching Hospitals NHS Trust.

Catherine Lacey is a clinical psychologist who currently leads support for staff working in community services at Guy's and St Thomas' NHS Foundation Trust in London. Working as a Clinical Psychologist for 10 years in 2 countries, Australia and the UK, Catherine has a passion for supporting staff in physical health settings. She has previously worked clinically in spinal, physical rehabilitation, women's services and renal care settings. She is also a Schwartz Round facilitator. These varied experiences have shaped her knowledge of healthcare systems, the day-to-day work in these areas and the impact on staff within them. Throughout her career she has had an interest in compassion-based approaches. She has undertaken training in Compassion Focused Therapy (CFT) and Compassion Focused Staff Support (CFSS) and primarily uses these models when working with staff in one-to-one therapy and group contexts.

Dr Joanna Levene is a consultant clinical psychologist and head of Specialty for the Physical Health Psychology Service in Nottinghamshire Healthcare NHS Foundation Trust. She also holds local and regional strategic roles, focused on improving physical and psychological health care. Joanna works clinically in cancer and palliative care services, where she runs reflective practice groups for healthcare staff working in these settings. She has a particular interest in integrating physical and mental health care, sharing psychological skills and knowledge with health and care staff, and improving staff well-being.

CONTRIBUTOR BIOGRAPHIES

Dr. Kate Lucre is a Birmingham-based compassion focused therapist and supervisor specialising in the use of CFT for complex attachment and relational trauma for groups and individuals. She is the supervision coordinator for the Compassionate Mind Foundation and also runs workshops for the Foundation and across the UK on CFT for Groups and Compassion Focused Staff Support and Supervision. Kate offers CFT supervision in groups and individually, including a monthly international Supervision Group for therapists involved in the provision of CFT groups. She has published the only data on Compassion Focused Group Psychotherapy for people who would attract a diagnosis of personality disorder and has recently completely a 7-year research programme evaluating a 12 month CFGP program. Kate is also involved in a number of UK wide research projects developing and evaluating Compassion Focused Staff Support Initiatives. You can see some of her past presentations at https://www.researchgate.net/profile/Katherine_Lucre2.

Dr Liz Matias is a senior clinical psychologist working in a Psychosis community mental health team. She has extensive experience of delivering staff support interventions in a variety of mental health settings including forensic inpatient units and community mental health teams. Liz has a specialist interest in collective narrative practices, namely the Tree of Life, largely inspired by the work of Angela Byrne in East London using the approach within mental health settings. Since joining South London and Maudsley NHS trust, she has further developed her interest in the Tree of Life. In 2017 she had the privilege of being trained by Ncazelo Ncube-Mlilo, a key founder of the approach, to become an advanced Tree of Life facilitator. Over the past five years she has led on initiatives to develop Tree of Life interventions for both service users and staff teams. Her work alongside Dr Julie Fraser with the Professional Tree of Life led to the approach being offered as a Trust-wide staff support intervention since 2019.

Dr Claire McDonald is a principal clinical psychologist and clinical lead for Staff Support at King's College Hospital NHS Foundation Trust in London. She helped to develop and coordinate a tiered, multidimensional and award-winning Staff Support Programme throughout the pandemic, which included offering support to staff, teams, managers and within the broader organisational context. Within her role, she leads the Trust Schwartz Round programme and the Staff Psychology Service within the Occupational Health and Wellbeing Department. Dr McDonald developed an interest in supporting NHS staff teams at the Maudsley Hospital in London where she adapted the Professional

Tree of Life model and piloted the concept of a 'Team Tree' intervention to help promote well-being and resilience within teams. Dr McDonald maintains a busy private practice in London, specialising in working with adults with a broad range of difficulties. She is trained in several evidence-based therapeutic approaches including Cognitive Behavioural Therapy and related third wave approaches, Narrative Therapy, Schema Therapy and EMDR.

Dr Raselle Miller is a clinical psychologist specialising in the promotion of equality, diversity and inclusion. She believes in the creation of inclusive anti-racist organisations across the globe. Raselle has held various posts in NHS adult specialist clinical health and mental health services over the last 15 years. She currently works at Guy's and St Thomas' NHS Foundation Trust, where she leads on creating culturally accessible well-being services for NHS staff from global majority communities. Raselle obtained her Masters in Psychology and Doctorate in Clinical Psychology from the University of East London, and her Postgraduate Diploma in Mental Health Practice from Middlesex University, London. She has had further training systemic, narrative, racial and intergenerational trauma and cognitive analytic therapy. Her clinical and research interests are staff support, global psychological techniques, quality of life and relational responses to treatment and care.

Dr Lisa Monaghan has trained with Jaakko Seikkula's Finnish team and is a trainer in Dialogic Practice, a Consultant Clinical Psychologist and a Narrative & EMDR therapist and accredited Mediator. Lisa has worked in both the NHS and third sector and helped to set up and run the first UK national open dialogue service: Dialogue First. She has worked in mental health and care settings for 23 years and has spent 12 years as the Lead Psychologist in inner and outer London Learning Disabilities Team's, as well as working on acute inpatient wards as the Principal Psychologist (male & female acute and older adult acute wards). Lisa is now the Trust Strategic & Clinical Lead for Staff Psychological & Well-being Service for University College London Hospital Foundation. Having taught on Doctorial Clinical Psychology courses and examined for the Peer Supported Open Dialogue training course, she has also undertaken multiple research projects in open dialogue, adapting models of different populations and psychopharmacology. Throughout her career, Lisa has developed an understanding of the importance of the stories of people's lives and how healing can occur when these are listened to with authenticity and compassion. Her passion is for collaborating with others wishing to share skills and learn together within all professional and personal arenas, as she strives to engage a wider audience in the social justice issues surrounding our current mental health services and our difficult social climate.

Rachel Morley is a consultant clinical psychologist who currently works as a senior psychosocial practitioner in the British Red Cross helping to embed trauma-informed approaches to staff support. Previously she led a NHS trauma service for asylum seekers and refugees in Glasgow and is very committed to the importance of reflective practice being part of staff support and well-being.

Dr Esther Murray has been a health psychologist for 14 years, initially working in cardiac care both in service improvement and psychological interventions for patients, later going on to a career in academia. Her early research was in chronic pain and its effect on doctor-patient communication. Esther has previous experience in psychological intervention in cardiac care and training NHS staff in communication skills. Esther is the first researcher in the UK to explore the concept of moral injury in medicine, and since being invited to present on the topic of Moral Injury at the Institute of Pre-hospital Care Performance Psychology Symposium in June 2017, Esther has been invited to present at national and international conferences for both healthcare professionals, educators and students. Esther also delivers training on the topic to London Ambulance Service's Advanced Paramedic Practitioners, the Counter Terrorism Specialist Firearms Officers of the Metropolitan Police and is a regular contributor to London HEMS Clinical Governance Days. Esther has recorded podcasts for WEM, St Emlyns, The College of Paramedics and for the London Advanced Paramedics and East of England Ambulance Service, she also delivers well-being workshops at the Royal London Hospital for staff in theatres and at the Royal College of Emergency Medicine and the Intensive Care Society. Her co-edited book The Mental Health and Wellbeing of Healthcare Practitioners (Wiley Blackwell) came out in summer 2021.

Dr Adrian Neal is consultant clinical psychologist and head of Well-being for Aneurin Bevan University Health Board (ABUHB). Adrian qualified as a Clinical Psychologist in 2003 and for the first 10 years worked within NHS England Community and Acute Adult Mental Health Services. He was also a part-time Lecturer Practitioner on the Coventry and Warwick Universities Clinical Psychology Doctorate. More recently, after completing an MSc in Organisational Psychology, he has specialised in Occupational Health and Wellbeing within the public sector. Moving to Wales in 2014 as part of his role as Head of Well-being within ABUHB he has been involved in collaborative projects across the Welsh Public Sector, including Welsh government. Adrian views NHS organisations as immensely complex, often toxic, and highly political, and believes that psychosocial factors (especially leadership) are the cornerstone to organisational culture, health, and well-being. Adrian co-leads the innovative Leading People leadership programme within ABUHB and is Past Co-chair of the Leadership and Management Faculty (DCP, BPS) and Past Chair of DCP Wales. Adrian is an Academic supervisor at Cardiff and Cardiff Metropolitan universities and has published academic articles and book chapters relating to mental health, occupational health, organisational culture and well-being.

Dr Anika Petrella is a researcher within the Cancer Clinical Trials unit at the University College London Hospitals (UCLH) NHS Foundation Trust. As part of the BRIGHTLIGHT research team, Dr Petrella focuses on the area of teenager and young adult cancer care and has a specific interest in helping young people cope with cancer. During the first wave of the COVID-19 pandemic, she led on an evaluation of the UCLH staff Psychological and Welfare Service. Dr Petrella established a cohort of clinical and non-clinical staff and monitored their use of available resources provided by the Trust and the impact of COVID-19 on well-being.

Dr Rachel Potter is a consultant clinical psychologist working in a large Health Board in South East Wales. Since qualifying Rachel has worked within NHS community services with adults with intellectual disabilities. Areas of special interest include supporting adults with Down's syndrome who develop dementia, supporting the implementation of the Positive Behaviour Support framework and adapting Dialectical Behaviour Therapy for adults with intellectual disabilities. In 2017 Rachel moved to a clinical lead role within an intensive community support team working with adults with intellectual disabilities who are engaging in behaviours that can be experienced as challenging. Much of Rachel's work is with staff teams and systems and this has resulted in her developing an interest in supporting and sustaining compassionate care within healthcare settings. Rachel was one of the original founders of the Taking Care Giving Care Rounds and continues to support the development and implementation of Compassionate Practices. Rachel lives in Cardiff and enjoys gardening, singing in a choir and spending time with her niece and nephew.

Dr Sherry Rehim is a clinical psychologist currently in the role of Lead Psychologist for Staff Wellbeing in Cancer and Surgery services at Guy's and St Thomas' NHS Foundation Trust. She joined the Trust in 2020 and was involved in developing the Staff Wellbeing Service in the context of a rapid Covid-19 response. Prior to this, Sherry worked in NHS services that work with people who have experienced complex trauma, specialising her knowledge and skills in the area of trauma, race and culture. She worked in the Child and Family Refugee Service at The Tavistock and Portman NHS foundation Trust before moving to the Looked after Children Service to focus her work with Unaccompanied Asylum-Seeking Children. Whilst having trained in specific trauma-focused interventions such as Eye Movement Desensitization and Reprocessing (EMDR) and Narrative exposure therapy (NET), her work is largely influenced by systemic, community, liberation and narrative therapy approaches.

Dr Neil Rees is consultant clinical psychologist and trust lead psychologist for Staff Health & Wellbeing at Guy's & St Thomas' NHS Foundation Trust. He joined the Trust a few months before the COVID-19 pandemic hit the UK. His role is to develop the staff well-being strategy and response for the organisation, managing a psychological interventions service for staff alongside more preventative and organisational initiatives. Neil's clinical career has focused on working with systems related to healthcare contexts ranging from adult clinical health psychology and sexual health, to paediatric palliative care and paediatric liaison, in community and hospital settings. These roles have all involved supportive consultation to NHS staff. He has also worked on a voluntary basis with the British Red Cross as part of the Psychosocial Support Team which deploys overseas to support British citizens and Foreign and Commonwealth Office staff affected by emergency situations. For 19 years he worked on the Professional Doctorate in Clinical Psychology at the University of East London where for 15 years he was Clinical Director and then Joint Programme Director. He was responsible for overseeing the clinical skills and professional development of trainee clinical psychologists, as well as ensuring that their health and well-being was prioritised.

Laura Simms brings over 30 years of healthcare experience to her role in the People Directorate of the English NHS. Her deep passion for compassion and inclusion was ignited during her student nurse training in the 1980s and paved the way for her clinical and healthcare leadership work, including as executive director of a palliative care social enterprise community interest company. Laura remains committed to working towards a diverse, compassionate, inclusive, fair, and joyful NHS and society. Having worked with the art, science, and practice of compassion for several years, amid the pandemic, Laura co-founded the Compassion Practice Collective www.compassionpractices.net to liberate compassion globally, and for all.

An advocate of empowering and mobilising others through the power of 'human' leadership, Laura also confesses to peddling courage and compassion at every opportunity, creating the conditions in which others can flourish. Practising both coaching and leadership mentoring, Laura is inspired and curious about the power of the arts and humanities in 'people' work. As a graduate of the NHS Leadership Academy Nye Bevan Programme, The School for Health and Care Radicals (now Change Agents), INVITAS, and an alumna of Saïd Business School, Oxford and Birmingham Universities, Laura is still growing and developing as a human and as a leader.

Laura speaks and writes on compassion for inclusion https://www.nhsemployers.org/articles/compassion-inclusion-and-link-belonging and compassion in the context of loss, grief and a complex world.

Dr Alister Scott is a leadership consultant, thinker-doer and catalyst behind a range of initiatives, including – with Laura Simms and Benna Waites – CompassionPractices.net, which provides practical how-to methods for people to bring more compassion into their organisations, their systems and their personal lives. As of August 2022 the site has over 500 professionals signed up and the founding team have convened a Core Enabling Group to explore how to enable more people to experience and facilitate the Compassion Practices so as to achieve the 'inspiring, shared purpose beyond self': to liberate compassion globally. Alister's commitment to compassion deepened when he was 'broken open' by the death of his wife Sarah in 2016 at the age of 50.

Alister is the co-author, with Neil Scotton, of the acclaimed *Little Book of Making Big Change Happen*. He advises senior leaders and teams internationally on leadership, systemic change and movement building and appears on a range of podcasts. His doctorate at the Science Policy Research Unit at the University of Sussex investigated what makes experts relevant to society's biggest challenges, tracing debates back as far as Aristotle, with his idea of phronesis – knowledge in service of society.

Alister has made it his mission to enable big positive change, helping to:

- rewild a beautiful site in Fermanagh, N Ireland in 1988, before the term rewilding had been invented;
- achieve World Park status for Antarctica for 50 years, in 1991;
- persuade one of the UK's largest pension funds, USS, to adopt an ethical, engaged investment policy in 1999;
- influence the UK government and the whole of Europe away from GM foods in 1999; and
- support many other leaders to achieve extraordinary things since the turn of the century.

Dr Jon Taylor is a consultant forensic psychologist and psychotherapist who has worked in range of prison, secure hospital and community forensic settings for almost 30 years. With a keen interest in developing a rich understanding of the role of trauma and adversity in the lives of those who develop offending behaviours, Jon is committed to promoting and modelling a compassionate and co-operative approach to all aspects of forensic service provision. Jon is a member of the Compassionate Mind Foundation and cofounder of the CFT forensic special interest group.

Dr Sadie Thomas-Unsworth is consultant clinical psychologist and clinical lead for the BNSSG Healthier Together support network which is a local mental health and well-being hub for staff working across health and social care. Alongside that, Sadie leads the staff support team within a large acute hospital trust. Sadie developed an interest in staff support through her clinical work in Paediatric Palliative Care and Paediatric cancer in which she saw first-hand the impact of the work on healthcare colleagues. In particular, she became interested in how we can support staff after distressing events to help them feel connected with one another and the values that brought them into their job. Sadie is particularly influenced by ACT/CFT and Systemic approaches and how they can inform our work with health and social care staff. Sadie is co-chair of the ACP Health and Wellbeing Network and Treasurer of the BPS Paediatric Psychology Network.

Cathy Thorley has worked in a London National Health Service for more than 25 years. After training as an Occupational Therapist, she later qualified as a Systemic Family Therapist in 2005 and a Systemic Supervisor in 2009. Cathy is the Clinical Lead for Peer Supported Open Dialogue (POD) in her Trust, and she is involved in a major UK trial comparing POD with treatment as usual. As well as working with families she also teaches and offers individual and group supervision, reflective practice, and consultation, drawing on dialogical principles, in many different contexts including staff support. With the support of colleagues, Cathy set up and managed a multi-disciplinary team offering an Open Dialogue style service (Dialogue First) taking referrals from GPs across England. This is the only service of its kind to be offered in England and she continues to be part of that team. Cathy has a particular interest in trauma and is an EMDR consultant. She trained as an Open Dialogue trainer in Helsinki and has been a tutor on the peer-supported Open Dialogue training since 2016. Cathy also teaches and supervises dialogically on compassionate leadership trainings. Cathy is grateful to be able to work dialogically in many contexts and feels enriched by this both personally and professionally.

Dr Karen Treisman, MBE, is a clinical psychologist who has worked in the National Health System and children's services. Karen has also worked cross-culturally in both Africa and Asia with groups ranging from former child soldiers to survivors of the Rwandan Genocide. She also is the author of 10 books, 5 sets of therapeutic card decks and 6 therapeutic soft cuddly toys.

Karen has extensive experience in the areas of trauma, parenting, adversity and attachment, and works clinically using a range of therapeutic approaches with families, systems and children in or on the edge of care, unaccompanied asylum-seeking young people and adopted children. Karen also specialises in supporting organisations and systems to move towards becoming, and to sustain adversity, culturally and, trauma-informed, infused, and responsive practice. This work focuses on creating meaningful and multi-layered cultural and paradigm shifts across whole systems. This was the focus of Dr Treisman's Winston Churchill Fellowship Travel Award which involved visiting several places in the USA to further study whole system and organisational approaches to trauma-informed and trauma-responsive care, and this topic is the focus of Dr Treisman's book *A Treasure Box for Creating Trauma-Informed Organizations: A Ready-to-Use Resource For Trauma, Adversity, and Culturally Informed, Infused and Responsive Systems.*

Karen is the founder and director of Safe Hands and Thinking Minds and within this is a consultant, trainer, speaker and assessor to a variety of local authorities, residential and nursing homes, schools, prisons and organisations. Karen is also an expert witness and regularly undergoes a variety of assessments for court. Additionally, Karen is also a reviewer for numerous academic journals and an international speaker and trainer.

Professor Mike Wang is emeritus professor of Clinical Psychology in the Centre for Medicine, University of Leicester, and former Director of the NHS-funded Leicester Doctoral Postgraduate Clinical Psychology Training Course. He is a former Chair of the Division of Clinical Psychology of the British Psychological Society and is currently Founding Chair of the Association of Clinical Psychologists UK. He holds numerous visiting professorships with overseas universities including India and China. He has more than 40 years' experience as a qualified clinical psychologist. He has been Fellow of the British Psychological Society since 1999 and is also a Fellow of the Royal Society of Medicine. In 2015 he was awarded the Humphry Davy Medal by the Royal College of Anaesthetists for his contribution to the understanding of accidental awareness during general anaesthesia.

Throughout his academic career he has maintained an Honorary Consultant role in the NHS, treating patients with anxiety disorders, depression, PTSD and obsessional compulsive disorder. He was born and raised in the north of England and is of mixed ethnic heritage.

Dr Benna Waites qualified as a clinical psychologist in Oxford in 1993 and has worked for three trusts in London and two Health Boards in Wales. Since 2001 she has been a Head of Health Psychology Specialty, then a Head of Adult Psychology and since 2006 a Head of Psychology which she job shares. Alongside her professional lead role, she works within the Continuous Improvement team (ABCi) where she set up and now leads the in-house leadership programme – Leading People. She has chaired the national Health foundation funded Psychology for Improvement work which has overlapped significantly with Employee Well-Being. She is involved in work developing national strategy on psychological safety and is a qualified Psychological Safety Index practitioner. Having grown up in London and Manchester, Benna now enjoys living in the Herefordshire countryside with her partner and three sons where she enjoys walking, gardening, cooking and eating!

Andrea Wood works as a psychosocial practitioner in the British Red Cross, offering reflective practice, supervision, 1:1 support and training within Refugee Support Services, International Family Tracing, Independent Living including High Intensity Users, and external organisations. She previously worked within

International Family Tracing. She is an integrative psychotherapist specialising in trauma, attachment, loss and change; former chair of the British Association of Dramatherapists and chair of Conference at the Centre for Child Mental Health, an international consultant for the British Council in the Middle East; a published author and editor of more than 40 books for educational professionals on trauma informed, attachment aware practice.

About the Editor

Dr Harriet Conniff is a mother and clinical psychologist who has worked in paediatrics and adult health settings for much of her career, mainly in intensive care and respiratory medicine. Throughout, she has been responsible for providing support to healthcare staff in different ways. Harriet feels passionately about this work and is continually learning from staff she is privileged to work with and her colleagues in the field of staff health and wellbeing. Harriet is systemically trained, specialising in the solution focused approach and finds the latter, as well as a systemic consultation model, particularly useful in staff support working.

In 2018 she gained a post leading on Staff support across the Evelina Children's Hospital and Women's Services part of Guy's and St Thomas' NHS Foundation Trust (GSTT) which was the first known staff support psychology post to work at this scale outside of Occupational Health domains. She now also works strategically at an organisational level in this large Acute Trust with 25,000 staff. She lives in London, her hometown, which she loves for its diversity, and she replenishes her energies by travel to mountains and the sea.

www.ingramcontent.com/pod-product-compliance
Ingram Content Group UK Ltd.
Pitfield, Milton Keynes, MK11 3LW, UK
UKHW020031040426
469662UK00007B/31